WAGING
WAR
on the
AUTISTIC
CHILD

WAGING WAR
on the
AUTISTIC CHILD

The Arizona 5 and the Legacy of
Baron von Münchausen

ANDREW J. WAKEFIELD

Skyhorse Publishing

Skyhorse Publishing books may be purchased in bulk at special discounts for sales promotion, corporate gifts, fund-raising, or educational purposes. Special editions can also be created to specifications. For details, contact the Special Sales Department, Skyhorse Publishing, 307 West 36th Street, 11th Floor, New York, NY 10018 or info@skyhorsepublishing.com.

Skyhorse® and Skyhorse Publishing® are registered trademarks of Skyhorse Publishing, Inc.®, a Delaware corporation.

www.skyhorsepublishing.com

10 9 8 7 6 5 4 3 2 1

Library of Congress Cataloging-in-Publication Data on file.

Cover design by Matthew Fetter
Cover photo: iStockphoto

Print ISBN: 978-1-63220-307-6
eBook ISBN: 978-1-5107-0539-5

Printed in the United States of America

This book is dedicated to fellow travelers, including John Walker-Smith, Arthur Krigsman, Lenny Gonzalez, Federico Balzola, and all those who have come to realize that the bowel bone's connected to the brain bone. You were right.

CONTENTS

PART II

PROLOGUE

What is the loss of job, career, professional license, honors, colleagues, and country against that of a child's voice? How do the very public denigration of one's science and the epithet of "child killer" from Bill Gates weigh against the intractable pain of intestinal inflammation? For me the answer lies in the fact that, whereas the former are mostly artifact—contrivance—the latter are symptoms of a ruthless disease. The former are self-serving, vulnerable to political expedients and the vain whims of respectability. On the other hand, chronic pain that is denied a cry for help can drag a child into Hell and keep him there.

As an academic gastroenterologist, I have now been researching the complex and intriguing interaction among bowels, immune system, and brain for seventeen years. For much of that time, the scientific process has been derailed by vested interests acting not on behalf of affected children, but rather for the protection of vaccine manufacturers and incompetent governments. Despite this, the evidence—reviewed in this book—is overwhelmingly in favor of a major gastrointestinal contribution to autism. Over fifteen years ago, I proposed that for many children with autism, their disease might actually start in the intestine; the current science leads me to believe this now more than ever before.

I sometimes ask myself whether if this had just been one child—one Lorenzo—or even a handful of damaged children, would I have had the temerity, the arrogance, to pit myself against such odds. The question is redundant: irrelevant in view of the massed, mute choir of the world's autistic children, eclipsed only by the failure of science and medicine, in silent complicity, to take up the yoke—to be relevant, to find autism's causes, and to stop the epidemic. Nonetheless, I still wonder.

In the meantime, an extraordinary web of deceit and calumny has been woven. Traveling aboard Rupert Murdoch's runaway media train, journalist Brian Deer was instructed to "find something big" on MMR. Deer created a story so heartwarming to public health, so reassuring to doctors that clever people shut out reason, suspended logic, and slept with their dissonant dreams.

Deer's story of me, the evil doctor, meant Medicine could be exonerated, public health policy had no hand in the autism catastrophe, and vaccines truly are a miracle. Some are still dreaming. In summary, in the wake of his 2004 "exposé" on the work of a team of doctors at the Royal Free Hospital, Deer filed a complaint with the UK's General Medical Council, and in one of the most perverse rulings in the history of that organization, I and one other colleague had our medical licenses pulled. Dr. Kumar, the chairman of the adjudicating panel, profited before, during, and after his damning decision from undisclosed stock in MMR manufacturer GlaxoSmithKline. In a further tonic to the bottom line, he urged compulsory MMR vaccination of UK children at a medical conference within weeks of passing sentence on my colleagues and me.

Deer's ego basked in the fame and recognition that his "revelations" had brought. While he might have hoped that parents "exploited" by me would hail him as a savior, this did not happen. Quite the opposite: their contempt for Deer led him into new avenues of invective and attacks against these same parents. On a global scale, parents were questioning more and more the safety and necessity of certain vaccines. The public relations wrecking crew that followed in the wake of Deer's offensive needed more lubrication for their heart-and-minds machine. This came, perhaps coincidentally, soon after the now discredited heir-apparent to the News Corp Empire, James Murdoch, joined the board of GlaxoSmithKline (GSK) to protect that company's image in the media. Allegations of scientific fraud against me—and me alone—were made by Deer in respect of the *Lancet* paper—first in the *Sunday Times*. Since these articles did not have the desired effect of quelling support and putting an end to the vaccine safety debate, they were repeated, this time in the *British Medical Journal*, with its imprinteur of a proper medical journal, and in a supportive editorial by the editor-in-chief, Dr. Fiona Godlee. Among his many mistakes, these articles were Deer's greatest. He, and I presume the *BMJ*, had taken the view that I was zero risk for legal redress; they could say what they liked without the risk of being sued. They were wrong—they had reckoned without the autism community, whose generosity and fighting spirit have made litigation possible. Through my lawyers I have now extended an invitation to Deer and Godlee to enjoy some good ol' Texas hospitality. With it comes the opportunity to tell the history of the last fifteen years as it was. That's it in a nutshell, except to say that in the wake of his disgrace, James Murdoch has now resigned from the board of GSK, apparently to focus his attention on operations in the US.

Meanwhile, this book grasps the nettle of alleged child abuse in the all too familiar setting of ASD, associated with gastrointestinal and immune disease. Part of the recent history has been concerned with the growing number of such cases. It is hoped that the book appalls and enlightens in equal measure.

This is not a run-of-the-mill dependency case. There are no allegations of substance abuse, physical abuse, sexual abuse, domestic violence. Unfortunately, whether you want to call it Factitious Syndrome by Proxy, Münchausen Syndrome by Proxy, or simply medical child abuse, all of these children have been subjected to egregious medical abuse at the hands of their parents.

. . . Dr. Mary Sanders, Dr. Susan Stephens, and Dr. Albert Jacobson will all tell you that these children have been subjected to numerous medical examinations, medications, invasive procedures, hospitalizations, social isolation, and developmental delays[1] because these parents have provided false, exaggerated, and incomplete information to numerous medical professionals.

Dr. Stevens [sic] and Dr. Jacobsen will tell you that, contrary to the parents' consistent reports to countless providers and medical professionals, these children do not have autism. They do not have mitochondrial disorder. They do not have antibody disorders. They do not have multiple food and environmental allergies.

Dr. Mary Sanders, a Ph.D. psychologist from Stanford University, who is an expert in the diagnosis of Factitious Disorder by Proxy, will tell you that both parents suffer from Factitious Disorder and that is because they have falsified the medical records that have caused the children to receive unnecessary and harmful treatments and diagnoses.

Finally and perhaps most telling, Barbara Woods, a CPS supervisor, and Dr. Albert Jacobson . . . will tell you that since the children came into the department's custody out of home care, the last four-and-a-half months, they have had no medications, no hospitalizations, no invasive procedures, no diet restrictions. They have been taken out of isolation, put into regular classrooms in a public school system and, other than one incident of strep throat and one incident of bronchitis, none of the children has displayed any signs or symptoms of illness or any behavioral issues that are out of the norm for children of their ages. In fact they have been thriving. They are doing well in school. They are socializing with peers, and they are enjoying a regular diet.

Accordingly the department will prove by more than the preponderance of the evidence that these parents certainly at the time of removal and indeed at this time, are unable to provide safe, effective and proper parental care and control for these children.

Ms. Jo Wamboldt for the Arizona Department of
Economic Security et al.
Oct. 27, 2010

Your honor, one of the central themes in this case, which our evidence will show, is that with treatment, children can recover. They can recover from autism, from functional antibody deficiency. They can recover from lead toxicities, or they can recover from or simply grow out of food allergies or food sensitivities. What is left to be answered is this: Does that mean that they never had the illness or diagnosis in the first place?

Tanya Imming, Esq., for the mother.
Oct. 27, 2010

Our evidence will show that [the parents] are far superior to minimally adequate, and we should be celebrating them and the children's recovery like thousands of other parents—thousands of parents. The testimony will show that they follow these [biomedical] protocols and have seen good results with their children and seen their children move towards recovery.

So our case is that simple. The parents followed the doctors' recommendation, and the kids improved and these are upstanding citizens. They are wonderful parents and we need to get their children back to them as quickly as possible.

Jennifer Kupiszewski, Esq., for the father.
Oct. 27, 2010

In the face of a disease process that beguiles the medical profession, there is a tendency, affirmed in autism's unfortunate history, to blame the patient or the patient's parent(s). This book is about a further emergent crisis faced by parents with children on the autism spectrum, that is, allegations of systematic child abuse in the form of Münchausen syndrome by proxy (MSBP), also known in the United States as factitious disorder by proxy (FDBP).

Make no mistake, the battles for autism and the soul of medicine—what remains of the latter—are writ large in this small-town story. It centers upon the current progressive themes of autism: environmental toxicity from heavy metals and vaccines, intestinal disease and food allergy, mitochondrial disorder and oxidative stress, and biomedical treatments and recovery. It is a story that sets the old guard against the new; institutionalized nihilism against an optimism borne out of fresh insights; and, in the view of many, ignorance against enlightenment. But here, there is also abuse and much more.

At its heart this is the story of one family and its struggle with the spectrum of autism in not one but five children. . . . A family seeking and finding answers in the eye of the storm and a revolution in medicine. Other families have suffered a similar fate and more will unless change comes.

For this story to be told by me, and if, therefore, it is to have any credibility, readers must understand the lies of Brian Deer the UK journalist, and all the proxy lies of those whom he has infected. Deer is a deliberate distraction, but one who must be addressed. The current frenzy, an exposé of Murdoch's News International—Deer's employer—shows that its journalists, sanctioned from on high, have managed to violate the code of journalistic ethics—a feat in itself. This should surprise no one. Each lie, like another finger in a towering levee, leaking as it strains to hold back a septic tide, is ultimately futile. And those fingers are having to pull back: the CDC's front man and vaccine researcher Dr. Paul Thorsen is subject to an extradition order for embezzlement of millions of research dollars from the CDC and, therefore, the US taxpayer—the "Dane Drain."[2] Dr. Paul Offit the vaccine millionaire has apparently been caught lying to the media.[3] And the major agencies—the CDC, the National Vaccine Advisory Committee (NVAC), and the National Institutes of Health's Interagency Autism Coordinating Committee (IACC)—have changed their position on the need to perform vaccine safety research and, specifically, investigation of the vaccine-autism link.[4] In a recent landmark publication, it has become clear that the US Vaccine Injury Compensation Program has been awarding compensation for vaccine injuries whose outcome includes autism since the program's inception in the late 1980s.[5]

And of course, everything that you will read here is, inevitably, my interpretation of the facts—you will form your own opinion.

INTRODUCTION

It was while in Phoenix at a lecture and book signing engagement in the summer of 2010 that I first heard of the Arizona 5. Mention of this family—which included five children with an autism spectrum disorder (ASD) who were under threat of removal from their parents by Child Protective Services (CPS)—came up during a charged dialogue about the increasing hostility of Arizona's CPS toward autism families, especially those using biomedical therapies to treat affected children. Apparently, the allegation of Münchausen syndrome by proxy (MSBP), a rare form of child abuse, was being leveled at these particular parents by a singularly motivated bureaucracy, the Arizona Department of Economic Security (ADES).

The story, as it was told to me in 2010, appeared to revolve around a conflict between this family and doctors from Phoenix Children's Hospital (PCH). On one side, there were two parents who believed that their children's illnesses were physical rather than psychological in origin and that, as such and in common with other physical diseases, these illnesses could be investigated, treated, and possibly ameliorated. Ranged against them was a group of doctors, supported by psychologists, bureaucrats, and litigators, who believed that the children were healthy but abused—abused by parents whose shared psychopathology manifested itself in gratification each time doctors prodded, probed, and prescribed for any of their children.

The parents' perspective had been shaped not just by an intuitive sense that their children were suffering but also by experience, day after day, year after year, of a succession of related symptoms involving abnormal behaviors, intestinal distress, and immune reactions that led them to seek medical help. In addition, by virtue of the Internet and the epidemic of ASD, they had been able to share and compare their experiences with numerous other parents, many of whom had witnessed the benefits of biomedical treatment for their own children who had similar physical and behavioral problems. Subsequently, and almost certainly as a direct consequence of biomedical treatments, the Arizona 5 children had improved both physically and behaviorally. In the eyes of some, this recovery—albeit partial—was taken as absence of a problem in the first place. ADES and its agents interpreted the parents' story, from the diagnoses of ASD right through to the children's recovery, as a grand and convoluted lie—a lie that needed to be exposed lest the children suffer further abuse or even death at their parents' hands.[1]

The forces ranged against the parents of such children have been and remain formidable: Some doctors believe that the label of autism is itself abused—a "designer disease" worn by aspiring families as today's *haute couture*.[2] Others are at an ideological impasse, believing that vaccines are mankind's benign salvation. And then there are those who are motivated to protect a substantial revenue stream to individual pediatricians, feeding, in turn, a ruthless multi-billion-dollar business. Here, in the allegations of child abuse, was an even more insidious breach in the soft, vulnerable underbelly of normal, loving American families struggling for all they are worth.

Or was it? Was there merit to the case put forward by the ADES? Although exquisitely rare—even more so in both parents—real and potential harm to children has been reported in the setting of proxy illness contrived by their parents. Had diligent, caring doctors—thorough and exhaustive in their process of diagnostic due diligence—happened upon five abused children of two parents who together craved autism, bowel disease, and other diagnoses in their children? Although not impossible, it would have been a first.

As I sat and talked with other parents and at least one doctor who knew the family well, the significance of this narrative as a story of our time—a microcosm, surely, but one upon which such families might collectively stand or fall—became clear. The genius of Dr. Seuss' moral allegories gave us *Horton Hears a Who*: Whoville, a tiny town on a tiny speck of dust, faced annihilation at the hands of some bad creatures because no one believed that the Who folks existed, since no one could hear them . . . no one, that is, except Horton the elephant. To survive they needed to be heard. And in the end, despite the collective clamor of the Who community, it was just one additional voice—no more than a "yopp" from JoJo, the tiniest Who of them all—that made them heard and saved them. I don't know when the "yopp" will come for the autism community, so in the meantime, I will contribute this story to the growing collective clamor.

This book is presented in five parts: the first, which is necessarily more technical, deals with the issue of bowel disease in many children with autism; this is a matter that is central to an analysis of the Arizona 5. The second part provides a brief review of the history of MSBP. The children are introduced in the third part with a detailed review of their medical histories. Part four provides the case made against the parents by ADES, its informants, its agents, and its legal counsel, as well as the case's deconstruction. Part five concludes with a summary analysis of the case.

From here on, evidence is king—factual evidence that trumps opinion, speculation, and circumstance. It is to the evidence that we now turn.

PART I

Chapter 1

AUTISM SPECTRUM DISORDER, GASTROINTESTINAL DISEASE, AND MÜNCHAUSEN SYNDROME BY PROXY

INTRODUCTION

The past fifteen years have seen a steadily increasing if somewhat reticent acceptance of a high prevalence of gastrointestinal (GI) symptoms and associated inflammatory GI pathology in patients with autism spectrum disorders (ASDs).[1] Since its first description in 1943, autism has not lacked for strong clinical indicators of a significant GI connection[2]—clues that were largely subsumed into this disorder's psychiatric legacy and consequently ignored. The reticence seems to have emanated from the continuing dominant influence of psychological/psychiatric viewpoints of autism and, for some, an aversion to engaging in the GI-related vaccine-autism debate. Despite this, the GI-autism connection is gaining increasing acceptance, not the least of which because of the observation that treatments directed at the associated GI abnormalities may produce both short-term[3] and sustained[4] symptomatic improvement.

Increasingly, however, in pursuit of a diagnosis for their children's genuine physical ailments and therapeutic relief thereof, parents of children with ASD have found themselves subject to allegations of child abuse, including MSBP. This invidious situation has arisen largely for three reasons: 1) *conflation:* GI symptoms are common to both autism and the rare cases of genuine factitious illness in children, 2) *ignorance:* healthcare professionals and the judiciary are unfamiliar with the facts of the published GI-autism science, and 3) *antagonism:* frequently, although not invariably, parental reluctance to vaccinate their children due to the perception of past or possible future harm from this procedure clashes with medical orthodoxy.

This same orthodoxy tends to be skeptical of—and even hostile toward—stories of clinical improvement following, for example, exclusion diets. Such treatments may then be represented as potentially harmful and abusive. These three factors operate against a rapidly changing autism landscape—both in terms of the emerging science and as a rapidly unfolding socioeconomic nightmare with the inevitable political duck-and-cover response. In the setting of ASD, the cumulative effects of *conflation*, *ignorance*, and *antagonism* mean that, as Professor William Long observed in his detailed, critical review of MSBP, this label "has, over the years, taken on a sinister and dangerous role, harming more than it helps."[5]

This effect is illustrated in a case study of one family that will be presented later in this book. The purpose here is to deal with the issue of GI disease in autism and how, in relation to this disease, parental health-seeking actions and subsequent clinical management should be clearly distinguished from MSBP. It seeks to stress how current knowledge of the autism-GI connection—while incomplete—makes it mandatory that in the presence of an ASD diagnostic due diligence is applied rigorously before even entertaining a possible "diagnosis" of MSBP. This report borrows from recent experience of MSBP-related litigation in Arizona to identify sources of error, diagnostic oversight, and invalid opinion in order to help develop investigative and legal approaches that may help to avoid future injustice and professional malpractice. First, however, it will be helpful to outline the changing landscape of autism that must in the future inform the medical and legal processes.

THE CHANGING LANDSCAPE OF AUTISM

Table 1 on the next page presents a summary of the major shifts in perception that have occurred or are occurring within the mainstream of medical science with respect to the origin and epidemiology of ASD. The views cited were not historically, nor are they currently, universally held. However, the current views are part of the peer-reviewed scientific literature and are the subject of medical and scientific debate to a sufficient enough degree that they merit due consideration and expert opinion in dealing with this issue in a legal setting. Moreover, disagreement between historical and current views does not mean that the former views were necessarily wrong. Although the word "autistic" has remained, the disorder itself has changed both in its clinical presentation and epidemiology, providing potential insights into the environmental cause(s) that is driving the current epidemic.

TABLE 1. Shift in perception related to ASD

Historical view	Current view
A rare psychiatric condition of constant prevalence	A common medical disorder of increasing incidence that is epidemic in Westernized countries[6]
Major genetic contribution	A disorder in which many genes may contribute to susceptibility but no consistent or reproducible gene findings are available, despite extensive research
Minor environmental (e.g., infectious) contribution to cause[7]	Major environmental contribution to cause[8]
No evidence of environmental toxic cause	Substantial and growing evidence of environmental toxic cause[9]
Regressive pattern of onset in a normally or near-normally developing child—extremely rare[10]	Regressive onset is emerging as a major pattern of disease[11]
Congenital disorder (child is born with autism)	Acquired (child develops autism)
Intestinal symptoms/disease absent or irrelevant[12]	Intestinal symptoms/disease common and relevant to neurological disease
History and symptoms of immune problems not relevant	Affected individuals frequently have associated immune disorders[13]
Childhood vaccines may rarely[14] play a role, if at all	Growing evidence of major contribution from childhood vaccines[15]
Biomedical treatments including exclusion diets are unhelpful and based upon pseudoscience	Biomedical treatments, including diets, can lead to sustained improvement in physical and behavioral symptoms
A lifelong disorder not associated with recovery	Clinical improvement and loss of ASD diagnosis can and does occur.

PREVALENCE OF GI SYMPTOMS IN ASD

GI problems in individuals with ASD provide an important insight into the changing landscape of this disorder. A 2010 paper titled "Evaluation, Diagnosis, and Treatment of GI disorders in individuals with ASDs: A Consensus Report"[16] represented a session convened under the auspices of the Department of Pediatrics of Harvard Medical School. This report states that "the preponderance of data were consistent with the likelihood of a high prevalence of gastrointestinal symptoms and disorders associated with ASDs."

The accumulated data on prevalence of significant GI symptoms in this population also reveals the discordance between rates in retrospective studies involving analysis of historical patient records (low prevalence of GI symptoms) and prospective case-control studies (high prevalence compared with neurotypical control groups). This arises out of a significant ascertainment bias in the retrospective studies, largely as a result of a historical disinterest among psychiatrists and psychologists in such symptoms in patients with ASD. The reported prevalence of GI symptoms in ASD ranges from 17–59% in retrospective studies[17] to 50–84%[18] in prospective studies of *current* GI symptoms, and to 91%[19] in prospective studies of those with a past or current history of significant GI symptoms. In the few studies that included appropriate neurotypical control populations, the prevalence of GI symptoms was between 0% and 25%. In accord with the consensus report, evidential weight should be placed upon prospective studies that have included appropriate control groups.

NATURE OF GI SYMPTOMS IN ASD

As with neurotypical children, obvious symptoms of GI distress in ASD include diarrhea, constipation, alternating constipation and diarrhea, abdominal bloating, anorexia, failure to thrive, and vomiting. In addition, clinicians experienced in the GI management of affected children recognize and have reported the often idiosyncratic and previously misinterpreted behavioral symptoms in nonverbal children and those with otherwise impaired communication skills that are indicative of underlying GI disorders. Attention was drawn to this in 2001[20] and has since been confirmed by Horvath and Perman,[21] Krigsman et al.,[22] and Buie et al.[23] Buie et al. have tabulated behaviors that may be markers of abdominal pain or discomfort in individuals with ASD (reproduced on the next page in Table 2). These behaviors should alert the clinician to a possible underlying GI pathology that requires further investigation and certainly before such behaviors are considered to be psychosomatic or induced by others.

TABLE 2. Behaviors That May Be Markers of Abdominal Pain or Distress

Vocal Behaviors	Motor Behaviors	Changes in Overall State
Frequent clearing of throat, swallowing, tics, etc.	Facial grimacing	Sleep disturbances: difficulty getting to sleep, difficulty staying asleep
Screaming	Gritting teeth	Increased irritability (exaggerated responses to stimulation)
Sobbing for "no reason at all"	Wincing	Noncompliance with demands that typically elicit an appropriate response (oppositional behavior)
Sighing, whining	Constant eating/drinking/swallowing ("grazing" behavior)	
Moaning, groaning	Mouth behaviors: chewing on clothes (shirt sleeve cuff, neck of shirt, etc.), pica	
Delayed echolalia that includes references to pain or stomach (e.g., child says, "Does your tummy hurt?" echoing what mother may have said to child in the past)	Application of pressure to abdomen: leaning abdomen against or over furniture or kitchen sink, pressing hands into abdomen, rubbing abdomen	
Direct verbalizations (e.g., child says "tummy hurts" or says "ouch," "ow," "hurts," or "bad" while pointing to abdomen)	Tapping behavior: finger tapping on throat.	
	Any unusual posturing, which may appear as individual postures or in various combinations: jaw thrust, neck torsion, arching of back, odd arm positioning, rotational distortions of torso/trunk, sensitivity to being touched in abdominal area/flinching	
	Agitation: pacing, jumping up and down	
	Unexplained increase in repetitive behaviors	
	Self-injurious behaviors: biting, hits/slaps face, head-banging, unexplained increase in self-injury	
	Aggression: onset of or increase in aggressive behavior	

Buie T., et al. *Pediatrics*. 2010;125:S1-S18.

A functional behavioral assessment would be useful in interpreting these behaviors.

Motor behaviors may be markers of pain or discomfort arising in other parts of the body.

Parents also report a variety of behaviors leading up to, associated with, and exacerbated by bowel movements. These include increasing anxiety and distress, increased hand flapping, self-injury, hyperactivity, and pain posturing. While moving their bowels, children may adopt a variety of postures such as squatting on top of the toilet seat in order to maximally flex the hips and increase intra-abdominal pressure, thus aiding evacuation. Despite difficulty passing stool, it may be loose (does not hold its shape in the toilet bowl), discolored (yellow), of highly offensive odor, and containing undigested food.

VISCERAL PERCEPTION IN ASD

Beyond the symptomatic presentation of GI disorders that is constrained and altered by impaired communication, clinical experience strongly suggests that, along with other sensory modalities, pain perception is abnormal in patients with ASD.[24] This is likely to influence the symptomatic presentation of conditions that typically cause pain. In the patient with autism, perception of different modalities of pain may be affected in different ways and this, in turn, may reflect the activities of different pathways and neurotransmitter systems. For example, in the individual with ASD, while there may be an apparent reduction in pain sensitivity (hypoalgesia) for a burn injury, visceral (abdominal organ) pain arising from GI inflammation or intestinal distention may be normal or abnormally heightened. This is evident in certain genetic disorders involving the autonomic (involuntary) nervous system such as familial dysautonomia (FD). Patients with this rare condition, in which the autonomic nervous system malfunctions, have decreased pain and temperature perception whereas visceral pain pathways are intact.[25] In light of the growing evidence for autonomic dysfunction in ASD,[26] the sensory disturbances in FD and ASD may have an overlapping pathogenesis.

Bursch et al. draw attention to the possibility of a heightened perception of visceral pain in ASD when describing two male teenagers with features strongly indicative of previously undiagnosed ASD who suffered severe abdominal pain for which no obvious organic cause was identified.[27] Caution is required since pathology may have been overlooked or underestimated. While in the first case, GI investigations were undertaken, they were by no means exhaustive and could not have ruled out mucosal inflammation, particularly in light of what is now known about the GI disease in autism. In the second case—an eighteen-year-old boy with a clear history of hypoalgesia to hot pain stimuli and hypersensitivity to milder tactile, olfactory, and auditory stimulation—pressure studies of his upper GI tract (antroduodenal manometry; see explanation below) showed brief simultaneous pressure increases in all nearby sites associated with regurgitation. The genuine and debilitating pain suffered by these two patients in the absence of obvious *major* pathology suggests that their visceral pain response may have been adversely heightened (dysasthesia) as a component of their autistic disorder. Relatively small disturbances in pressures within the intestine may, for example, have elicited disproportionately severe pain. It is recognized that patients with irritable bowel syndrome (IBS) and normal results on studies of intestinal motility may experience pain—visceral hyperalgesia—in the presence of normal peristalsis[28] (the rippling motion of muscles in the digestive tract that propels food forward).

INTESTINAL DYSMOTILITY

In addition to altered pain perception (nociception) in ASD, reduced intestinal motility, where the normal peristalsis[29] of the intestine is faulty and transit of intestinal contents is delayed, is indicated by the frequent history of gastroesophageal reflux (GER) and constipation. In the autism literature, studies of intestinal motility are notably absent despite the apparent frequency of this problem. Definitive studies of intestinal motility are usually undertaken in specialist GI centers where there is an expertise in measuring intestinal pressure (manometry) using standardized techniques for recording detailed bowel motility patterns.[30] Patients are usually referred to such centers after they have been investigated for common GI disorders elsewhere.

Chronic intestinal pseudo-obstruction (CIP) is a rare disorder of GI motility where intestinal peristalsis becomes altered and inefficient. Symptoms of CIP include recurrent episodes of nausea, vomiting, distention, and constipation in the absence of a mechanical GI obstruction. The majority of cases are associated with abnormalities of the intestinal musculature or neural networks within the wall of the intestine.[31] Manometry is frequently required in the differential diagnosis of motility disorders including CIP. Because of the rarity of CIP and the need for diagnostic expertise, Cucchiara et al. stress that GI manometry is an investigation that should be preceded by an extensive diagnostic evaluation to exclude other disorders mimicking CIP. They make the point that in patients with signs of intestinal dysmotility, barium contrast studies and endoscopy of all of the GI tract as well as laboratory studies *must always*[32] be part of the diagnostic evaluation.

In the investigation of obscure abdominal pain and other GI symptoms in children, both CIP and MSBP may become part of the differential diagnosis. However, even in specialist centers, the differential diagnosis between MSBP and CIP may be problematic. Cucchiara et al.[33] diagnosed MSBP in four of twelve children undergoing GI manometry studies for possible CIP. However, of their four cases of MSBP, prior imaging studies had identified disordered intestinal transit in two patients. In a third patient, X-ray evidence of air-fluid levels (indicative of obstruction) in the ileal (final section of small intestine) region during episodes of vomiting and abdominal pain was reported. Importantly, GI manometry was performed at a time when the children were asymptomatic and abnormalities may have been missed. The diagnoses of MSBP were made based upon an apparently unstructured evaluation of the mothers' behavior and prompt disappearance of symptoms following separation from "maternal interventions." As reported, this situation is unsatisfactory. Episodic symptoms suggestive of obstruction are, by their nature, interspersed by asymptomatic periods when tests may be normal. If the prior abdominal imaging studies were performed when the patients were symptomatic, then the features of delayed transit and localized intestinal obstruction take on a greater diagnostic significance. In addition, there was no reference in the Cucchiara report as to the nature of any "maternal interventions," the removal of which apparently led to symptomatic improvement in the child.

It is evident from their findings, however, that prior investigations in the twelve children had failed to identify what turned out to be celiac disease in two cases, intestinal malrotation in two cases, Crohn's disease in two cases, and congenital chloride-losing diarrhea in one case, indicating that these prior investigations were inadequate, having failed to identify pre-existing disease in the majority of cases, all of which had manifested as possible CIP.

While this study, published in 2000, provides some useful pointers for investigation prior to manometry, it fails to specify the laboratory studies that the authors consider necessary in this patient group. In addition, capsule endoscopy (a technique that has revolutionized the ability to visualize the small intestine) was only licensed by the FDA for use *in adults* in 2001 and was not used in children until later. Extensive clinical experience of capsule endoscopy in children with ASD has revealed widespread low-grade pathology such as mucosal micro-erosions that would likely be beyond the limits of barium contrast studies to detect (Krigsman, A., personal communication). We would now recommend that capsule endoscopy should be added to the list of extensive investigations that are required before GI manometry is undertaken and certainly before a diagnosis of MSBP is made in such cases.

Finally, in support of their diagnoses of MSBP, Cucchiara et al. report the "strong suspicion" that in two cases a parent had illicitly administered either opioids (morphine-like) or anticholinergic drugs (blocks the neurotransmitter acetylcholine)—recognized causes of impaired intestinal motility. This conjecture is inconsistent with the finding of "normal gastrointestinal motility" that is explicit in their report. Moreover, deliberate poisoning is readily investigated by dope testing employing, for example, urine analysis using high-pressure liquid chromatography (HPLC) and mass spectroscopy (MS), neither of which appear to have been performed. Where suspected poisoning is considered to be the cause of GI symptoms, this should necessarily be investigated in toxicological studies.

GI symptoms are reported to be a common feature in cases where MSBP has been either alleged or confirmed according to the respective authors.[34] Some of these cases are clear-cut, involving, for example, diarrhea, vomiting, and failure to thrive associated with confirmed, deliberate poisoning.[35] Other explanations are less satisfactory. From a review of the case reports it is not clear what GI investigations, if any, have been undertaken, and the majority of these reports are therefore unhelpful.

In order to identify clinical criteria that might help to discriminate between CIP and MSBP in toddlers, Hyman et al. compared medical records of eight pediatric condition falsification (MSBP) victims to those of fourteen children with CIP. They concluded that clinical features suggestive of MSBP in children presenting with chronic and severe digestive complaints include: [36]

- daily abdominal pain
- illness involving three or more organ systems
- an accelerating disease trajectory
- a reported history of preterm birth
- absence of dilated bowel on X-ray
- normal antroduodenal (antro refers to the distal part of the stomach, the antrum) manometry
- no urinary neuromuscular disease

Viewed in the context of ASD, one can see how, using this symptom profile, an inappropriate suspicion of MSBP might easily arise: in children with ASD, daily abdominal pain is not unusual; there is frequently illness involving three or more organ systems (e.g., brain, gut, immune); preterm birth is associated with factors such as maternal hemorrhage that are associated with a greater risk of ASD;[37] while fecal impaction is not uncommon on a plain abdominal X-ray, dilated bowel loops are not reported frequently in ASD; and finally, there are no data on antroduodenal manometry in this group of children (studies are required). While, for example, primary and secondary incontinence are common in children with ASD, this has been assumed to have a behavioral/developmental basis and formal studies of urinary neuromuscular function have not been performed.

In conclusion, it is inappropriate to apply these criteria in the evaluation of ASD children for possible MSBP.

INTESTINAL VOLVULUS

As a further note of caution, ignoring GI symptoms in children with possible CIP and/or chronic intractable constipation, where MSBP may be suspected, may be fatal. Intestinal volvulus is a surgical emergency that occurs when a loop of intestine twists in such a way as to comprise its blood supply. The presenting symptoms of volvulus may mimic those of underlying CIP. Left untreated, volvulus may result in intestinal gangrene, perforation, peritonitis, and death. In a retrospective chart review, Altal et al. identified eight patients between two and twenty-two years of age at the time of diagnosis with colonic volvulus who also had CIP and chronic idiopathic[38] constipation (CIC).[39] All patients presented with worsening of abdominal distension and pain. The mean duration of symptoms of colonic volvulus before seeking medical help was 4.2 days (range 1–7 days). Water-soluble contrast enema was the single most useful investigation for confirming the diagnosis. All patients required surgery. In this series of cases, there was no mortality associated with colonic volvulus. They conclude that "clinicians should be vigilant and include volvulus in the differential diagnosis of the acute onset of abdominal distension and pain in patients with CIP and CIC. Delay in diagnosis can result in bowel ischemia (inadequate blood supply) and perforation."

PAIN-ASSOCIATED DISABILITY SYNDROME

Another rare diagnosis that overlaps with CIP and with which many physicians are unfamiliar is pain-associated disability syndrome (PADS).[40] This term is used by some to describe patients with chronic pain—neither feigned nor self-induced—whose restriction in daily activities "appears disproportionately severe for the observable pathology." Since GI symptoms in the absence of obvious pathology may raise the question of MSBP, this diagnosis requires further consideration. In seeking to identify factors associated with visceral PADS, Hyman et al. reviewed the records of forty patients, ages seven through twenty-one years, including eighteen males, with GI symptoms severe enough to prevent school attendance or eating for two months or more. Patients had failed the "usual treatments" and lacked a satisfactory organic explanation for the severity of the pain.

The dominant symptom was abdominal pain in thirty patients, regurgitation in five patients, nausea in three patients, and chest pain in two patients. All patients complained of pain or discomfort, and disordered sleep was a problem for thirty-nine patients.

Prior evaluations had, in fact, led to a disease diagnosis in twenty-four patients (60%).[41] It is not certain how, in light of these diagnoses, the perception of pain was judged by the authors to be disproportionate. Significantly, however, the authors have drawn attention to how additional psychosocial and behavioral factors may lead to stress and autonomic disturbances that enhance the pain response. The potential relationship between autonomic disturbance and altered pain response has been referred to above in the context of ASD, where behavior is *de facto* abnormal. It is striking, therefore, that in the report of Hyman et al., developmental disorders were present in no fewer than twenty-two patients (55%). These included receptive or expressive language disorder (fifteen), attention-deficit disorder (ADD) (three), PDD (two), and mild mental retardation (two). Eating disorder and psychosis were not found. This prevalence of developmental disorder is very high and suggests that there is something intrinsic to the developmental disorder that is associated with or contributes substantially to the risk of an exaggerated pain response, an occult GI pathology, or both. In light of the current recognition of subtle organic GI pathology in both ASD (see above) and ADD,[42] and autonomic disturbances that are likely to influence pain perception, the observations of Hyman et al. are likely to be highly significant and reinforce the position that extreme caution should be exercised when considering MSBP in the differential diagnosis of abdominal pain in children with developmental disorder.

Contributing to the perception that organic pathology may be present in these patients is the fact that in 50% of the patients in the study of Hyman et al., acute febrile illness was cited as a possible triggering event for GI symptoms. This is also reported in ASD where GI and/or behavior symptom onset is reported, not infrequently, to follow a febrile reaction to infection or vaccination.

The take-home message is that an apparently exaggerated visceral pain response in children with developmental disorders may not be exaggerated at all.

CONSENSUS

The GI-autism consensus paper[43] provides a useful summary of the mindset that should guide both clinical practice in dealing with ASD patients with possible GI disorders and the courts in consideration of what is a reasonable and necessary approach to such patients:

- Individuals with ASDs whose families report GI symptoms warrant a thorough GI evaluation.
- All of the common (and we would add "and less common") GI conditions encountered by individuals with typical neurologic development are also present in individuals with ASDs.
- The communication impairments characteristic of ASDs may lead to unusual presentations of GI disorders, including sleep disturbances and problem behaviors.
- Caregivers and healthcare professionals should be alert to the presentation of atypical signs of common GI disorders in patients with ASDs.

The burden of responsibility is upon doctors to anticipate and exclude a GI disorder in children with ASD prior to involving CPS unless there are compelling grounds for doing so over and above the possible GI disorder. In the context of suspected MSBP, Thompson wrote:

> Gastroenterologists must be alert to complaints of abdominal pain, constipation, diarrhoea or vomiting when the tests are negative and the observed behaviour of the patient does not fit the complaint.[44]

Physicians should beware. An additional level of discrimination must be applied in the evaluation of children with developmental disorders, where it is essential that in the face of unexplained symptoms where it is quite possible that, for obvious reasons, the observed behavior may not fit the complaint, medical evaluation and testing should be comprehensive.

TABLE 3. Diagnostic Evaluation of Gastrointestinal Symptoms and Disorders in Individuals with ASDs

Symptoms	Possible Associated Gastrointestinal Disorder	Definition	Diagnostic Evaluations to be Considered
Sleep disturbance	GERD	Parental/ provider report	(1) Diagnostic trial of proton-pump inhibitor; (2) pH probe, EGD
Self-injurious behavior, tantrums, aggression, oppositional behavior	Constipation, GERD, gastritis, intestinal inflammation	Parental/ provider report	(1) Abdominal radiograph; (2) diagnostic trial of proton-pump inhibitor or PEG 3350; (3) pH probe, EGD, colonoscopy
Chronic diarrhea	Malabsorption, maldigestion	≥ 3 loose stools daily for > 2 wk	(1) Stool analysis for occult blood, enteric pathogens, ova/parasites (*Giardia* or *Cryptosporidium*), *Clostridium difficile*; (2) consider PEG 3350 if overflow diarrhea is a possibility; (3) lactose breath test (or measure lactase-specific activity), EGD, colonoscopy
Straining to pass stool, hard or infrequent stool	Constipation		(1) Abdominal radiograph to look for fecal impaction; (2) diagnostic trial of PEG 3350
Perceived abdominal discomfort: pressing abdomen, holding abdomen and crying, problem behaviors related to meals	Constipation, GERD, intestinal inflammation, malabsorption, maldigestion	≤ 2 hard stools per week (Bristol stool score)	(1) Diagnostic trial of proton-pump inhibitor or PEG 3350; (2) abdominal radiograph; (3) lactose breath test (or measure lactase-specific activity); (4) pH probe, EGD, colonoscopy
Flatulence and/ or bloating	Constipation, lactose intolerance, enteric infection with *Giardia* or *Cryptosporidium*		(1) Abdominal radiograph; (2) diagnostic trial of PEG 3350 or lactose restriction; (3) lactose breath test or EGD (measure lactase-specific activity)

(Continued)

TABLE 3. (*Continued*)

Symptoms	Possible Associated Gastrointestinal Disorder	Definition	Diagnostic Evaluations to be Considered
Any or all of the above	FAP, IBS	FAP: abdominal pain without demonstrable evidence of anatomic, metabolic, infectious, inflammatory, neoplastic, or other pathologic condition	(1) Behavioral soothing; (2) diet enhancements with fruits, fiber, sufficient fluids; (3) increase in routines for sleep and toilet time
		IBS: FAP associated with alteration in bowel movements	

Buie, T., et al. *Pediatrics.* 2010; 125:S1-S18.

Chapter 2

GASTROINTESTINAL DISEASE IN ASD

Where MSBP is suspected or alleged, further consideration of this diagnosis should be largely mitigated if not completely redundant in the presence of a demonstrable organic disease that would better account for the child's symptoms and, therefore, the parents' actions. Organic disease in this setting refers to a disease affecting a tissue or organ(s)—where incontrovertible evidence indicates it was not induced by deliberate poisoning—that could give rise to the child's symptoms. Diarrhea and/or abdominal pain arising in the setting of colonic inflammation due to Crohn's disease or food allergy are examples.

The first chapter dealt with the frequency and nature of GI symptoms in a large proportion of patients with ASD. The following two chapters seek to build the bridge between symptoms and underlying organic disease. The current chapter describes what is known about the frequency of disease in patients with ASD and GI symptoms and the associated microscopic features of damage to the intestinal lining. The emerging importance of intestinal bacterial ecology—the microflora—and changes in intestinal function will be reviewed also. This chapter also deals with controversies—real and contrived—surrounding intestinal diseases in these children.

The first thing to say is that although the frequency of inflammatory intestinal disease varies from study to study, subtle, mild-to-moderate inflammation coupled with swelling of areas of discrete immune (lymphoid) tissue—similar to enlarged tonsils—are common findings in this patient group. The latter finding, which is known as lymphoid nodular hyperplasia (LNH), is frequent in those ASD patients undergoing lower GI endoscopy (Chapter 2, Table 4). The combination of inflammation and LNH are consistent not only with the children's symptoms but also with the involvement of some form of food-allergic disorder to the intestinal disease. Clinical experience also indicates that this disease is treatable, with treatment leading to symptomatic improvement for many children. Physicians should therefore maintain a high index of suspicion of bowel disease and be proactive in the endoscopic and biopsy examination of ASD patients.

Inflammation in this setting refers to an increase in the numbers of inflammatory cells in the tissues of the intestinal lining. These may be acute inflammatory cells—those associated with the formation of pus and abscesses—called neutrophils. Alternatively, chronic inflammation is associated with an increase in the numbers of inflammatory cells such as lymphocytes, plasma cells (antibody-producing cells), and macrophages. Macrophages, the largest cells in the immune system, function, among other things, like the clean-up crew, clearing up debris from sites of tissue injury. A further cell type that is prominent in the inflammatory process associated with ASD is the eosinophil. This cell is important in food-allergic disorders and certain infections and will be discussed further in the next chapter.

Acute and chronic inflammation may coexist, which is a situation referred to in the colon as chronic active colitis. The relative amounts of acute and chronic inflammation may relate to the activity of the disease at any particular point in time. The disease course in, for example, ulcerative colitis and Crohn's disease may involve longstanding chronic inflammation interspersed with flares of additional acute inflammation when the disease is more active. Finally, many parents will be familiar with the terms "nonspecific" and "indeterminate" in reference colitis. These interchangeable terms simply refer to a colitis for which the microscopic findings are not diagnostic of either Crohn's disease or ulcerative colitis.

Inflammatory pathology in ASD can, like Crohn's disease, affect the digestive system anywhere from the mouth to the anal canal. Until relatively recently, pediatric gastroenterologists were able to visualize and biopsy from the top end, only the esophagus, stomach, and the first part of the small intestine (duodenum and proximal jejunum). From the bottom end, access was limited to the rectum, colon, cecum, and (depending on the skill of the doctor) the last part of the ileum (terminal ileum). More recently, some physicians have used capsule endoscopy to visualize the small intestine in ASD children (see Part 1, Chapter 1) and have come to appreciate that, in fact, the majority of the disease may be located here (Krigsman, A., personal communication). A current limitation of the capsule technique is that, while it provides a visual image of the small intestinal lining, it does not provide a tissue sample for microscopic analysis.

For the physician undertaking both upper and lower intestinal endoscopy, multiple biopsies of the mucosa are essential to ensure disease is not missed and the full extent of disease can be documented.[1] In fact, seven or more biopsies of the colon should be taken routinely because the disease may not be evident to the naked eye, and it can only be documented by examining tissues under the microscope; this situation is well recognized and referred to in the large intestine as "microscopic colitis." Under the microscope, lesions consist of a focal, mild-to-moderate acute and/or chronic inflammation. Focal active colitis, often with LNH and small ulcers, may be found.[2] Table 4 summarizes the microscopic findings of larger reported series. While the natural history of the mucosal disease is not known, clinical experience indicates that it responds favorably to treatments used routinely in Crohn's disease and ulcerative colitis. These include anti-inflammatory medications such as 5-amino salicylates (asprin-like drugs) and immune-modulating medications such as the steroid prednisolone. However, while some cases with established inflammation may improve or disappear over time, others may progress or present at a later age with a pattern much closer to that of[3] Crohn's disease (Krigsman, A., personal communication). This presents the possibility that, at least for some children, the bowel disease in autism may be an early phase of Crohn's disease, and there is the potential for early intervention.

TABLE 4. Summary histopathological findings in studies of autistic spectrum disorders

Investigators	No. of subjects + age (average in months & range)	Upper GI inflammation (%)	LNH, no. (%)	Ileitis (%)	Colitis (%)
Wakefield et al.[4]	60 72 (36–192)	NA	93%	Active ileitis* 8%	88%
Horvath et al.[5]	36 68 ± 24 (mean and standard deviation)	Esophagitis 69% Gastritis 22% Duodenitis 69%	NA	NA	NA
Krigsman et al.[6]	146 63 interquartile range; 43	NA	72%	36%	69%

(*Continued*)

TABLE 4. (*Continued*)

Investigators	No. of subjects + age (average in months & range)	Upper GI inflammation (%)	LNH, no. (%)	Ileitis (%)	Colitis (%)
Balzola et al.[7]	122 16 (4–30)	Gastritis 36% Duodenitis 18%	45%	64%	100%
Gonzalez et al.[8]	68 (22–122)	Esophagitis 19.4% Gastritis 94% Duodenitis 100%	NA	NA	100%
Torrente et al.[9]	25 36 (12–60)	Gastritis 52%	NA	NA	NA
Torrente et al.[10]	25 77 (30–151)	Duodenitis 64%	NA	NA	NA
Kushak et al.[11]	111 (upper endoscopy) 89 (lower) 14–240	Esophagitis 20% Gastritis 12% Duodenitis 10%	16%	NA	Colitis 12% Eosinophilic colitis 14%
Anthony et al.[12]	75 (upper endoscopy) 182 (lower)	Esophagitis 15% Gastritis 24% Duodenitis 25%	None 14% Mild 21% Moderate 30% Severe 35%	NA	Acute 47% Chronic 71% Eosinophilic 41%

*Chronic ileitis was considered difficult to assess in the presence of LNH.

CONTROVERSIES IN INFLAMMATION

It is evident that reporting of the rates of inflammation in the intestines of ASD children varies widely, being high in the majority of studies but considerably lower in, for example, the study of Kushak et al. (Table 4). Does this automatically mean that one study is right and the other wrong? While this is possible, from experience it is unlikely; where intestinal inflammation is subtle—as it is in many children with ASD—difference in opinion among pathologists on the inherently subjective interpretation of biopsy changes is the rule rather than the exception.[13] If one sticks with the strict textbook definition of inflammation—an increase in inflammatory cells within the tissue—as referred to above, then certain questions arise. The first is: "An increase compared with what?" This matter is relatively easy to address. Comparison with similar biopsies from children without intestinal disease will provide a benchmark for what the normal number or density of these cells should be. This exercise, a qualitative comparison with normal biopsies, was undertaken in the *Lancet* study that originally described enterocolitis in children with ASD.[14]

The second qualitative question is: "Do different pathologists, blinded to the origins of the biopsies, agree on the findings?" This comparative exercise was undertaken on three separate occasions[15] at the Royal Free Hospital School of Medicine in order to assess for disease in ASD children. As an example of this, I wrote on September 28, 1998, to Professor John O'Leary, professor of histopathology (which concerns the microscopic examination of tissues for evidence of disease) at St. James's Hospital in Dublin, setting out the basis for an independent, blinded review. "[Dr.] Anthony will be sending you 10 cases (normal and autistic children) which are coded, for your assessment. . . . The data from your assessment will be compared with that obtained in our own laboratory and reported accordingly."[16]

The outcome of this exercise was duly reported in the *American Journal of Gastroenterology* in 2000, and the agreement among different observers was high,[17] providing further reassurance that our discovery was real.

The third question is: "To what extent can the qualitative findings be confirmed by objective quantitative data on inflammation in these tissues?" In other words, are the actual counts of inflammatory cells greater in the intestines of children with ASD than the counts in non-ASD controls? This question was answered in follow-up studies from the Royal Free group and others.[18] Two standard approaches to the quantitative assessment of inflammation were undertaken: the first involved labeling specific inflammatory cells with antibody markers that were distinguished by a color reaction in the tissue section. This technique was applied to tissues from children with ASD and non-ASD children. All the samples were coded and then viewed under the microscope. The microscopist, who didn't know the code and therefore which biopsy came from which group of children, counted each individual colored cell in a predetermined area of tissue. This process was repeated over many different areas for each child's biopsies. The density of cells was calculated and, ultimately, the code was broken and the scores for the two groups were compared.

The second technique involved extracting the individual immune cells from the biopsies, antibody-labeling them with a fluorescent probe, and firing them through a laser beam that caused the cell to emit a signal that the machine (a flow cytometer) recorded for each labeled cell. These two techniques, which eliminated any bias on the part of the observer, confirmed that biopsies from children with ASD fulfilled the criteria for inflammation in a high proportion of cases—more so, in fact, than was evident microscopically.[19] Specifically, immune cells were isolated from the duodenal, ileal, and colonic biopsies of fifty-two ASD children, twenty-five microscopically normal children, and fifty-four children with inflammatory disease of the intestine. The latter two groups of children were developmentally normal. Adjacent biopsies were assessed by microscopic examination without any knowledge on the part of the pathologists as to the study aims. In all three regions of the intestine—duodenum, ileum, and colon—chronic inflammatory cells were significantly increased in ASD children compared with developmentally normal, non-inflamed control groups,[20] reaching levels similar to inflamed controls. There was also a prominent mucosal eosinophil (allergy cell) infiltration of the intestinal lining in affected children that was significantly lower in those on a diet that excluded the wheat protein gluten and the cow's milk protein casein, while lymphocyte (chronic inflammatory cell) populations were not influenced by diet. The importance of this finding will become evident in the next chapter and in the analysis of the role of food allergy and the benefits of dietary exclusion in children with ASD and the Arizona 5 in particular. The follow-up studies to the original report in the *Lancet* confirmed the presence of an inflammatory bowel disease in children with ASD, with features that distinguished this disease from other well-recognized GI conditions.

It is notable that some years ago, in conversation with Dr. Tim Buie, the pediatric gastroenterologist who works with Dr. Kushak and heads the team at Mass General, he commented that their pathologists acknowledge an increase in inflammatory cells in colonic biopsies but "not enough to call colitis."[21]

This statement is inconsistent with the textbook definition of colitis and may, at least in part, account for the reported differences in disease frequency. As far as I am aware, there are no reports from Dr. Buie's group that have used objective techniques for quantifying inflammatory cells in the relevant biopsies.

THE REAL CONTROVERSY

One major barrier to the objective consideration of intestinal disease in these children is that many people consider that this disease is inextricably linked to the issue of whether vaccines cause autism. This means that some, in order to discredit the vaccine association, have determined that the bowel disease needs to suffer a similar fate.

Perverse objectivity—the deliberate misrepresentation of the evidence— plumbed new depths in a series of articles by journalist Brian Deer. These articles were commissioned by and published in the *British Medical Journal* (*BMJ*) where Deer's analysis was strongly endorsed as "proof of fraud" by editor-in-chief Dr. Fiona Godlee. As Deer was to claim in a recent radio broadcast, "[Wakefield] has now been branded by the *British Medical Journal* a fraudster. They described his work as an elaborate fraud. . . ."[22]

Describing the basis of my apparent fraud, Deer stated, ". . . he also went through the results manually altering test results and diagnoses and histories of the children so to create the appearance that there was a link between MMR and autism."[23]

And in doing so, apparently, I had deliberately and wilfully deceived my colleagues—senior academics who have published thousands of clinical and research papers but who appear to have been asleep at the switch on this high-profile occasion. The focus of Deer's obsession was unambiguous: "It's squarely an allegation against Wakefield. He did it."[24]

So there it was: I was accused of altering the clinical histories and test results in autistic children in order to manufacture a disease—a disease described in the *Lancet* in 1998 in order to fabricate a case against the MMR vaccine. In a well-orchestrated and elaborate public relations rollout, the news of my malfeasance spread around the globe, focusing mainly on major news outlets in the United States, where I am currently working to resolve the issue of vaccine safety and the causes of ASD. A mainstream media that thrives on pharma dollars, in a torrent of incontinent abandon, portrayed fraud as fact.

The problem is that Deer made his allegations in the full and certain knowledge that his claims were false. His deception was intended as a smoke screen— an attempt to discredit at any cost those who had fired the first round in the vaccine-autism debate. On the contrary, the objective documentary evidence proves beyond a shadow of a doubt that I did not falsify the data—no one falsified data. The findings are real, and they were accurately reported in the *Lancet*. Bear with me while I describe the pedantic diagnostic process—one of which Deer was fully aware.

Before his retirement in 2000, Professor Walker-Smith's Department of Paediatric Gastroenterology was the busiest in Europe and arguably the best in the world. Biopsies taken for routine diagnostic purposes from all children undergoing endoscopy under his care at the Royal Free went to the Department of Pathology where they were reviewed under the microscope by the duty pathologist. The duty pathologists were not specialists in pediatric intestinal diseases. They might have had an interest in brain disease or breast cancer, but not in inflammatory bowel disease in children; they happen only to have been on the duty rota that day. As unsatisfactory as this may seem, it is the normal practice in National Health Service (NHS) hospitals. From this routine review, a report was generated that went into the children's clinical records.

Next came an audit of these diagnoses by Professor Walker-Smith and his team, who met with a senior pathologist on a regular basis to review all of the biopsies of patients from the previous week. This audit had been part of Professor Walker-Smith's routine clinical practice for many years and had given him an unparalleled experience of the appearances of bowel disease in children. This process of oversight made it much easier to observe the emergence of new patterns of disease, particularly those that are subtle or complex. At the General Medical Council (GMC) proceedings, Professor Walker-Smith was asked to put this into context for his patients with ASD. He obliged:

> We saw a very clear pattern emerging with these children. There seemed to be some, on the clinical side, degree of similarity between the clinical features. These were the severe abdominal pain, often manifesting as screaming. They were the presentation, usually with diarrhoea, but then at times there were episodes of constipation . . . and [they] did have a similarity between them when they were abnormal; and perhaps, principally, the histology which was not grossly abnormal but did show evidence of both chronic inflammation and episodes of acute inflammation as instanced by cryptitis, etc.[25]

Professor Walker-Smith was able to describe how, earlier in his career, he had gone through a similar exercise in careful observation in the description of key features of celiac disease in children.[26] He concluded, "So there is nothing new in my career in doing this kind of exercise."[27]

Given the fact that Royal Free pathologists had little or no experience in bowel disease in children, it was not surprising that there were instances where they had overlooked or misinterpreted inflammatory changes in the biopsy tissues from these cases.

The discrepancy between some of the routine reports and Professor Walker-Smith's own impression of disease led him to instigate a further level of scrutiny. This exercise was also stimulated when I asked him to present our initial experience with these children to a clinical research meeting in December 1996—fourteen months before the publication of the *Lancet* paper—at the Wellcome Trust, a large medical charity, in London. He wanted to make absolutely certain that his impression of disease in these children was valid before making any public statement. As he elaborated to the GMC:

> **This was totally unrelated to Andy Wakefield**[28]. . . . This was a personal initiative which I took myself. . . . I selected Dr Paul Dhillon. Dr Paul Dhillon . . . a co-author of the paper, was an experienced histopathologist who knew about gastroenterological disease and inflammatory bowel disease in particular. He had no particular expertise in children per se, but he was an expert in inflammatory bowel disease.[29]

Professor Walker-Smith chose Dr. Dhillon over other pathologists at the Royal Free because, as he went on to say, "[He] had much more experience, as indeed I believe I myself had from my years of looking down a microscope twice a week with histopathologists."[30]

He went on to explain the diagnostic process:

> What I asked him [Dr. Dhillon] to do was if he would pull out the histology of the first seven children that we had investigated, autistic children, and would he gather together the slides of those children and look at them, without any of the clinical information being provided to him. I would then meet with him and we together would look together down the microscope at the histological findings. . . .[31]

Professor Walker-Smith confirmed that Dr. Dhillon had had nothing more than the slides in front of him: no records, no diagnoses, and no knowledge of the children's clinical findings. At the GMC, his legal counsel asked Professor Walker-Smith about the advantages of reviewing all the biopsies at one time in this way. He described it as "Immense . . . I had not realised quite so clearly, how similar these pathological features were until I, with my own eyes, actually saw these seven children. . . . It was a very valuable exercise to put all these children together."[32] As for the bowel disease in these children, he reiterated, "I saw with my own eyes these changes."[33]

The [disease] changes that the Professor Walker-Smith saw and that Dr. Dhillon confirmed were, by December 1996, assimilated into a presentation for the forthcoming Wellcome Trust meeting. Professor Walker-Smith's notes began:

Entero-colitis and Disintegrative Disorder Following MMR
A Review of the First Seven Cases

I wish today, to present some preliminary details concerning seven children, all boys, who appear to have entero-colitis and disintegrative disorder, probably autism, following MMR. I shall now briefly present their case history.[34]

By this stage, there was little doubt in the mind of Professor Walker-Smith—indeed the minds of most of the senior authors—that MMR vaccine had played a significant part in this story. In his presentation notes, Professor Walker-Smith then set out the details of his own audit of the clinical histories and tissue findings for each child. The relevant behavioral and intestinal pathology findings were documented by him and the latter was confirmed as indeterminate (nonspecific) colitis in each case.

The entire series of biopsies taken from the twelve *Lancet* children were reviewed by Dr. Dhillon in the manner described above, latterly in the company of Dr. Anthony, an experimental pathologist, and me. From a personal perspective, I found this to be an invaluable learning experience. Dr. Dhillon's findings were recorded on a standardized form that he had designed for the purpose (see Figure 1). In his statement to the GMC, Dr. Dhillon described this process in detail, stating, "For my research review of slides, I was not given any clinical details about the children who had provided the samples. I made microscopical observations and recorded these observations using the system described above. The observations were given to Dr. Wakefield."[35]

I duly transcribed the pathologists' findings into what was to become the *Lancet* paper. Minor changes were made by the senior authors in the final drafting, when all of the pathology assessments—those of Dr. Dillon, Dr. Anthony, and Dr. Davies, another senior histopathologist from the Royal Free—were compared. Dr. Davies was later to write in the *BMJ* in support of this diagnostic approach: ". . . ANY study of histopathology has more credence, with reduced inter- and intra-observer variation, when a systematic review, using defined structured criteria over a short time-frame, is performed."[36] In fact, quite independently of Dr. Dhillon, Dr. Davies and Dr. Murch convened a separate review of the relevant children's biopsies in November 2007, following the circulation of a draft of the *Lancet* paper.[37] According to Dr. Murch, those present at this review were entirely satisfied with the descriptions of the biopsies.

Dr. Dhillon's diagnoses, based as they were upon a "systematic review using defined structured criteria," were faithfully reproduced in the *Lancet*.[38]

Crucially, as far as Deer's allegations are concerned, Professor Walker-Smith affirmed in his testimony that, if there was a change between the routine pathology report and the final diagnosis reported in the *Lancet*, it arose out of the exercise that he carried out with Dr. Dhillon[39] not as a result of fraud on my part.

It was the result of this exacting process—the discovery of a potentially novel disease syndrome—that was reported in the *Lancet* paper. Discovery is a raison d'être for tertiary referral centers—centers of excellence—and one reason why they are so important.

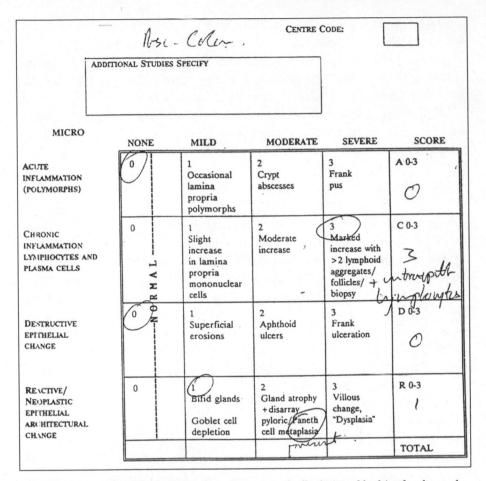

FIGURE 1. Dr. Dhillon's histopathology form, specifically designed by him for the analysis of ASD children's biopsies. Asc. Colon = Ascending Colon Biopsy. This biopsy from Child 9 in the *Lancet* paper was scored as normal by the duty pathologist. The biopsy actually showed a marked increase in chronic inflammatory cell infiltrate, with inflammation of the surface layer of cells (epithelium) (Row 2, Columns 4 and 5, indicating "+ intraepithelial lymphocytes") and architectural changes typical of chronic inflammation (Row 4, Columns 1, 2, and 5, indicating Paneth cell metaplasia as "present").

And the process was also of direct clinical relevance to the children's well-being, as Professor Walker-Smith described in his testimony: "I had a clear duty, once I had new information which was relevant to the patient, to communicate that information to the relevant people or, in some cases, to consider using anti-inflammatories, which I had not done hitherto."[40]

Finally, once I had put the paper together in draft form, including these rigorously confirmed findings, it was circulated to all authors for their modification and approval. And when the proofs of the article were received from the *Lancet* several weeks in advance of publication, they too were circulated to all senior authors so that their respective contributions could be rechecked.

These are the origins of the "changes" that Deer and the *BMJ* have accused me of making in the course of perpetrating scientific "fraud." The story that Deer told and Dr. Godlee affirmed bears no resemblance to these facts.

Referenced below and available to Deer at the time of writing his articles, are the specific descriptions of this diagnostic process in published papers from the *Lancet* 1998 paper[41] and two papers published subsequently in 2000[42] and 2004.[43]

January 2011 was not the first time that Deer had paraded his ignorance in the *BMJ*, having written a letter in 2010, presumably with the help of his source, Professor Tom MacDonald of Barts Hospital, titled "Wakefield's 'autistic enterocolitis' under the microscope."[44] There, he went after the testimony of Dr. Susan Davies, one of the *Lancet* authors and a pathologist who worked clinically with Professor Walker-Smith and was later to act as his dedicated pediatric GI pathologist. In seeking to expose Dr. Davies as a weak link in the claim to bowel disease in the *Lancet* children, he got off to a shaky start by describing her as the ". . . lead pathologist on Wakefield's study."[45]

She pointed out Deer's error in a response to the *BMJ*, in which she also rebuked him for his "misrepresentation . . . and lack of understanding of the process in studies involving histopathology."[46]

She offered Deer an insight into the gradual realization of the inflammatory disease that I had originally suspected was ailing these children and detailed the painstaking process of disease discovery:

> As to the severity of any pathology, there was a gradual awareness by those attending the regular clinicopathological conferences [Professor Walker-Smith's weekly meetings] that we were identifying subtle changes in some of the mucosal biopsies from autistic children. Subtle does not always indicate insignificant: the focal features of cow's milk protein enteropathy may be misinterpreted as normal; the hidden pathogen in immunodeficient syndromes is identified only by close scrutiny; the presence of Helicobacter pylori [the bacterium that causes stomach ulcers] in gastric biopsies was previously not recorded, as they were considered insignificant. . . . The significance of any minor changes cannot be determined at the outset; the natural history evolves and/or may be altered by any therapy, but the changes must first be recognised.[47]

And recognized they were, although not by Deer. But driven by an agenda that has come to define his fragile ego, these insights did not trouble him.

Inspired by how easy it was to publish pro-MMR material in the *BMJ*, he plunged headlong into his commissioned articles with abandon.

As for editorial oversight of the *BMJ* articles, it is clear that in her enthusiasm for Deer's attempted exoneration of MMR vaccine, Editor-in-Chief Dr. Godlee did not check the facts, which were referred to both in my book *Callous Disregard: Autism and Vaccines—The Truth Behind a Tragedy*, published by Skyhorse Publishing in May 2010, and my complaint to the UK's Press Complaints Commission about Brian Deer's brand of "journalism."

The relevant documents, including Professor Walker-Smith's presentation notes, the transcript of his sworn testimony before the GMC, the relevant sections of Dr. Dhillon's statement to the GMC, and the published papers that described the diagnostic process, were available to Deer and the editors of the *BMJ* well in advance of publication.[48] They knew or should have known that their allegations were false. It is clear that the *BMJ* acted recklessly in failing to check these facts adequately before making their damaging allegations.

Ironically, the folly of Deer and Godlee will be remembered as a turning point in the whole vaccine-autism debate—the moment at which they provided an unwitting opportunity to bring down the house of cards.

But in the meantime, the damage done to children suffering from ASD and GI disease, deprived of adequate medical care and (as this book seeks to illustrate) discriminated against on so many levels, is incalculable. The extent of Deer's empathy was recorded outside the GMC hearing when a mother, protesting in our support, showed him a picture of her son, naked but for his shorts and covered in feces from a poorly fitting ileostomy appliance. His entire colon had been surgically removed due to disease. Deer's considered opinion was "That's just diarrhea." His perception of the parents conveyed a similar lack of humanity: "The festering nastiness, the creepy repetitiveness, the weasly, deceitful, obsessiveness, all signal pathology to me [*sic*]."[49]

And with rhetorical misanthropy he added, "And they wonder why their children have problems with their brains."[50]

INTESTINAL INFLAMMATION IN ASD

So, with that history out of the way—at least for now—what *is* the nature of the intestinal disease in autism? Inflammation in the upper GI tract may affect the esophagus (eosinophilic[51] or refux-type esophagitis), stomach (focal gastritis[52]), duodenum (duodenitis[53]), and jejunum (jejunitis). The characteristics of the gastric (stomach) and small intestinal lesions distinguish them from other common forms of intestinal inflammation[54] such as Crohn's disease.

LYMPHOID NODULAR HYPERPLASIA

Lymphoid nodular hyperplasia is a tissue reaction in the specialized foci of immune cells (lymphoid nodules or Peyer's patches in the small intestine) in response to antigens (these are molecules—usually a protein, peptide, or carbohydrate—capable of eliciting a specific immune response) from food or microbes such as viruses and some bacteria. Historically it has been associated with infections such as *Helicobacter pylori* (the bacterium that causes stomach ulcers,[55] rotavirus[56] and adenovirus,[57] and immunodeficiency states[58]). More recently it has been linked to rotavirus vaccination[59] and is emerging as a hallmark lesion in children with non-IgE-mediated food allergy.[60]

LNH is common in the ileum and colon of children with both ASD and GI symptoms. Under the microscope, pathologists from Mount Sinai Hospital in New York[61] identified ileal LNH in 93 of 127 (73%) patients of Dr. Arthur Krigsman. Colonic LNH was observed in 46 of 143 (32%) of his ASD patients. LNH of both the ileum and the colon was present in 32% of patients.

Of the ninety-eight patients in Dr. Krigsman's series who had confirmed ileal and/or colonic LNH, seventy-eight (80%) also had ileal and/or colonic inflammation. Overall, those with LNH were over three times more likely to have inflammation indicating that the presence of LNH predicts inflammatory disease. Younger children who had regressed or arrested after normal early development had a greater risk of LNH when compared with those children with early onset autism.[62]

A second study from Dr. Anthony and colleagues at the Royal Free Hospital, involving 148 children with ASD and 30 non-ASD controls, found that the prevalence of endoscopic and microscopic LNH was significantly greater in ASD children when compared with the control group—in the ileum (90% vs. 30%) and colon (59% vs. 23%)—whether or not controls had coexistent colonic inflammation. As judged by the doctor performing the endoscopy, the severity of ileal LNH was significantly greater in ASD children when compared with controls, with moderate to severe ileal LNH present in 68% of ASD children when compared with 4 of 27 (15%) controls. In this study, the presence and severity of ileal LNH was not influenced by either diet or age at colonoscopy. Isolated ileal LNH without evidence of pathology elsewhere in the intestine was a rare event, occurring in less than 3% of children overall.[63]

Other markers of inflammation may be abnormal in ASD patients. In inflammatory conditions such as Crohn's disease, intestinal immune cells (lymphocytes) secrete chemical mediators (cytokines) that play an extremely important role in the inflammatory response, acting either to promote or limit particular aspects of this response. It is the profile of these cytokines—the balance between those that promote inflammation and those that limit it—that is disturbed in inflammatory bowel diseases. Analysis of immune cells from the lining of the colon,[64] small intestine, and blood[65] of children with ASD and GI symptoms showed a marked imbalance in these cytokines with a strong proinflammatory response. Not only was the proinflammatory cytokine level (e.g., tumor necrosis factor-alpha [TNF-α]) elevated, but, unusually and distinct from other common forms of intestinal inflammation, the anti-inflammatory cytokine level (interleukin-10 [IL-10]) was way down in these same children. With no buffer to the production of TNF-α in the form of IL-10, the immune imbalance appeared to be even more profound in these children than, say, in Crohn's disease. This particular finding—the cytokine imbalance—is emerging as one of the more consistent immunological findings in the ASD population and may indicate a novel disease process in these children.[66]

In addition to demonstrable inflammatory pathology in many children with ASD and GI symptoms, there are also functional abnormalities that indicate the presence of significant intestinal disease.

BRUSH BORDER ENZYME ABNORMALITIES

The small intestine is lined with specialized cells that secrete digestive enzymes for breaking down carbohydrates, proteins, and fats prior to their absorption into the body. Deficiencies in these enzymes reflect small intestinal dysfunction that presents with symptoms of diarrhea, gaseousness, pain, failure to thrive, and pale bulky stools associated with undigested fat. Levels of these enzymes are commonly low in patients with diseases of the small intestine, including children with ASD. Horvath et al.[67] demonstrated low activities of the brush border disaccharidase (paired complexes of sugars) enzymes (lactase, maltase, sucrase, palatinase, and glucoamylase) in twenty-one of thirty-six (58%) children with ASD and GI symptoms. The most frequent finding was a low lactase level, which was present in fourteen of thirty-six patients (39%). Ten children had decreased enzyme activities in two or more enzymes. Children with low enzyme activities had loose stools, gaseousness, or both. These findings of functional defects in the epithelium are consistent with the visual evidence of small intestinal inflammation that have been seen in affected children using capsule endoscopy in Dr. Krigsman's clinical practice (Krigsman, A., personal communication).

From Mass General Hospital for Children, Kushak et al. measured intestinal disaccharidase activities in 199 individuals with autism to determine the frequency of enzyme deficiency.[68] All patients had duodenal biopsies that were evaluated microscopically and assayed for lactase, sucrase, and maltase activity. Frequency of lactase deficiency was 58% in autistic children age five years or under and 65% in older patients. In the younger age group, boys with autism had a nearly twofold lower lactase activity than girls with autism. Inflammation in the duodenal biopsies was only found in 6% of their cases, that is, far fewer than had enzyme deficiencies. It appeared that lactase deficiency without accompanying intestinal inflammation is common in autistic children. The authors proposed that impaired digestive enzyme activity may contribute to abdominal discomfort, pain, and the aberrant behaviors of ASD. Since most children with ASD and lactose intolerance were not identified by clinical history or biopsy changes, intestinal malfunction is even more prevalent in this population than is evident from the patients' symptoms and endoscopic and microscopic evidence of disease.

The Mass General group has also studied the relationship of patients' symptoms to disaccharidase activities, comparing this in autistic and non-autistic individuals. Specific activities for lactase, sucrase, maltase, and palatinase were studied in duodenal biopsies from 308 patients with ASD and 206 non-autistic controls undergoing endoscopy on suspicion of GI disease. Disaccharidase activities were analyzed for all patients according to the patients' presenting symptoms including diarrhea, abdominal pain, food sensitivity, failure to thrive, constipation, gastroesophageal reflux, or a combination of symptoms.

In the analysis of Kushak et al., ASD patients with diarrhea demonstrated significantly lower maltase activity than did neurotypical children with diarrhea.[69] Frequency of lactase deficiency in patients with failure to thrive was significantly higher in those with ASD (80%) compared with the non-autistic group (25%). Palatinase deficiency was also more common in ASD patients with diarrhea (28%) compared with the non-autistic patients with the same intestinal pathology (11%).[70] The emerging link between GI symptoms and functional GI abnormalities is valuable information; it may provide not only novel treatment options but also ways of assessing their benefits.

INTESTINAL PERMEABILITY IN AUTISM

The intestine is lined by a continuous layer of cells (epithelial cells)—operating as a barrier—that under healthy circumstances lets some molecules in and keeps others out. Intestinal permeability (IP) refers to the passive inward transport of small-to-medium-sized molecules across the small intestinal mucosa, and its measurement provides a reflection of one aspect of this barrier function. One method of assessing permeability due to the movement of molecules *between* the epithelial cells of the intestinal lining (paracellular transport) is to measure the fractional urinary excretion of non-metabolized sugars such as lactulose and mannitol. In the healthy small intestine, permeability for larger sugars (e.g., disaccharides like lactulose) is much lower than it is for smaller sugars (e.g., monosaccharides like mannitol), resulting in a lower urinary ratio of large-to-small sugars. Diseases of the small intestine such as Crohn's disease and celiac disease are associated with inflammation, increased permeability, and, consequently, an increased urinary lactulose-mannitol ratio. An increase in IP is often referred to as "leaky gut."

Leaky gut appears to be relatively common in children with autism. Several studies have now confirmed increased IP in a high proportion of individuals with ASD. D'Eufemia and colleagues from Rome, Italy, first reported abnormally high IP in Italian patients with ASD in 1996.[71] Increased IP was detected in nine of the twenty-one (43%) patients with autism but in none of the forty controls. In a second study, Horvath et al. identified abnormally elevated IP in nineteen of twenty-five (76%) ASD children. More recently, de Magistris et al. reported abnormally high IP in thirty-seven of ninety (41%) children with ASD compared with 5% of two hundred healthy controls—a difference that was statistically significant.[72] A report from Horvath et al. suggests that leaky gut in ASD may be improved by treatment with the pancreatic hormone secretin.[73]

INTESTINAL MICROBIOLOGY

The importance of human intestinal bacteria—the microflora—in health and disease cannot be overstated. Providing a somewhat humbling perspective to the cohabitation of bug and man, Collins and colleagues from McMaster University in Hamilton, Ontario, recently observed that "There are approximately 10^{14} bacteria in the human gastrointestinal tract and their combined metabolic activity exceeds that of the liver."[74]

At a recent lecture on the rapidly expanding field of metabolomics (analysis of the products of the body's metabolism in health and disease), the audience was informed that, from the metabolic standpoint, we—you and I—are actually nine-tenths bacteria and one part human!

Collins and colleagues continued in their justifiable homage to intestinal microbes by comparison of our vital statistics: "The number of bacteria [in the colon] exceeds the number of cells in the human body by a factor of 10 and the number of genes exceeds that of the human genome by a factor of 10–100."[75]

And then, as a testament to the vital but precarious balance in which we live codependently with our bugs, the authors pointed out that this "remarkable ecosystem" is separated from the human body by a single layer of cells—the intestinal epithelium. Ranged on one side of this microscopic barrier is 80% of the body's immune system and on the other, billions of bugs, both working in harmony in healthy individuals.

Our bacteria are essential for normal health, playing crucial roles in the development, education, and regulation of the immune system, production of vitamins, detoxification of metabolic byproducts and drugs, and more—much more. And what Collins and his colleagues were really getting to in their article is that our bacterial microflora interact with our brains in a bidirectional exchange that can go awry—and when it does, the functions of both systems are adversely affected.

Dysbiosis is a state of living with an intestinal flora that has potentially harmful effects. This situation can occur when the immune system of the mucosa is not functioning properly, as in inflammatory bowel disease (e.g., ulcerative colitis) and HIV infection and other immunodeficiency states.

Against this background, disturbances in the intestinal microflora with pathological overgrowth and behavior of certain bacterial species—dysbiosis—are emerging as a forerunner in the gut-brain connection in ASD. In 1998, Ellen Bolte, the mother of a child with autism, proposed a role for intestinal dysbiosis with anaerobic (existing in the absence of free oxygen) clostridial bacteria (the family of organisms responsible for tetanus and gas gangrene) in autism, specifically via the potential neurotoxic effects of clostridial byproducts.[76] *Clostridium bolteae*, a subspecies of this particularly noxious clan, apparently took her name accordingly.

In order to investigate the role of intestinal dysbiosis vis-a-vis clostridia in autism further, Finegold et al.[77] examined the fecal flora of children with late-onset (regressive) autism compared with developmentally normal controls. In the fecal flora of children with regressive autism, clostridial counts were high when compared with controls. The number of clostridial species found in the stools of children with autism was greater than in the stools of control children. Children with autism had species of *Clostridium* not found in controls, whereas controls contained species not found in children with autism. In all, there were twenty-five different clostridial species that distinguished patients with ASD and healthy controls. In gastric and duodenal specimens, the most striking finding was the total absence of non-spore-forming anaerobes (non–oxygen requiring) and microaerobic bacteria from control children and significant numbers of such bacteria from children with autism. Finegold et al. concluded that their studies "demonstrate significant alterations in upper and lower intestinal flora of children with late-onset autism and may provide insights into the nature of this disorder."[78]

Ellen Bolte's original hypothesis was a further compelling parental insight into autism's organic origins. Her concept of neurotoxicity associated with clostridial dysbiosis was to receive further validation from the thesis work of graduate student Jody Wall at Ohio State University.[79] Using gene amplification technology, Wall examined the presence and quantity of both beneficial bacteria (*Bifidobacterium*, *Lactobacillus*) and pathogenic bacteria (clostridial species, including Bolte's eponymous bug *Clostridium bolteae*) in children aged 3–9 years with ASD compared with age and gender-matched controls. In order to establish the baseline for differences between the microflora in these two groups, only children who had no prior use of antibiotics or probiotics were included. ASD stool samples revealed significantly lower amounts of lactobacilli[80] and higher amounts of *C. bolteae*[81] than those of controls. Interestingly, the bug count correlated with certain GI symptoms: children who had lower amounts of *Bifidobacterium* had significantly more bloating[82] and flatulence,[83] and children with higher amounts of *C. boltae* had significantly more episodes of bloating[84] than other children.

Using standard bacterial culture technology at the University of Arizona, Professor Jim Adams and colleagues have recently confirmed this depletion of bifidobacteria in children with ASD and a strong correlation between GI symptoms with autism severity. Children with ASD had lower levels of species of bifidobacteria[85] and higher levels of species of *Lactobacillus*,[86] but similar levels of other bacteria and yeast, using standard culture growth-based techniques; it is worth noting that the more severe the GI symptoms, the worse the autistic behaviors. Adams and colleagues reinforced the growing perception that autism's symptoms are exacerbated by or even partially due to the underlying GI problems, including the makeup of one's gut bacteria.[87]

Given these fundamental differences in intestinal microflora between children with ASD and their neurotypical counterparts, the question arises as to whether the effects of diet on behavior are direct or mediated through the effects of diet on gut bacteria. In 2009, Li and colleagues acknowledged that "The ability of dietary manipulation to influence learning and behavior is well recognized. . . ." But he went on to observe that these effects were ". . . almost exclusively interpreted as direct effects of dietary constituents on the central nervous system."[88]

They went on to challenge the biological basis of a relatively novel paradigm by proposing that diet influenced bacteria and that bacteria, in turn, changed our behavior. Specifically, Li et al. examined the possibility that shifts in bacterial diversity in the intestine due to dietary manipulation could influence memory and learning. Laboratory mice fed on chow containing 50% lean ground beef for three months displayed improved working[89] and reference memory[90] when compared with mice fed on standard rodent chow. The beef-fed animals also displayed slower speed in seeking food[91] as well as reduced anxiety level in the first day of testing.[92] Molecular analysis of the gut flora demonstrated significantly higher bacterial diversity in the beef-fed group when compared with mice receiving standard chow. The observed correlation between dietary-induced shifts in bacterial diversity and mammalian behavior indicate a potential role for gut bacterial diversity in cognition—a fascinating, if challenging, insight into the fact that no mammal is an island.[93]

But what was not known in 2010 was that the bacterial colonization of the gut impacts mammalian brain development as well as subsequent behavior. Using measures of motor activity and anxiety-like behavior, Diaz Heijtz et al. demonstrated that germ-free mice born and raised with no gut bacteria display increased motor activity and reduced anxiety when compared with mice that have a normal gut flora. The authors documented that the behavioral pattern was associated with altered expression of genes in the brain known to be involved in motor control and anxiety-like behavior. Their results suggest that the process of microbial colonization of the gut initiates gut-brain signaling mechanisms that affect brain development in areas of motor control and anxiety behavior.[94,95]

We do not and cannot live in a germ-free environment; coexistence is required for life—ours if not theirs. Our bugs and the way in which we acquire them may make us more of who we are as sentient beings than we care to imagine.

But how do bugs do what they do? One possibility is that the effects of gut bacteria are mediated by the chemicals that they produce. One example from the arena of current autism research is a chemical called propionic acid (PPA), a short chain fatty acid that is a metabolic byproduct of gut bacteria and is also used as a common food preservative. In a series of elegant studies, Derrick MacFabe, MD, and colleagues from London, Ontario, have shown that PPA, when injected into the cerebrospinal fluid that bathes the brain, can cause behavioral abnormalities and changes in the brain similar to those reported in autism. Compared with controls, rats treated with PPA in this way displayed impaired social behaviors. Analysis of the brain tissue of PPA-treated rats revealed oxidative stress[96] and neuroinflammatory responses similar in character to those reported in some patients with autism.[97,98]

And the field abounds with similar insights into the fundamental importance of bacteria in the gut-brain crosstalk. Abnormal stress responses in germ-free mice improved or normalized following gut colonization with normal intestinal bacteria.[99] From Collins' laboratory at McMaster University came the fascinating observation that disturbance of the gut microflora with antibiotics led to mild inflammation, increase in the pain neurotransmitter *substance P* in the intestine, and an increased pain response, and visceral hyperalgesia in mice.[100] This effect was attenuated by probiotic administration. It appears that bacteria influence the perception of intestinal pain, with normal bacteria potentially keeping it in check. It is enormously tempting to draw a line between the apparently excessive pain response observed clinically in some children with ASD and the emerging evidence for disturbances in their intestinal microflora.

Finally, it is my personal belief that autism at the level of the central nervous system is a dysautonomia: a disorder of regulation of autonomic responses that control not only vital subconscious functions such as heart rate, intestinal motility, and temperature regulation, but also higher functions such as the state of arousal including emotional responses to external stimuli. I believe that autism has an epicenter in the brainstem,[101] the nuclei of the vagus nerve that are "ground zero" for autonomic regulation. The vagus nerve is the tenth cranial nerve. It is long, beginning at its nuclei in the medulla of the brainstem, and it supplies nerve fibers to, among other places, the abdominal organs. Through the vagus nerve from the intestine, these brainstem nuclei can detect and monitor gut bacteria and their effects. It may be that, in turn, during critical phases of brain growth and development, gut bacteria can modify these nuclei and the higher brain centers that they serve and regulate.

TREATMENT APPROACHES TO GI DISEASE IN ASD

It is not the intention here to provide an exhaustive list of possible biomedical approaches to autism but instead to outline a few guiding principles. When considering the merits of treating GI symptoms or specific GI pathology in ASD patients, it is important to bear in mind that orthodox practitioners are frequently comfortable treating the behavioral symptoms of this disorder with psychotropic medications that have not been subjected to randomized controlled clinical trials and that are not approved for use in children or for use in autism.

It is also important to recognize that the physician, in treating the symptomatic and health consequences of the GI disease, is not treating the patient's autism. Autistic behaviors may improve as a consequence of GI-directed treatment, but this may change simply because the patient is no longer in pain or no longer has diarrhea. Trials of dietary intervention using a gluten-free/casein-free exclusion protocol have, however, used endpoints of behavior and cognitive functioning and not scores of GI symptoms.[102] Despite this, there is some evidence that the diet is affecting the GI system as well.[103] Anthony et al. observed a reduction in acute inflammation in children on a gluten-free/casein-free diet when compared with those on an unrestricted diet in an audit of 148 consecutively investigated children with ASD. The diet did not appear to influence either chronic inflammation or LNH (unpublished observations).[104]

Few controlled trials of therapy are available. Nonetheless, based upon symptoms, treatments may include drugs that reduce stomach acid, control intestinal inflammation, increase intestinal motility, or otherwise address constipation.

In seeking to test the hypothesis that removal of anaerobic bacteria such as clostridia might be beneficial in ASD, Sandler et al. noted objective cognitive improvement in autistic children in an open label[105] study of oral vancomycin,[106] an antibiotic that acts locally in the intestine. Children regressed again following cessation of therapy, suggesting that any dysbiosis and associated toxic sequelae were likely to be secondary to underlying intestinal pathology rather than the primary problem but that bacterial products were contributing to the behavioral features of autism. It seems likely, therefore, that the evidently dysfunctional mucosal immune system in affected children creates an environment that favors a dysbiosis that would be ameliorated only temporarily by vancomycin.

MEASLES VIRUS IN THE INTESTINE

One important matter that deserves a paragraph is the finding of measles virus in the intestinal tissues. In addition to being a respiratory pathogen, measles virus infects and damages the intestine. It can cause long-term disruption of the immune system, inflammation, and longstanding infection. It may also cause autism.[107] The finding of measles in the GI tract of children with ASD was proposed in 1995 and was first reported by Professor John O'Leary in collaboration with Royal Free doctors in 2002.[108] Using state-of-the-art gene amplification technology, measles virus genetic material was found in seventy-five of ninety-one (82%) children with regressive autism and GI disease compared with five of seventy (7%) developmentally normal children. Specifically, the virus was detected by Professor O'Leary in the swollen lymphoid tissue of the terminal ileum, although in my own laboratory using a less sensitive technique, we were unable to detect measles genetic material. These molecular approaches were guided by the earlier detection of measles virus protein in these same tissues that was not found in the inflamed colon.[109] Professor O'Leary's findings came under attack in US vaccine court based upon a report by Dr. Stephen Bustin, who was acting on behalf of vaccine manufacturers in the UK MMR litigation. Professor O'Leary subsequently took part in a triangulated analysis among the laboratories of Dr. Bill Bellini at the CDC, Dr. Ian Lipkin at Colombia University, and his own lab in Dublin.[110] They were set the task of analyzing the same genetic material from biopsies of ASD children provided by Dr. Tim Buie from Mass General Hospital for Children. While the technical aspects of the study were commendable, with all three labs reporting virtually identical results, the case selection was not. The measles virus was found in one of twenty-five cases and one of thirteen non-autistic controls. However, Dr. Buie's biopsies came from only five children whose relevant symptoms had started after MMR vaccine. Furthermore, biopsies came from either colon or ileum—while only the latter biopsies were relevant. No information was provided on whether, in the five key cases, the biopsies were from the ileum—they might all have been irrelevant. And no information at all was provided on whether or not the children had intestinal inflammation as in the Royal Free cases. In other words, the study was a bust, and the painstaking molecular analyses that mitigated Bustin's attack on the O'Leary lab were all in vain. Nonetheless, accompanying newspaper headlines widely lauded this salvation of MMR vaccine while regrettably, Dr. Lipkin went on the record stating, "The work reported here eliminates the remaining support for the hypothesis that autism with GI complaints is related to MMR vaccine exposure."[111]

Dr. Lipkin's statement went far, far beyond the limitations of his published findings in what was perceived by many as a betrayal of the science and vaccine-injured children. Furthermore, persistent intestinal infection by measles virus, although an obvious starting point for our research, is but one mechanism among many by which this virus could cause or trigger autism.

CONCLUSIONS

GI symptoms require thorough investigation in children with developmental disorders on the autism spectrum. Until proven otherwise, they reflect physiological dysfunction and intestinal disease.

Where disease and dysfunction are present, they should be treated thoroughly and appropriately in the recognition that issues of safety should be paramount and that much remains to be learned about the optimal approach(es) to a complex problem.

The contemplation of a diagnosis of MSBP in an ASD child with the possibility of GI disease without thorough investigation of symptoms, recognition of diagnosed disease, and implementation of appropriate treatment is the path to professional negligence.

Finally, in the words of some of the more conservative interested parties, "More than 50% of autistic children appear to have GI symptoms, food allergies, and maldigestion or malabsorption issues. We need large, evidence-based studies to be done in order to fully understand the gut-brain association in autism."[112] This knowledge is salutatory albeit somewhat humbling since such problems have been largely ignored in the past.

Notwithstanding the need for huge investment in the further understanding of this fascinating field and compelling clinical challenge, in 2010, when one Arizona family was facing destruction at the hands of CPS—however well meaning its agents may have been—a great deal *was* known. In particular, a great deal was known about the problems with bowels, bugs, and diet in ASD and its clinical manifestations. Another crucial piece of this puzzle, and one that is highly relevant to the Arizona 5, is the role of food allergy.

BUGS, BATTERIES, AND BEYOND

Our bacteria are more than beneficial fellow travelers. Beyond the byways of the intestine they—or their remnants—live and operate as a life force within our cells. Somewhere in the mists of time, certain bacteria—*proteobacteria*—took up residence in primitive cells, providing them with the ability to generate energy from sugars and oxygen. The eukaryotic cell—a complex, membrane-bound structure with its genetic material contained within a nucleus—emerged and assembled into progressively more and more complex structures—from blobs to bodies. Without these bacterial remnants known as mitochondria, life as we know it would not exist. Mitochondria are the structures responsible for energy production in a cell. It goes without saying therefore, that mitochondrial dysfunctions that limit a cell's energy supply can have profound effects on health.

The discovery of "mito" disorders is relatively recent, with Ronald Luff having described the first sufferer of mito disease in 1959.[113] Four years later and consistent with their bacterial ancestry, mitochondria were discovered to have their own genetic blueprint or mtDNA. Aberrations in this blueprint account for more than forty different diseases. In addition, mutations in the cell's own nuclear DNA can lead to mitochondrial dysfunction, broadening the spectrum of mito disease considerably. The common denominator for these diseases is the inability to efficiently burn food and oxygen to produce energy. This, in turn, leads to impaired cellular function, oxidative stress, with damage and possible death of cells. The wide variety of associated pathologies includes seizures, digestive disease, paralysis, blindness, heart disease, and neurodevelopmental disorders such as autism. Those systems most susceptible to damage are those that require the most energy. Under resting conditions, this includes the brain and the heart and skeletal muscles, and under conditions of stress such as infection and vaccination, the immune system appears particularly vulnerable.

Recent attention has focused upon the axis of suboptimal if clinically silent mitochondrial dysfunction combined with immune system challenge, leading to developmental regression and autism in a previously healthy child. This scenario was put under the spotlight following publication of the case of Hannah Poling, a young girl who developed autism after receiving nine vaccines on the same day followed by fever, seizures, and profound and lasting regression.[114]

Her case report, written by her father, a pediatric neurologist, and published in the *Journal of Child Neurology*, was coauthored by a government witness in the Vaccine Injury Compensation Program (VICP), Dr. Andrew Zimmerman from Johns Hopkins. The fact that the authors readily acknowledged the role of vaccination in Hannah's neurological injury meant that the government had little option but to concede the case, ultimately to the tune of approximately $20 million over Hannah's lifetime.

And Hannah's single-point mutation in her mtDNA—one shared by her healthy mother—was clinically silent until she was exposed to excessive, overwhelming vaccination. There is absolutely no evidence—none at all—that she would have inevitably experienced illness associated with this mutation had she not been vaccinated as she was. Indeed, it is not even certain that her mtDNA mutation has any relevance at all to her mito dysfunction, which could simply have been caused by excessive vaccination.

While the case established the mito-vaccine-autism precedent, it was—in classical "public health speak"—dismissed as exquisitely rare and not relevant to the broader vaccine-autism debate. It was only a matter of time before this vain hope was dashed by a series of publications showing that not only were mito disorders common in the ASD population,[115] but they were common in the population as a whole. Previous estimates of 1 in 4,000 of the population had to be revised to 1 in 200 after Elliot and colleagues published their "revolutionary" findings on the analysis of cord blood samples from newborn children in the *American Journal of Human Genetics*.[116] If vaccines are bad for those with vulnerable mitochondria, public health vaccine policy is in need of a major overhaul.

In an excellent literature review of the current status of mito dysfunction in ASD, Dr. Daniel Rossingnol and Dr. Richard Frye highlighted features of such dysfunction in the general population of children with ASD and reported its characteristics in children with ASD and mito disease.[117] Eighteen publications representing a total of 112 children with ASD and mito disesase were identified. The groups were compared with published literature of two general populations: ASD children without mito disease and non-ASD children with mito disease. The prevalence of mito disease in those with ASD was 5.0% (3.2–6.9%)—much higher than was found in the general population (~0.01%). The prevalence of abnormal laboratory markers of mito dysfunction (e.g., carnitine and ubiquinone), including measures of impaired aerobic metabolism (e.g., raised lactic acid), was high in ASD and much higher than the prevalence of mito disease itself.

Their overview suggested that children with ASD have a spectrum of mito dysfunction of differing severity. The prevalence of developmental regression (52%), seizures (41%), motor delay (51%), gastrointestinal abnormalities (74%), female gender (39%), and elevated lactate (78%) and pyruvate (45%) was significantly higher in the ASD group with mito disease than in the general ASD population. Crucially, 79% of mito disease cases were not associated with genetic abnormalities, raising the likelihood of secondary mitochondrial dysfunction.

Mitochondria are vulnerable to environmental toxins such as thimerosal.[118] The discordance between the high rate of mito dysfunction—well in excess of that of mito disease due to genetic abnormalities—speaks to the distinct possibility of secondary mito damage due to environmental toxicity.

In Rossingol and Frye's review, they found that treatment studies of mito dysfunction in ASD children were limited, although improvements were noted in some studies with carnitine, coenzyme Q10 and B vitamins. The potential importance of the findings despite the various limitations of the studies, including small sample sizes and biases, reinforces the need for systematic, large-scale science.

The combination of mutations in mtDNA and nuclear DNA that might confer vulnerability to mito dysfunction in the wrong environmental circumstances might be present in as many as one in fifty children. World expert on mito disorders Dr. Douglas Wallace, former professor of molecular medicine and director of the Center for Molecular and Mitochondrial Medicine and Genetics at the University of California, Irvine, and now the director of the Center for Mitochondrial and Epigenomic Medicine and Michael and Charles Barnett Chair of Pediatric Mitochondrial Medicine and Metabolic Disease at Children's Hospital of Philadelphia, explained that "Mitochondrial dysfunction is a major underlying risk factor for human disease."[119]

The implications for vaccination strategies are not lost on Dr. Wallace, who is also the father of a young man with autism and a member of the Scientific and Medical Advisory Board of the United Mitochondrial Disease Foundation.[120] In April 2010, Dr. Wallace told the Vaccine Safety Working Group of Health and Human Services' National Vaccine Advisory Committee that over-vaccination of people with mito disorders was a deep concern.

"We have always advocated spreading the immunizations out as much as possible because every time you vaccinate you are creating a challenge for the system," Dr. Wallace testified. "And if a child has an impaired system that could in fact trigger further clinical problems."[121]

National immunization programs have been founded on the false and dangerous premise that one-size-fits-all, and the erroneous view that vaccines are safe because the science has been done to prove it. Dr. Wallace seems to dissent from the public health view: "We do not know what is not safe. We do not know the actual risk of a person with light mitochondrial disease has and being challenged either by vaccination or by a severe infection."[122]

Based upon next to no evidence, the CDC claims that multiple simultaneous vaccinations are safe "for children with normal immune systems," even though it also acknowledged that "usually simultaneous vaccination is incompletely studied at time of licensure."[123] Despite this evident contradiction, what constitutes a "normal immune system" in the presence of a mito gene weakness is anybody's guess.

Mito disorder and oxidative stress were to feature in the case of the Arizona 5. When considering the evidence presented later in Part 3, it is important to remember that at the time the case was heard, the discoveries of Poling, Oliviera, Elliot, and others were in the public domain, the government had conceded Hannah Poling's vaccine injury, and Dr. Wallace had made clear his views on vaccine risks in the presence of a mito disorder. At the very least the literature supported the possibility that mito disorder, oxidative stress, intestinal damage, autistic regression, and vaccines were precariously aligned, standing like a row of dominoes in a kindergarten at 08:59:59 on a Monday morning. The image of an integrated chain of cause and effect was coming into focus and could not be ignored, even at the highest levels within the US federal health agencies.

Chapter 3

A FEAST OF CONSEQUENCES: WILLIAM THOMPSON AND THE GREATEST MEDICAL FRAUD IN HISTORY

Sheila Ealey, an elegant and articulate African American mother, sat on the sofa next to her teenage son, Temple, in the drawing room of their New Orleans home. After Hurricane Katrina had destroyed their previous house and everything in it, Sheila and her husband, Ron, had worked tirelessly to rebuild a beautiful and cultured home for their family. They had succeeded.

Temple, now seventeen, should have been at school or on the practice field. But at fifteen months of age he had mistakenly received two doses of the MMR vaccine, one directly after the other. The second shot was intended for his twin sister, Lucinda. It was Sheila who noticed the missing shot and challenged the practice nurse, who immediately admitted to the error and documented it in Temple's chart. It was a frightened and angry mother who walked out of the doctor's office that morning with her screaming infant son and his unvaccinated twin sister. Lucinda is now a beautiful eleventh-grade scholar, fluent in three languages, a classical pianist with a beautiful singing voice who carries an unspeakable burden in her heart. For Temple it ended with that fateful visit to the doctor. By the following day, the thriving, happy, babbling boy was gone, never to return.

Tears poured down Sheila's cheeks. Never before, outside the privacy of the family home, had she let her emotions take over in this way. In an interview with Polly Tommey, whose story of her son Billy was so very similar to that of Sheila Ealey, she could contain her grief no longer. When Sheila's catharsis abated, there remained a prolonged, heavy silence punctuated only by small, childlike noises from Temple at her side.

Sheila's and Polly's stories overlapped in one further aspect that did not make it into the documentary for which we were shooting that day in Louisiana. The medical records containing the evidence incriminating the MMR vaccine in their damaged children had been stolen—Temple's from his temporary home in Austin, Texas, where they had taken refuge from Hurricane Katrina, and Billy's from a laboratory in the north of England that was involved in testing samples from children with autism. The records at the respective doctor's offices had simply gone missing, never to be recovered. There would be no litigating in either case in the absence of these records. As Sheila remarked, "The person who stole them already knew that."

As for the documentary, on that day with the Ealeys we were capturing one of the consequences—the "feast of consequences"[1]—that portrayed the street-level view of the worst medical fraud in history, one perpetrated by scientists at the Centers for Disease Control and Prevention (CDC) against the children of America.

BACKGROUND

The association between the MMR vaccine and autistic regression in previously developmentally normal children first hit TV screens on the *Susan Powter Show* in 1995 when California mom Cindy Goldenberg described how her son Garrett regressed shortly after his MMR vaccine, a fate that was to subsequently spread to other children like a canyon fire in the teeth of El Niño. In the same year, I started hearing identical reports, including the presence of prominent digestive issues in affected children, while working as an academic gastroenterologist at the Royal Free Hospital Medical School in London. The first children with this condition were subsequently reported in the *Lancet* in 1998. By 2000, a possible causal association between vaccines and autism had become a profound public concern.

Following the publication of the findings described in the *Lancet* article above, a series of questions arose. These included the obvious issue of why only a minority of children experience regression into autism when the vast majority of children receive the MMR vaccination. Smoking causes lung cancer, so why don't all smokers develop cancer? The answer often lies in the fact that the risk is *modified* by other factors associated with the exposure. For example, the outcome from exposure to many infections is modified by *age of exposure*. Children who experience measles under one year of age are more likely to have a complicated disease course than those who first experience this virus after their first birthday.

Similarly, the risk of meningitis from the dangerous and recklessly licensed MMR vaccine containing the Urabe AM-9 mumps strain was associated with age of exposure.[2] Children vaccinated at a younger age were at greater risk.

I shared with CDC scientists my research team's working hypothesis that younger age at first MMR may be a risk factor for autism. I did so at a science symposium on autism at Cold Spring Harbor Laboratories on Long Island, and as part of a congressional review of vaccines and autism, conducted by the Honorable Dan Burton and the Office of Government Reform. Five CDC scientists, Frank DeStefano, Coleen Boyle, Marshalyn Yeargin-Allsopp, William Thompson, and Tanya Bhasin—the Gang-of-Five—took up the challenge. The role of Dr. William Thompson, PhD, a senior scientist from the CDC's Immunization Safety Branch, was "to lead or co-lead" [these] safety studies." He later confirmed that the MMR safety study was "carried out in response to the Wakefield (1998) *Lancet* study that suggested an association between the MMR vaccine and an autism-like health outcome."

Let's get the gnarly stuff out of the way. The CDC's Gang-of-Five conducted a case-control study in which they compared two groups of children. One group had autism (cases) and the other group did not (controls). They compared these two groups for age at first MMR vaccination. They also examined whether the autism risk was greater in children receiving the MMR vaccine before and after age cutoffs of eighteen, twenty-four, and thirty-six months. Thompson confirmed in a later statement to Congressman Bill Posey,

> We hypothesized that if we found statistically significant effects . . . we would conclude that vaccinating children early with the MMR vaccine could lead to autism-like characteristics or features.

THE ANALYSIS PLAN

Through 2000–2001 the Gang-of-Five developed an Analysis Plan, a protocol that sets out the rules by which the study would be conducted, how data would be collected and analyzed, and, in this case, a timetable for completion of the study and submission for publication. The Analysis Plan is part of the *scientific process*. At the CDC, where he had worked for seventeen years, Thompson was widely respected by his colleagues as an epidemiologist and statistician. He was closely involved in drawing up the Analysis Plan and was the principal scientist responsible for the associated statistical analyses. In a money-laundering ring, he would have been the equivalent of the accountant—the last person you would want plea-bargaining with the Feds.

Once an Analysis Plan is locked, you stick by it. You don't deviate from that plan, particularly when you discover results that are not to your liking—which, as Thompson confirms, is exactly what happened:

> In this paper we deviated from what we agreed to up front. (Thompson on a telephone call with Brian Hooker)
>
> We failed to follow the final approved study protocol. (Thompson's statement to Bill Posey)

And deviation from the Analysis Plan—changing the scientific process—is, in these circumstances, fabrication[3] and therefore scientific fraud.

Lest the reader think that this was an isolated infraction, a blip on the otherwise unblemished radar of CDC vaccine safety research, think again:

> Thompson conceded to me that whenever CDC sees an effect that they don't want to report about vaccine injury, what they do is they get the scientists and they put them in a room where they work and work until they are able to get that effect to go away. (Dr. Brian Hooker in interview)

Foremost among such incidents was the CDC's infamous Verstraeten study of thimerosal, the mercury-based preservative present in many vaccines through the 1980s and 1990s and still present in many flu shots—shots that are given to pregnant women and children from six months of age. In a "data-raking" exercise of shameless proportions, CDC officials and others squeezed a hugely significant adverse effect of thimerosal down to zero. While Thompson was not involved in that study, the experience with Verstraeten set the bar for his MMR–autism investigation.

> The goal was to not deviate from the analysis plan to avoid the debacle[4] that occurred with the Verstraeten Thimerosal Study published in *Pediatrics* in 2003. (Thompson's statement to Congressman Bill Posey)

The only difference between the Verstraeten study and the subsequent DeStefano MMR study was that now we had a whistleblower to expose the fraud.

THE DATA

For their study, the Gang-of-Five took information on study children from two sources: the primary source of information was a child's *school record*, available for all children, which provided data on date of birth and race.[5] Additional information was available from children's birth certificate records, available for just over half the children—those born in the state of Georgia. The reason for using these additional records from a smaller number of children was to examine for possible *confounding*. Hold up! What's that?

Confounding

If you were to analyze the association between alcohol consumption and lung cancer, you would find one. Does this mean that drinking alcohol causes lung cancer? No. If you take into account, or adjust for, the cigarette smoking habit, then the apparent effect of alcohol goes away. It was confounded by the real risk—cigarette smoking. The apparent effect of alcohol was observed because, at the population level, more people who smoke cigarettes also drink alcohol.

Does early MMR cause autism, or is it confounded by some other factor? Possible confounding factors such as a child's birth weight and gestational age, and maternal factors such as age and parity, were available in the Georgia birth certificate records.[6] Adjusting for these factors in the smaller group allowed the Gang-of-Five to determine whether the real risk factor lay in these maternal or birth characteristics rather than early exposure to MMR. It didn't; as stated in the published paper, "there was little or no confounding effect from these factors."[7]

Based on this finding, there was no scientific basis to ever refer to these Georgia birth certificate data again; they were irrelevant. The results presented in the published paper should have been confined to the *total* group and the information contained in these children's school records. Yet the paper presents quite the opposite: in reporting their results, the authors rely heavily on the irrelevant and misleading Georgia birth certificate data and omit crucial findings from the total group.

Why would they have relied on the data from the smaller group? Because the smaller the numbers the lower the statistical power. The *statistical power* of a study is its ability to detect a statistically significant risk, in this instance between early MMR and autism, if that risk genuinely exists. In order to conceal the risk that *was* evident in the total group, they defaulted to the smaller group with lower statistical power, where the statistical significance was lost.

What They Found and How They Made It Go Away

A. A SIGNIFICANT RISK IN THE TOTAL GROUP

One of the first things that Thompson did in the fall of 2001 was to plot a graph of age at first MMR against percentage of children vaccinated. This graph is shown below. Children with autism are represented by the solid line and children without autism by the broken line. If there is no link between age at first MMR and autism risk, then these two lines should track together, whatever the age at first MMR. They do track together until fifteen months, and then they separate and remain apart.

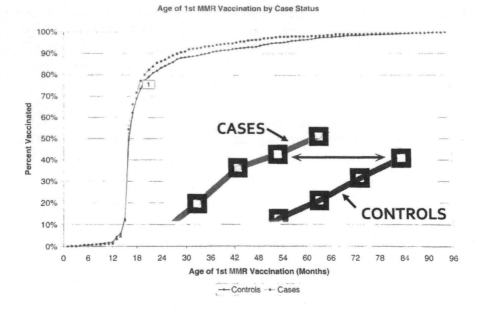

The finding rocked Thompson back on his heels. Children with autism had received their MMR earlier than those without autism. As Thompson himself confirmed, the graph showed a smooth, linear function—it was real and compelling evidence of a causal association. This graph, which should have undoubtedly appeared in the final paper, was concealed and never again intended to see the light of day. Years later it resurfaced when Thompson provided copies of the original data outputs to Dr. Brian Hooker and me.

B. A SIGNIFICANT RISK IN AFRICAN AMERICAN CHILDREN

Thompson then analyzed the data by race. Remember, data on race was to come explicitly from the children's school records, available for the total group. Like Hooker, Thompson found a highly significant autism risk in African American children who received their MMR on schedule (twelve to eighteen months) compared with those receiving it after thirty-six months. In his statement to Bill Posey, Thompson wrote:

> For the NON-BIRTH Certificate Sample, the adjusted RACE effect statistical significance was HUGE. (OR = 2.94 [95%CI 1.48–5.81). That is the main reason why we decided to report the RACE effects for ONLY the BIRTH Certificate Sample.

Further analysis confirmed that the risk was confined to African American boys, a finding that was later confirmed by Dr. Brian Hooker to whom Thompson initially confessed. This underscored the significance of the findings since autism is known to be four to five times more common in boys. There is no record that any of his colleagues ever challenged the validity of Thompson's findings. But they did have to deal with a major threat to their credibility as the last word on vaccine safety and that of the entire childhood immunization infrastructure.

Thompson's statement to Posey confirms how they planned to resolve this thorny issue:

> All the coauthors met and decided sometime between August 2002 and September 2002 not to report any RACE effects for the paper." The decision that the findings should not go beyond the walls of the CDC was reaffirmed on January 12, 2004, in a planning meeting for an upcoming presentation of the findings to the Institute of Medicine, when Thompson noted, "Race Differences (internal use only).

A decade later Thompson issued a public statement[8] after he had been "outed" as a whistleblower confirming the fraud and regretting that "key results were deliberately omitted from The Paper."

C. A SIGNIFICANT RISK IN CHILDREN WITH ISOLATED AUTISM

When designing the study, the Gang-of-Five posed themselves the question: "If early MMR vaccine is a risk for autism, in which children would we be most likely to detect this effect?" Their answer was "children with no other associated developmental issues." These included children of all races with no developmental delays in the first year of life, no cerebral palsy, no birth defects, no hearing or visual problems, and no mental retardation as judged by an IQ of less than 70. They called this group *isolated autism*, and this is exactly where they found the risk. In a conversation with Brian Hooker, Thompson declared,

> You see that the strongest association is with those without mental retardation . . . the effect is where you would think that it would happen. It is with the kids without other conditions, without the comorbid conditions. And you know, honestly, I looked at those results . . . I'm just looking at that and I'm like, oh my God. I cannot believe we did what we did. But we did. It's all there. It's all there.

The complete data sets and analyses provided by Thompson confirmed, once again, that the children at greatest risk included those vaccinated according to the CDC's schedule. These data were simply omitted from the paper.

Destruction of Documents

Thompson alleges that documents were destroyed for the specific purpose of concealing the race data. In his statement to Posey, Thompson states:

> Sometime soon after the meeting where we decided to exclude reporting any RACE effects, also between August 2002 and September 2002, the coauthors scheduled a meeting to destroy documents related to the study. Dr. Coleen Boyle was not present at the meeting even though she was involved in scheduling that meeting. The remaining four coauthors all met and brought a big garbage can into the meeting room and reviewed and went through all our hard copy documents that we thought we should discard and put them in the large garbage can.

Brian Hooker, lawyer Jim Moody, and I wrote an official complaint to the Office of Research Integrity (ORI), the body with research oversight over the CDC, demanding an investigation into the research misconduct. Alarmingly, ORI handed off the complaint to the CDC for internal investigation. Thompson was interviewed as part of this process. He confirmed the contents of his statement to Bill Posey:

> The Inquiry Committee asked each interviewed respondent about the alleged meeting. [Thompson] stated that the meeting was scheduled with all coau-

thors present, in order to dispose of any documents related to race so that there would be no evidence that the group had done them, and that during that meeting those present made collective decisions about what to throw out. (CDC Inquiry Committee, Draft Report, 2015)

Thompson makes it clear that in his opinion, the *intent* in destroying the documents was to cover the tracks that led back to a highly significant autism risk in African Americans following MMR on schedule.

Not surprisingly, the three coauthors still at the CDC—Boyle, Yeargin-Allsopp, and DeStefano—expressed a different view:

The other CDC authors all denied recalling or participating in any such meeting and denied destroying any relevant records. (CDC Inquiry Committee, Draft Report, 2015)

If it can be established forensically that there was such a meeting and that "relevant records" from the study *were* destroyed then, notwithstanding the fact that the coauthors would have lied, then the issue to be considered is one of *intent*. The merits of any argument about whether or not the authors committed a felony should rest upon their *intent* in destroying those documents. If, as Thompson claims, it can be established that the *intent* was to conceal a risk of harm to children, it is hard to imagine the legal bloodshed that would ensue.

As to the forensics, Thompson supplied us with agendas for research meetings held to review the DeStefano autism–MMR study, spanning 2002 and including the period in question—August to October of that year. Hard-copy data outputs of the study results are available for these meetings, wherein Thompson regularly updated his coauthors on the study analyses. Two key data outputs merit further consideration: the first is for September 2002 for a meeting for which, unusually, no agenda was produced. Written in Thompson's hand across the top of the first page is "Handwritten notes from coauthor—September 2002."

Within the document are three handwritten notes or annotations made by the unnamed coauthor, all specifically highlighting the high autism risk in African Americans. The document coincides with the time that the coauthors state no meeting took place. Not only is it clear that a meeting *did* take place, but the finding of greatest concern to the coauthors is specifically highlighted three times in the document from this meeting.

Next comes the data output from October 2002. Here, the offending data on African American children are completely gone—disappeared. Only the race data on the Georgia birth certificate group are presented. In an interview for our documentary, Brian Hooker remarked on this finding: "There was a dramatic difference in the results presented before and after the time that Thompson alleges that the coauthors met to destroy the data."

Now you see it, now you don't. The very finding that Thompson insisted was the one that led to the imperative to destroy the documents was suddenly gone. Brian Hooker reflected on the significance of this finding: "If I did not have the documents from before the time that the coauthors met to destroy the data, there would have been nothing to suggest that the findings ever existed."

This was, I believe, fully the intention of the authors in destroying the records and is entirely consistent with the events as described by Thompson. Moreover, never at any time up to the revelation of the fraud did Thompson's coauthors or superiors question the scientific validity of his findings over the four-year period that he spent analyzing this study. Their only concern appears to have been keeping the findings "for internal use only."

Everything alleged by Thompson is supported by the contemporaneous evidence. What makes him such a valuable witness is that, on the DeStefano issue, he refused to speculate or to make allegations for which there were not "hard records." Any jury faced with the question "Did Thompson's coauthors lie about destroying documents?" must on the balance of evidence come down in Thompson's favor.

Throughout the entire period of the study, Thompson was confident in his scientific findings and perplexed by the intention to conceal them. But, as he said by way of explanation to Hooker, "My bosses wanted to do certain things and I went along with it. In terms of chain-of-command, I was four out of five." He added, "I have a boss who's asking me to lie."

But when it came to destroying crucial study documents—ones that led back to the fraud—Thompson took out insurance: "However, because I assumed this was illegal and would violate both FOIA [Freedom of Information Act] laws and DOJ [Department of Justice] requests, I kept hard copies of all my documents in my office, and I retained all the associated computer files."

Without these documents there would be no exposé, no documentary, and no overt imperative for the CDC to stop their disastrous practices. In fact, it is hard to believe that Thompson was not laying a trail of breadcrumbs from very early on in the hope that, sooner or later, the fraud would come to light. In a handwritten meeting note from 2002, when the autism risk from early MMR was evident from their data, he wrote, "Fix data." As a scientist, I cannot believe that this is something another scientist would write in the normal course of events. I believe it was part of Thompson's trail of breadcrumbs—a deliberate reference to an order from a senior coauthor—that led back to the crime. Now it will be up to his coauthors to provide all their corresponding documents and computer files when this matter comes to court, as surely it will. In the draft report of the CDC's internal investigation, however, the committee found no reason to consider this most serious matter—a possible felony—any further:

> The inquiry found no evidence beyond the conflicting statements of the coauthors regarding the alleged meeting and . . . no evidence of destruction of documents that should have been retained. (Draft CDC Inquiry findings, 2015)

On the basis of "no evidence," the CDC has no intention of pursuing this matter any further. But the evidence exists; it has simply not been examined—all the more reason for this matter to go before Congress and the courts.

Thompson alleges that a decision was taken not to report highly significant race data for the whole group. On the balance of the evidence this must be true since, for the whole study, group race data were collected, race analyses were planned and conducted, significant race findings were obtained, and yet no race data for this group are presented. In a long e-mail to me and Brian Hooker, itemizing the CDC's misconduct—misconduct that he could confirm with "hard records,"—Thompson confessed, "We lied about the scientific findings . . . I was responsible for deceiving millions of taxpayers over the potential negative side effects of vaccines." He also warned, "The CDC can no longer be trusted to do vaccine safety work . . . the CDC can't be trusted to police itself."

The draft report of the internal inquiry makes this latter confession abundantly clear.

THE US CONGRESS

Indiana congressman Dan Burton, chairman of the Government Oversight Committee, is himself the grandfather of a vaccine-injured child with autism. Starting in 2000 he held a series of vaccine–autism hearings.

On three separate occasions, Thompson's coauthor Dr. Coleen Boyle delivered her characteristically reassuring testimony to Burton's committee on the progress—or apparent lack of it—of the DeStefano study. In April 2000 she told the committee: "Data collection is nearing completion, and the study results are expected later this year."

In April 2001, without the "expected" results, she stressed to the committee that, "substantial scientific review does not support" the MMR–autism link. She then confirmed in writing that, "A final report from the study will undergo peer review in the latter part of 2001."

Returning to Congress in 2002, now fully aware of the damning evidence of harm from early MMR vaccination, she made no mention of their findings, stressing only that, according to the IOM, the evidence favors rejection of a causal relationship between the MMR vaccine and autism. Now she reported that the analyses and manuscript should be completed by the fall of 2002. It turns out that at that time she was busy with her colleagues working to conceal their adverse findings.

THE INSTITUTE OF MEDICINE

As 2004 approached, the DeStefano study, now overdue for publication by nearly three years, was still a vexed issue for Thompson and his coauthors. Thompson explained: "The reason you don't see anything more on this study, it was five of us behind closed doors for two years."[9]

Clearly, concealing the adverse findings in a way that would elude detection was causing them no uncertain problem. Nonetheless, they faced a deadline: in February 2004 the findings were due to be presented to the Institute of Medicine (IOM), an "independent" scientific body that advises the government on matters of vaccine safety research. The independence of this organization on such matters is highly questionable (vaccine safety reviews are funded by the CDC), and their pro-CDC bias is self-evident in closed-session committee minutes subpoenaed by Congressman Burton. Nonetheless, Thompson, as the scientist who led the DeStefano study, was going to have to get up and present the findings, and he wasn't happy about it. Shortly before the meeting, he asked DeStefano if they should brief the CDC's director, Julie Gerberding, on their findings. The answer was clearly no, leaving Thompson in an increasingly invidious position. Finally, he defied protocol and wrote directly to Gerberding:

> Dear Dr. Gerberding . . . I'm sure you are aware of the Institute of Medicine meeting that will take place on February 9th. . . . I will have to present several problematic results relating to statistical associations between the receipt of MMR vaccination and autism.

In other words, if you put me up there, I'm going to tell the truth.

Despite alerting the CDC director to a major problem with MMR vaccine safety, Thompson received no direct reply from Gerberding. His warning, despite

being presented three years after its sell-by date, allowed Gerberding the opportunity to act out of an abundance of caution and announce to the IOM that
the CDC would not only recommend delaying MMR vaccination until after age
three years in US children but also conduct a larger, more comprehensive study
using, for example, the CDC's Vaccine Safety Datalink database in order to gauge
the reproducibility of the original findings. She did neither.

Several things did happen after Thompson's warning that reflect the true
character and integrity of the CDC hierarchy in 2004. Thompson was removed
from the roster at the IOM, to be replaced by DeStefano, who had no qualms
about falsely reporting that they had found no association between the MMR
vaccine and autism. That same month, the fraudulent DeStefano paper was
published to a fanfare of "study proves that MMR is safe," and on March 9
Thompson was put on administrative leave. Citing the list of reasons for their
disciplinary action against a senior scientist, his bosses complained of "inappropriate and unacceptable behavior in the workplace," which included,

> You criticized the NIP/OD [National Immunization Program/Office of Direc-
> tor] for doing very poor job of representing vaccine safety issues, claimed that
> NIP/OD had failed to be proactive in their handling of vaccine safety issues,
> and you requested that Dr. Gerberding reply to your letter from a congressional
> representative before you made your presentation to the IOM.

Citing the CDC's falsified evidence, the IOM produced a report of that
February 9 meeting. It declared that MMR vaccine was not associated with
autism and that no further investment in research into the link was recommended, and it admonished those who had been critical of CDC officials for not
doing their job properly.

OBSTRUCTION OF JUSTICE AND VACCINE COURT

At this time, approximately five thousand children were plaintiffs in the US
Court of Federal Claims, known in common parlance as Vaccine Court. In 1986,
in a trade-off to protect vaccine manufacturers from liability for damage caused
by their products, Congress had legislated for rapid and generous compensation
of those children who were collateral damage in the CDC's war on infectious disease. Citing the IOM report and the DeStefano study, the quasi-judges, or Special
Masters who preside over the administrative process of these "courts," appeared
to take pleasure in demeaning the plaintiff's parents and their medical experts as
they threw out all five thousand cases. So it was that up to one trillion dollars in

potential liability was avoided. If you need a "why?" for the fraud, you need look no further. Back in Atlanta, DeStefano got a good night's sleep.

Following publication of the DeStefano paper, the Gang-of-Five were to receive an award from the head of Health and Human Services for their scientific contribution. Ironically, it was Yeargin-Allsopp, an African American whose own father was apparently a close friend of Martin Luther King Jr., who collected the award. Standing right alongside her, basking in the reflected glory, was Gerberding. Sometime later, Gerberding was to receive an award of her own: a highly paid job at pharma giant Merck as head of their vaccine division. Clearly, they were pleased with the way she had handled the exoneration of their MMR vaccine. But not everybody was celebrating. Thompson told Brian Hooker, "It was the lowest point in my career that I went along with that paper. . . . I paid a huge price. . . . I became delusional because I was so paranoid about this being published."

As a direct result of shame and self-loathing that followed his participation in the fraud, Thompson tried to commit suicide twice that same year. On one occasion, heavily drugged, he drove out to the freeway to end it all. His attempt was thwarted when he ran into the back of another car, was arrested, and spent several nights in the Dekalb County Jail. Lest it be said that Thompson's value as a witness to the fraud is diminished by his ensuing psychological crisis, it should be noted that his scientific record to this point was outstanding.[10] While he had been, on occasion, outspoken on safety issues and critical of other staff members, he was very highly regarded by his bosses. Before and after the events of February 2004 his boss, Robert Chen, chief of the CDC's Immunization Safety Branch, had written a commendation for Thompson in which he set out the credentials required of someone to lead their "highly complex" vaccine safety studies: "Dr. Thompson possesses the unique combination of training, skills, and experience necessary to ensure that the scientific integrity of these studies will be of the highest caliber."

In November 2004, Chen considered that Thompson's "continued oversight of these studies is essential." In early 2004, Thompson had unraveled psychologically precisely and specifically because of his participation in scientific fraud.

2014

In a 2014 interview, Brian Hooker stated, "I was in my office at Simpson University, where I teach, when my phone rang. It had a 404 area code, so I knew it was the CDC. Lo and behold, it was Bill Thompson."

So started the revelation of the worst medical fraud in history. A decade had gone by since the fraud had been perpetrated, during which time an industry PR machine on steroids had rammed the CDC's schedule down the throats of the public in the face of sporadic measles cases—cases that all recovered and continued their lives as normal (because if they hadn't we would have certainly known about it). In the meantime, most likely due to their required vaccines, thousands of children were left permanently disabled by an encephalopathy—brain damage—that presented as autism.

I will leave it to Brian Hooker to tell this part of the story, one that was made possible by his invaluable interaction with Thompson and his resolute determination to see justice done. My role was to help persuade Thompson to become an official whistleblower, to get all of his documents to Congressman Posey, and to conduct a forensic review of these documents for our movie and the official complaint to the Office of Research Integrity. Finally, having dealt with vaccine whistleblowers since 1997, I was aware that such individuals are in danger as long as the only ones who know their identity are their enemies—those whose interests they threaten. Hooker had written two papers based on data that could have come only from an insider at the CDC, and at least one of the papers said as much. His coauthors believed that the documents had all been destroyed. As soon as Hooker's papers went to print, Thompson, the only possible source of the leak, was a marked man. For his own protection Thompson had to become a public figure as a matter of urgency. Hooker summed up the situation: "We thought we would be dredging a river for Bill Thompson."

In the weeks leading up to his public disclosure, Thompson texted my wife, Carmel, and me as we traveled to the University of Arkansas in Fayetteville to see our daughter. To Carmel he wrote, "I do believe your husband's career was unjustly damaged and this study would have supported his scientific opinion. Hopefully, I can help repair it." And to me: "I apologize again for the price you paid for my dishonesty."

There are many who are far more deserving of an apology.

Soon afterwards, Thompson ceased any direct communication. Having acted upon our advice and enlisted a whistleblower attorney, he was, quite rightly, told to say nothing further. His documents went to Posey, to whom he provided videoed testimony and a full statement. On July 29, 2015, from the floor of the House of Representatives, Posey summarized the fraud and the destruction of documents and urged his colleagues in Congress to hold hearings on this matter. At the time of writing, this was seven months ago and nothing appears to have happened.

THE HIATUS

Following Thompson's "outing," he followed up through his lawyer with a public statement confirming elements of the fraud and clearly identifying his coauthors as fellow conspirators. There followed a hiatus, a period when DeStefano and the others could not have known just what records Thompson had retained or what he had handed over. This was a dangerous time for the CDC since their inevitable attempts at denial and cover-up risked further exposure and compounding of their dishonesty. And this is exactly what happened. In the wake of the breaking news, on August 26, 2014, award-winning investigative journalist Sharyl Attkisson interviewed DeStefano. Flying blind, he claimed that there was a consensus among the authors about the deviation from the approved Analysis Plan: "I think at the time we had consensus among all coauthors that the birth certificate sample provided the more valid results because it could, uh, it had more complete information on, uh, on race."

No concerns had been raised at any stage from the initiation of the study to its conclusion that brought into question the adequacy and reliability of the race data from the school records. Moreover, as disclosed to Posey in his statement, Thompson is clear:

> We never claimed or intended that if we found statistically significant effects in the TOTAL SAMPLE, we would ignore the results if they could not be confirmed in the BIRTH CERTIFICATE SAMPLE.

Thompson confirms that the intention to conceal the risk of harm from MMR was deliberate. And switching data sets is forbidden once the data have been collected and analyzed and given a result that isn't welcome.

Attkisson pursued the issue of Thompson's concerns, asking, "Were you aware of any of [Thompson's] concerns? . . . Have you been aware before today of any of his concerns about this?" DeStefano was clearly struggling: "Uh, uh, yeah, I mean I've continued to see, uh, uh, see him for over the past ten years and we've interacted fairly frequently and, uh, uh, NO, I wasn't aware of this."

Relentless, Attkisson pressed DeStefano further on his denial: "So whoever he raised his concerns to, he didn't, he didn't raise it to you or anybody you knew of?"

"No" was the answer.

Thompson's contemporaneous concerns abound. In a record from the Gang-of-Five's meeting in preparation for the IOM, he asks, "What shall we do about race effect? Shows large effect for blacks, no effect for whites. . . ." And below, almost as a mantra to himself: "Stay calm. Don't over react. . . . [sic]"

In letters to his supervisor Dr. Melinda Wharton and Director Gerberding, he wrote, "Dear Doctor Wharton, I spoke to you regarding the sensitive results we have been struggling with in the MMR autism study." This was followed by threats to get himself a lawyer and remove his name from the draft manuscript. Really, Dr. DeStefano, Thompson had no concerns?

He also wrote, "Dear Doctor Gerberding, I will have to present [to the IOM] several problematic results relating to statistical associations between receipt of the MMR vaccine and autism." This apparent faux pas was actually followed by a reprimand by DeStefano *himself,* conveying threats to "fire" Thompson from the CDC.

DeStefano knew full well of Thompson's concerns. Already in a hole, as the interview progressed, DeStefano kept on digging, referring further to the birth certificate group:

> . . . and secondly, more importantly, [the Georgia birth certificate group] had information on important factors that, uh, had to be, you know, controlled for, particularly in studies of autism, in particular, it would be things like birth weight, the mother's age, the mother's education.

But their paper had confirmed that there was no significant effect from these factors. There was no scientific reason for them to dwell further on this irrelevant group.

DeStefano's dishonesty in his clumsy attempts to cover up the fraud is not a matter of my opinion alone. In response to Thompson's story going public, DeStefano also provided a quote for CNN on August 28, 2014. The CNN anchor summarized it as follows:

Dr. Frank DeStefano, lead author of the 2004 study, said he and his colleagues stand by their findings. DeStefano said all the study authors, including Dr. Thompson, agreed on the analysis and interpretation before the study was submitted for publication ten years ago.

In a text to Brian Hooker and me on August 29, 2014, Thompson wrote, "We are in the driver's seat now that Frank lied in his interview with CNN."

WHAT NEXT?

As I write, we are preparing to release a feature documentary, *Vaxxed: From Cover-Up to Catastrophe*, on this appalling episode in US medical history. It is but one in a litany of similar crimes with strong racial connotations, starting with the Tuskegee syphilis experiment; the experimentation and decimation of Yanomami Indians in the Orinoco basin with the Edmonston B measles vaccine, already withdrawn in the US due to its excessive reactivity; and the use of an experimental high-potency measles vaccine, one that caused delayed death in girls in developing countries, given without consent or concern to black and Latino children in South Central Los Angeles.

Now a series of actions are urgently required, actions demanded by the doctors, congressmen, lawyers, and scientists, including a Nobel Laureate, who were interviewed for our movie. These actions are:

1. Remove responsibility for vaccine safety research immediately from Health and Human Services (incorporating the CDC) and create an entirely independent entity to oversee and conduct this research. Thompson is absolutely adamant that the CDC is no longer fit to conduct vaccine safety research or to police itself.[11] A comparison of health outcomes in fully vaccinated versus never vaccinated children should be a priority for this new safety body.

2. Bring those who perpetrated this crime and those who allowed it to continue before the Oversight Committee on Government Reform and make them face criminal and civil prosecution in jury trials.

3. Push Congress to repeal the National Childhood Vaccine Injury Act, making drug companies liable for their defective products and allowing plaintiffs due legal process, such as discovery and a jury trial, which is currently denied to them. Without these measures, there is no incentive to ensure that vaccines are safe.

4. Enact a moratorium on any and all new vaccines.

5. Enact a moratorium on any state or federal vaccine mandates with repeal of all laws that remove philosophical, religious, and broad-reaching medical exemptions.

6. Give urgent attention to those children damaged by vaccines by first acknowledging and compensating them, and second by dealing with their medical issues and making adequate provision for their long-term care.

7. Delay voluntary vaccination against measles, mumps, and rubella until after thirty-six months in the first instance.

8. Separate the MMR vaccine out into the single vaccines.

9. Remove any and all toxins from vaccines.

10. Legislate that vaccines should undergo independent safety testing under the same rules that apply to pharmaceuticals.

POSTSCRIPT

Why is this the worst medical fraud in history? Because it was perpetrated by those who were charged with the responsibility of protecting the nation's most precious asset—its children. The potential risk of permanent harm to healthy children was mandated, and parents were denied any informed consent other than reassurance that the CDC's studies supported the safety of this vaccine. And like the odious Martin Shkrelly, the CDC effectively spat in the face of the US Congress. Confidence in the US Public Health Service may never recover.

Chapter 4

FOOD ALLERGY AND THE GUT-BRAIN AXIS

Category	Presenting condition
Gastrointestinal	
IgE-mediated	IgE-mediated food allergy
Non-IgE-mediated	Non-IgE-mediated food allergy Celiac disease Gastroesophageal reflux disease
Conditions of overlapping IgE-and non-IgE-mediated allergy	Eosinophilic esophagitis Eosinophilic gastritis Eosinophilic enterocolitis
Skin	
IgE-mediated	Extrinsic eczema (often associated with IgE-mediated food allergy)
Non-IgE-mediated	Intrinsic eczema
Respiratory	
IgE-mediated	Allergic conjunctivitis Allergic rhinitis Atopic asthma
Non-IgE-mediated	Non-allergic rhinitis Non-atopic asthma Recurrent or chronic rhinosinusitis Recurrent otitis media Adenoid hypertrophy

The issue of food allergy and its role in ASD will be discussed in some detail for four reasons: First, food allergy is common in children and becoming increasingly so. Second, from the clinical perspective, food allergy seems particularly prevalent in children with ASD. Third, it provides a prototypic mechanism for a link between the gut and the brain. And fourth, it is pivotal to the claim and counter-claim in the case of the Arizona 5.

Some of the strongest evidence for a plausible disease mechanism (pathogenesis) in ASD is emerging from studies that have focused not on the brain but on the intestine. Among the more consistent and compelling discoveries is that of GI pathology in some affected children with an associated chronic immune system activation and inflammation—a process that may be driven, in part, by some form of food allergy. Recognition of the contribution of food protein antigens—molecules that activate an immune response—to this inflammatory cycle in the form of food allergy are receiving growing attention. So is the possibility that an aberrant immune reaction to food, set up in the gut, can have immune and inflammatory knock-on (secondary or incidental) effects in the brain. Such a mechanism has been identified in celiac disease, and it is not a stretch for ASD by any means. Once again, this chapter seeks to describe what was known in 2010 and, therefore, what should have informed the medical profession, Child Protective Services (CPS), and the courts in their respective dealings in the case of the Arizona 5.

Adverse reactions to food, recognized from at least the time of Hippocrates over two millennia ago, come in many guises. Food-allergic disorders are common and are becoming more so, affecting in the region of 8% of children under three years old and up to 35% based upon parental reporting.[1] Nontoxic reactions may be immunologic reactions (allergic) or non-immunologic (e.g., food intolerances due to digestive enzyme deficiencies). Both immunologic and non-immunologic mechanisms may coexist. In turn, allergic reactions to ingested foods may be mediated through different axes of the immune system. Accordingly, they manifest differently and require different diagnostic approaches and treatment.

The stage for food allergy may be set during the earliest encounters between the infant's intestine and the food they eat. It has even been observed that, occasionally, initial sensitization to food proteins may occur in the fetus, presumably via the mother's diet.[2]

Alternatively, the sterile, immunologically naïve intestine of the newborn is bombarded with foreign proteins and other potential allergens from the moment of delivery. The optimal outcome of this encounter is the development of immunological tolerance—a state of non-overreactivity—to beneficial bacteria and foodstuffs. The evolution of this ecological optimization is limited by the immaturity of certain aspects of newborn intestinal physiology, including low out-put of sterilizing stomach acid, low digestive enzyme activity, and immune system immaturity, e.g., low levels of the antibody (IgA) that protects mucosal surfaces of the body such as the intestinal lining. The net effect of this immaturity is that the earlier the introduction of solid foods, the greater the likelihood of allergic reactions to these foods.[3] In addition, it is possible that immune perturbation from infection or vaccination may provoke allergy to previously innocuous foods.

It is not surprising that food allergies come in a variety of forms, given the complexity of the immune system and the extraordinary range of foreign substances to which the intestinal lining is exposed. Food allergic reactions mediated by IgE antibodies are those with which the public is most familiar. This is the immediate or anaphylactic type that is seen with, for example, peanut allergy. Symptoms caused by immediate GI hypersensitivity typically develop within two hours of consuming the offending food and often much sooner. They include nausea, colicky abdominal pain, vomiting, and/or diarrhea. These may be accompanied by skin reactions such as urticaria[4] (hives) and asthma. Repeated exposure leads to a degree of reduced sensitivity and less obvious clinical reactions, such as failure to thrive (poor appetite and low weight gain) and intermittent abdominal pain.

A second category is non-IgE-mediated or delayed-type food allergy, frequently due to dietary protein intolerance. This condition may present early in life and is associated with irritability, protracted vomiting and diarrhea, and consequent dehydration. Symptoms usually occur four to seventy-two hours after food ingestion. Because of the delay in the onset of symptoms, it may be difficult to link them to food. Re-exposure to the offending food(s)—commonly cow's milk or soy protein formulas in younger children and eggs, wheat, rice, oat, peanuts, chicken, turkey, and fish in older children—may lead to diarrhea (sometimes bloody), abdominal distention, and failure to thrive. Celiac disease, an immunologic intolerance to wheat gliadin (a protein present in wheat), is a specific disorder within the subset of non-IgE-mediated disorders. The third category involves mixed IgE- and non-IgE-mediated food allergies.

Non-IgE-mediated food allergy includes conditions in which inflammation of the intestinal lining is associated with swelling of the lymph glands (lymphoid nodular hyperplasia [LNH]; see Part 1, Chapter 2). Under the microscope, biopsies frequently show infiltration of the mucosa by immune cells called eosinophils (allergy cells).[5] As described in the previous chapter, these findings (LNH[6] and an eosinophilic inflammation[7]) have been reported in children with autism as part of their GI disease.

Eosinophilic esophagitis, gastritis, and gastroenteritis are examples of this form of food allergy. Clinically, allergic esophagitis presents most commonly from infancy through to adolescence and is associated with reflux, intermittent vomiting, food refusal, abdominal pain, irritability, and sleep disturbance. These symptoms do not typically respond to conventional reflux medication such as acid-blocking drugs.

In the latter two categories—IgE and non-IgE-mediated food allergies—GI symptoms such as diarrhea, abdominal pain, and failure to thrive usually predominate. However, food-allergic GI reactions may be accompanied by symptoms ranging from arthritis to asthma, migraine, cluster headaches, eczema, fatigue, heartburn, and behavioral disturbances—particularly in children. Alternatively, the GI disease may be "occult" or clinically silent and surprisingly, perhaps, the non-GI symptoms such as behavioral issues may be the *only* manifestations of intestinal food allergy.

THE DIAGNOSIS OF FOOD ALLERGY

As in all clinical encounters, in the diagnosis of food allergy, the patient's history and physical examination findings are paramount. The history should ascertain the nature of the symptoms, the identity and amount of the suspect food(s), the time to reaction from ingestion, whether the same reaction occurs with repeated exposure to that food, and when the last reaction occurred. Allergic shiners, coarse hair, and dry skin with or without eczema may be present. The physical examination should include anthropomorphic measures such as height and weight and a thorough general examination. Attention to signs of abdominal disease is an obvious requirement, whereas eliciting signs of neurological and behavioral deficits, although not as obvious, may be equally important for reasons that will become evident.

Beyond the history and examination, the differential diagnosis of food allergy generally follows one of two paths. If an IgE-mediated allergy is suspected, it can usually be confirmed by skin tests. Testing involves subcutaneous injection with small quantities of glycerinated extracts of common food allergens and measurement of any consequent skin reaction.[8] An alternative, the RAST (radioallergosorbent test) is a blood test performed in the laboratory that looks for IgE antibodies against specific foods.

Skin prick tests are negative in non-IgE-mediated food allergy, and until recently, specific testing had been relatively unhelpful in the identification of foods responsible for non-IgE-mediated reactions, facts that will be important in the later analysis of the Arizona 5. On its own, testing for the presence of alternative types of antibodies such as IgG (immunoglobulin G) to foods is not helpful for predicting a non-IgE-mediated food allergy. More recently, commercial laboratory testing has become available for food-related antibodies in the blood that form complexes with molecules called complement molecules that are also present in the blood. It is these complexes that are thought to promote the allergic inflammation and tissue damage.[9] Food-related immune complexes can be detected against a range of common foods using a sample of the patient's blood. It has been suggested that testing in this way can help the physician or nutritionist determine what foods should form part of any trial of dietary exclusion; however, further formal scientific study of the merits of this particular testing is required. Clinical testing for non-IgE-mediated food allergy has also progressed with the development of patch testing, the application of suspect foods to the skin in a series of Finn Chambers[10] that allow the measurement of any positive reaction following prolonged exposure.

If a non-IgE-mediated food allergy is suspected, upper and lower GI endoscopy and biopsy are necessary and may confirm the diagnosis by finding eosinophilic inflammation of the intestinal mucosa and/or a lymphocytic infiltrate in the lining epithelial cells.

Thereafter, the real test of whether a particular food(s) is responsible for the patient's symptoms is an allergy elimination diet followed by rechallenge with the suspect food(s). Ideally, this is done in circumstances where neither the patient nor the doctor is aware of when the food is eliminated or reintroduced. Resolution of symptoms following removal and their subsequent provocation upon re-exposure provides the definitive diagnosis.

The natural history of non-IgE-mediated food allergy is that it resolves over time.[11] The interval to recovery is highly variable; for example, some children grow out of a milk allergy in a matter of months while others may take eight to ten years.

FOOD ALLERGY AND NEUROLOGICAL DISEASE

In building the scientific argument for a link between the gut and the brain—and specifically abnormal immune reactions to ingested food and autism symptoms—a good starting point is a review of the evidence for gut-immune-brain interactions as a more general concept. Specifically in the context of a non-IgE-mediated food allergy, the best-studied example of the neurological knock-on effects of intestinal disease is untreated celiac disease. Celiac disease is an immune-mediated (allergic) disorder triggered by ingestion of wheat gliadin and related proteins in genetically susceptible individuals. This susceptibility is encoded in immune response genes designated DR3-DQ2 (present in 90–95% of celiac sufferers) and DQ8 (present in 5–10% of celiac sufferers). However, hereditary factors alone do not explain the development of celiac disease, and infectious triggers have been proposed. In the continued presence of gluten, the disease is self-perpetuating; if untreated, it can lead to severe complications such as lymphoma.

In addition to the characteristic intestinal changes, including small intestinal mucosal flattening, inflammation, and malabsorption, celiac disease is associated with various extraintestinal manifestations. These include neurological complications such as neuropathy, nerve inflammation (neuritis), ataxia (lack of muscle coordination), seizures, and behavioral changes. Celiac disease is a classical example of a disease in which a primary intestinal food allergy can lead to secondary brain injury.

It is important for families affected by ASD to recognize that neurological complications arising in the setting of gluten sensitivity may occur in the absence of GI symptoms, with the only signs of this cryptic gluten sensitivity being ataxia, dementia, seizures, or affective symptoms such as depression. In the setting of ASD, this may include behavioral symptoms that, given their prominence, mask any less obvious GI issues. Cryptic gluten sensitivity includes the situation where the patient suffers no overt GI symptoms but has antibodies against wheat gliadin and experiences extraintestinal symptoms that are often neurological in nature. For example, Dr. Marios Hadjivassiliou and colleagues from Leeds in the UK investigated patients with neurological disease of unknown cause for the presence of antigliadin antibodies.[12] Antibody levels in the blood were compared with those in patients with a specific neurological diagnosis such as stroke, multiple sclerosis (MS), and Parkinson's disease (PD).

Positive titers for antigliadin antibodies—as evidence of an immune response to gluten—were present in thirty of fifty-three (57%) patients with neurological disease of unknown cause compared with much lower proportions of the stroke/MS/PD group (5%), and healthy blood donors (12%). Interestingly, despite these patients having no GI symptoms, duodenal biopsies in twenty-six out of thirty antigliadin antibody-positive patients revealed mucosal pathology, including celiac disease in nine and non-specific duodenal inflammation in ten. Clearly, gluten sensitivity is common in patients with neurological disease of unknown cause and may be present without overt GI symptoms. Moreover, this gluten sensitivity may be causally related to the neurological disease.[13]

In pursuing this association further, Hadjivassiliou and colleagues focused upon patients suffering from ataxia, the most common neurological manifestation of celiac disease. Notably, ataxia is reported frequently by parents of children with regressive autism, being particularly prominent during the regressive phase[14] (see Part 3, Chapter 5). In some individuals with a genetic susceptibility to celiac disease and serological evidence of gluten sensitivity (antigliadin antibodies), gluten ataxia is the sole manifestation of their disease.

The authors identified twenty-eight patients with ataxia and antigliadin antibodies. Brain scans showed that six patients had evidence of cerebellar atrophy—shrinkage due to loss of nerve cells. Necropsies performed on two patients who died showed inflammation in the cerebellum and damage to the spinal cord. These observations led the authors to the conclusion that gluten ataxia occurs as a result of immunological damage to these areas of the brain. Of note, despite no GI symptoms, sixteen of the twenty-eight patients had GI pathology consistent with celiac disease with the presence of an alternative inflammatory disease in another two.

In a larger study, Hadjivassiliou identified a high prevalence of gluten sensitivity among 41% of a group of 132 patients with ataxia of unknown cause. In those with a genetically based ataxia and in healthy blood donors, the prevalence was low. GI symptoms were present in only a small minority (13%) of those with gluten ataxia. The authors concluded that gluten ataxia is the single most common cause of ataxia of unknown origin and urged that newly presenting patients with this condition get antigliadin antibody testing.[15]

So how might antibodies that develop against gluten in the intestinal lining cause problems in the brain? Hadjivassiliou's theory was that antibodies made against wheat proteins travel in the bloodstream to the brain, where they cross-react, possibly through a lookalike process of molecular mimicry, with brain proteins of a structure similar to those of wheat proteins. The authors suggested that in a similar manner to celiac disease, an autoimmune reaction occurs in the brain, particularly the cerebellum—the part that is principally responsible for controlling balance and coordination.

When the authors put serum (the antibody-containing part of the blood) from patients with gluten ataxia onto slices of human cerebellum in the laboratory, a strong antibody reaction was detected in specific cells unique to the cerebellum—Purkinje cells—for twelve of the thirteen patients tested. Commercial antigliadin antibody also stained human Purkinje cells in a similar manner. Purkinje cells, named after the Czech anatomist Jan Evangelista Purkyně, are like lights at a busy intersection; these cells effectively control the flow of information from the cerebellum.

Broadly, the study confirmed two things: first, patients with gluten ataxia have antibodies against cerebellar Purkinje cells; second, antigliadin antibodies cross-react with Purkinje cell–associated antigens.[16] The findings raise a subsidiary question: Does binding of these antibodies to the Purkinjie cells impair their health and function? One study that might advance the argument for a pathologic role of these antigliadin antibodies in causing ataxia would be to isolate them and inject them into an experimental laboratory animal to see if they reproduced the symptoms and brain damage described by Hadjivassiliou and colleagues.

Their observations also raise the tantalizing possibility that there may be target molecules in the brain that bind antigliadin antibodies as a precursor to immune damage. Alaedini et al. from Cornell University identified one of these molecular targets as Synapsin I, one of a family of brain proteins involved in regulating neurotransmitter release at synapses. Theoretically, therefore, antigliadin antibodies might upset brain function by interfering with neurotransmission.[17]

And anti-Synapsin I antibodies are not the only players. In fact, the major target of autoimmunity across the whole spectrum of gluten sensitivity is an enzyme called tissue transglutaminase (transglutaminase type II). Hadjivassiliou and colleagues described the binding of antibodies against this enzyme in the cerebellum and brainstem as well as in the intestines of patients with gluten ataxia. This binding was similar to that seen in patients with celiac disease, supporting the proposition that gluten ataxia, in common with celiac disease, is an immune-mediated disorder that starts with food allergy.[18]

From a clinical perspective, the deal-breaker for a gut-immune-brain interaction in the neurologic manifestations of celiac disease is whether removal of gluten from the diet, which is known to cause celiac antibodies to fall and eventually disappear from the blood, leads to an improvement in the clinical symptoms of gluten ataxia. Hadjivassiliou's team put this to the test in a study of forty-three patients with gluten ataxia. All were offered a strict gluten-free diet and monitored every six months. All patients underwent a battery of tests to assess their ataxia at baseline and after one year on the diet. Twenty-six patients (treatment group) adhered to the gluten-free diet and had evidence of elimination of antigliadin antibodies by one year. Fourteen patients refused the diet and were allocated to the untreated control group. Three patients had persistently raised antigliadin antibodies despite adherence to the diet and were therefore excluded from the analysis. After one year, there was a significant improvement in all of the ataxia tests in the treatment group compared with the control group. They observed that gluten ataxia responded to a strict gluten-free diet even in the absence of obvious intestinal disease. Crucially, they had identified a neurological disease that was treatable by diet. This made the correct diagnosis of gluten sensitivity in patients presenting with ataxia a vital step in their potential for recovery.[19]

CELIAC DISEASE AND AFFECTIVE SYMPTOMS

Beyond ataxia, celiac disease is associated with a range of psychological and behavioral problems. Reports on adult celiac sufferers indicate that between 30–69% have depressive symptoms,[20] and 42% have depressive disorders.[21]

Of the few studies that have focused upon young people with celiac disease, disorders of sleep and the ability to relax have been described in adolescents,[22] and the frequency of behavioral disorders and depressive problems was higher in children with untreated celiac disease when compared with those on a gluten-free diet and those without celiac disease.[23]

Where celiac disease is clinically silent due to a lack of GI symptoms, a careful history often reveals that, in many such cases, there is low-intensity comorbid illness associated with decreased well-being, which in children includes behavioral disturbances with a tendency to depression, irritability, and impaired school performance.[24] Fabiani et al. described an increase in weight and height velocity, appetite, and mood amelioration and an improvement in physical and school performance in adolescents whose celiac disease was apparently asymptomatic at diagnosis once they began following a gluten-free diet.[25]

From Finland, Pynönnen et al. reported that celiac patients had a significantly higher lifetime prevalence of a major depressive disorder (31% versus 7%) and disruptive behavior disorder (28% versus 3%) than non-celiac controls.[26] These differences were evident for the celiac group before a gluten-free diet but not after, suggesting that diet may reduce affective symptoms. The authors recommend that patients presenting with affective disorders and behavioral disturbances should be screened for gluten sensitivities.

CELIAC DISEASE AND AUTISM

The first report of autism occurring in association with celiac disease dates from 1971.[27] Barcia and colleagues subsequently reported an increased incidence of biopsy-confirmed celiac disease in their patients with pervasive developmental disorder (PDD) at a frequency that was three and a half fold higher than in the developmentally normal population.

Advancing the argument for a similar gut-immune-brain axis in autism would be supported by reports in which autism or autistic symptoms have occurred in some children with celiac disease and for these symptoms to have abated with a gluten-free diet. It is not necessary that all children with celiac disease have symptoms of ASD or that the bowel pathology found in many children with ASD overlaps with celiac disease. Proof of principle requires only that in well-described cases of celiac disease where autism symptoms are present that such symptoms resolve following the removal of gluten.

For example, Genuis et al. provided a detailed description of a five-year-old boy with regressive autism and chronic GI symptoms who not only had very high celiac disease antibody titers but also evidence of malabsorption with nutritional and vitamin deficiencies. A gluten-free diet led rapidly to relief of his GI symptoms and improvement in his behavior and cognitive function. Two and a half years later, he no longer had autism and his mother described him as " . . . doing incredibly well and [he] is so very happy."[28]

THE BOWEL AND BEHAVIOR BEYOND CELIAC DISEASE

The link between food allergy and behavioral disturbances goes beyond celiac disease; a link between certain foods and aberrant behavior has long been recognized, although support from well-designed scientific studies has only come more recently. In 1947, Randolf reviewed "the fatigue syndrome" of allergic origin as a common cause of irritability and abnormalities of behavior in children.[29] He described how this syndrome usually results from chronic food allergy involving sensitivity to more than one food, while "sensitivity to wheat and corn is encountered most frequently."[30]

He divided the affected children into two groups: first, the chronically tired, sluggish, and depressed child, and second, the hyperkinetic and hyperexcited child. Randolf commented: "Both are inclined to be irritable and fretful in their behavior and to be maladjusted in both the home and school. Their schoolwork suffers because of a characteristic difficulty in concentration and impairment of memory."[31]

Although food allergy is more commonly associated with a history of one or more GI symptoms, Randolf recognized that behavioral symptoms may be the sole allergic manifestation exhibited by a child. He also recognized the need to prioritize the allergy symptoms over the behavioral, stating: "When dealing with allergic children, the significance of psychic and emotional factors in the genesis of irritability and behavior problems may be judged to best advantage after the allergic reactions are brought under control."[32] Put another way, he is saying that we should exclude a medical disorder before assuming that the problem is all in the mind. There is a lesson here for some of those doctors whom we encounter later in this book.

By 1979, it was recognized that states of excessive excitability and fatigue associated with food allergy in children could be part of a continuous process operating in two stages rather than operating as two distinct sets of responses occurring in different children. This was characterized by a "high" or tension (hyperkinetic) stage followed by a "low" or fatigue stage, usually in that order but sometimes reversed. This phenomenon became known as the allergic tension-fatigue syndrome.[33] The observation that food intolerances, likely of an allergic origin, could be linked not only to behavioral changes in children but also to infectious environmental triggers had been reported some years earlier. In 1956, Daynes presented his findings of "Naughtiness, depression, and fits due to wheat sensitivity" to the Royal Society of Medicine in London.[34] He made the following observations:

> Typically a child between 1 and 5 years becomes naughty and difficult a few days after the onset of an acute infectious illness . . . such as measles or gastroenteritis. He is irritable, negativistic, and spiteful, sleep is disturbed and he wakes up in the night and often screams; his appetite is poor, he fails to gain weight, his abdomen is often distended and the stools may become bulky, pale and offensive. This condition, if left untreated, usually rights itself after a month or two, but it may last for much longer in which case slight petit mal attacks may develop in addition to worsening of the other symptoms. I have been placing these children on a gluten-free diet at the earliest opportunity and the symptoms respond dramatically, usually within two or three days. They relapse if a premature return to a normal diet is made. Study of over 40 cases has led me to formulate a syndrome – pre-coeliac syndrome.

Here we have an early report of an infection such as measles triggering likely food allergy. In addition, Daynes also described the first informal observation of clinical improvement following an exclusion diet followed by return of symptoms upon re-exposure, a wheat-withdrawal-rechallenge effect.

Some aspects of the relationship between food allergy and behavioral problems remain controversial. In order to make the case, the early observational studies required support from both controlled clinical trials and mechanistic science to underpin a plausible biological basis for interactions between food and behavior. This evidence has been provided by studies such as that by Egger et al., who examined seventy-six "overactive" children treated with a diet that was very low in substances capable of eliciting an immune response (oligoantigenic).[35] They reported:

> Sixty-two [children] improved, and a normal range of behaviour was achieved in 21 of these. Other symptoms, such as headaches, abdominal pain, and fits, also often improved. Twenty-eight of the children who improved completed a double-blind, crossover, placebo-controlled trial in which foods thought to provoke symptoms were reintroduced. Symptoms returned or were exacerbated much more often when patients were on active material than on placebo. Fortyeight foods were incriminated. Artificial colorants and preservatives were the commonest provoking substances, but no child was sensitive to these alone.

Sleep disturbances are a recurring theme in parental reports of food-related behavioral disturbances. Not only are they a prominent feature in children with food allergy and the incipient decline of children into autism, but also improvement in sleep is often the first sign of improvement reported by parents when the child with ASD starts the gluten- and casein-free diet. To confirm that sleeplessness in infants can be related to an undiagnosed allergy to cow's milk proteins, Kahn et al. studied seventy-one infants, including twenty with chronic insomnia, and thirty-one who suffered skin or digestive symptoms attributed to cow's milk intolerance, thirteen of whom also had insomnia. Control infants consisted of twenty with no history of sleep disturbance or milk allergy. Laboratory tests revealed allergic reactions to milk in all the infants in the first two groups. The sleep of the infants with insomnia normalized after cow's milk was eliminated from the diet. Insomnia reappeared when the infants in the first group were rechallenged with milk. The findings confirmed that food allergy is an important cause of sleep disturbance in infants.[36]

Laboratory studies have since provided some insights into possible mechanisms for this gut-brain interaction. For example, in 2003 Basso et al.[37] administered the egg protein ovalbumin to previously sensitized laboratory mice. Mice allergic to ovalbumin had higher levels of anxiety, activation of emotionality-related brain areas, and aversion to the ovalbumin-containing solution. Either administration of antibodies that neutralized IgE antibody or the induction of immune tolerance to ovalbumin prevented both the food aversion and the brain activation. These important findings established a direct relationship between brain function and food allergy, creating, as the authors described, "a solid ground for understanding the [cause] of psychological disorders in allergic patients."

MAST CELLS AND THE GUT-BRAIN AXIS

A key player not only in food allergy but emerging also in the link between ASD's environmental cause(s) and its devastating effect is the mast cell. Mast cells are present in most tissues characteristically surrounding blood vessels and nerves and are especially prominent near the boundaries between the outside world and the tissues, such as the skin, lungs, and digestive tract. The *Mastzellen*, or mast cell, was first described by Nobel Laureate Paul Ehrlich, a scientist born in 1854 in the German kingdom of Prussia. His doctoral thesis, awarded from the University of Leipzig in 1878, described mast cells on the basis of their unique staining characteristics in tissues and the large granules that they contain. They were so named from the German *Mast* (food) in the belief that these granules provided nourishment for surrounding tissues. Now more appropriately considered to be part of the immune system, their relationship to food has emerged in the alternative guise of mediators of food allergic responses—ironically, their granules are potentially toxic rather than nourishing.

Mast cells are one of the body's early warning systems—a system that can sometimes be difficult to shut down or override—causing more harm than good. Their profound and far-reaching effects are due, in part, to their tendency to "explode" on exposure to allergens, releasing their granules (degranulation) of highly reactive proinflammatory chemicals. With time, the complex role of these cells as an integral part of the immune/inflammatory response has emerged. In fact, so important is this role that animals lacking mast cells cannot develop inflammation.

Recognition of the importance of mast cells in ASD has come from Dr. Theoharis Theoharides and his team from Tufts University School of Medicine in Boston. His interest started not with autism but with a spectrum of rare disorders associated with excessive mast cell activity, collectively termed mastocytosis. Mastocytosis is associated with both food intolerances and disturbances in cognition and behavior. This evident gut-brain connection and the emerging parallels with autism led him to examine the prevalence of ASD in children with a diagnosis of mastocytosis. In a landmark observation, ASD turned out to be ten times higher in those with mastocytosis compared with the current prevalence of around one in one hundred children for ASD![38]

The Tufts University group is pursuing the theory that mast cells, principally those situated at the body's natural barriers such as the bowel-blood barrier and the blood-brain barrier, cause these barriers to leak when the mast cells become overly activated by, for example, food allergens. This, they propose, leads to the ingress of proinflammatory molecules into the brain and neuroinflammation.

Mastocytosis involves proliferation and activation of mast cells, which, in the skin, is evident clinically as a rash—urticaria pigmentosa (UP). Theoharides et al. reported a highly relevant clinical example of possible mast cell triggering in the setting of ASD. The authors described one child with UP, diagnosed at one year, whose UP worsened following routine immunization at three years. His exaggerated skin reaction was associated with concurrent developmental regression leading to a diagnosis of PDD-NOS.[39]

Dr. Theoharides and his team have contributed greatly to our understanding not only of the potential role of these cells in ASD but also how their excessive activation and harmful effects might be prevented with pharmacologically active foodstuffs. They are currently investigating whether inflammation in the brain can be reduced with naturally occurring flavonoids such as quercetin and luteolin, which act to stabilize mast cells and inhibit their release of inflammatory mediators.[40] It remains to be seen what beneficial effects these compounds might have in ASD.

FOOD ALLERGY AND ADHD

By 1998, elimination diets of low immunogenicity (low allergic potential) had been examined in at least seven controlled studies[41] and had demonstrated either significant improvement compared with a placebo of full-diet[42] or deterioration when rechallenge with offending foods was undertaken after a trial of diet.[43] Based upon these studies, Arnold suggested that the profile of a probable responder is a middle- or upper-class preschooler with atopy—a predisposition to allergic disease—and prominent irritability and sleep disturbance, with physical as well as behavioral symptoms.[44] Again, across the spectrum of associated behavioral abnormalities, sleep disturbance has emerged as one of the most prominent and consistent hallmarks of food allergy.

By 2010 from a Dutch team headed by Dr. Buitelaar in Nijmegen, robust data from a randomized controlled study had confirmed the efficacy of a restricted elimination diet in improving symptoms of ADHD. The diet group, which was allowed only certain foods,[45] was compared with an unrestricted diet control group. After nine weeks, eleven of fifteen (73%) in the diet group showed a decrease by 50% or more on parent rating scales compared with none of twelve (0%) in the control group. Similarly, with teacher ratings, seven of ten (70%) in the diet group showed improvement compared with none of seven controls.[46]

And by 2011, and therefore relevant to any future debate—medical or legal—on the effect of food on behavior, Buitelaar and colleagues had completed and reported a two-phase study consisting of food removal and a randomized double-blind food rechallenge. The study was substantially larger than their earlier one, involving fifty children in each of the diet and control groups. Not only was there a highly significant improvement of behaviors on diet but there was a similarly significant relapse rate once the restriction diet was stopped.[47]

The authors concluded by "supporting the implementation of a dietary intervention in the standard of care for all children with ADHD."[48] While the study did not examine the role of non-IgE-mediated food allergy in this relationship, it means that the debate over whether food affects behavior is effectively a done deal.

DOES FOOD ALLERGY PLAY A ROLE IN AUTISM?

The science of celiac disease has helped to establish a gut-immune-brain axis. The immunologic and inflammatory mechanisms that have been elucidated for such an axis are by no means exclusive—inflammatory cytokines may have a direct effect on mood and behavior, independent of autoimmunity, for example. What the research has established, nonetheless, is a plausible and coherent chain of potential cause and effect. Similarly, in order to establish a role for food allergy in autism symptoms, a number of links in the chain of causation need to be forged. Studies that would help include:

1. the demonstration of abnormal immune (e.g., antibody) responses to specific foods
2. an inflammatory reaction associated with this immune response
3. a cellular or biochemical neurological response to these immune/inflammatory events
4. modulation of the foregoing effects by an elimination diet and/or pharmaceutical control of the associated immune/inflammatory process

Inspired initially by anecdotal parental observations that various food intolerances influenced autism symptoms in their children, some interesting clinical observations have been reported. In 1995, Lucarelli et al. found high levels of antibodies to a variety of milk proteins[48] in patients with autism compared with developmentally normal subjects.[50] The authors then examined the effect of an exclusion diet free of cow's milk and other foods that gave a positive skin test (IgE-mediated allergy) in thirty-six patients. They reported a marked improvement in behavioral symptoms after a period of eight weeks on the elimination diet.

Beyond IgE-mediated food allergy, more substantial evidence has emerged of a role for non-IgE-mediated food allergy in autism in support of the popular and growing awareness that reactions to common foods like dairy and wheat can have neurological and behavioral knock-on effects.

In a logical progression that has paralleled the work of Hadjivassiliou and others in celiac disease, Vojdani et al. pursued the possibility that autism is associated with antibodies that develop against food proteins that then recognize and react with similar proteins in human neural tissues, leading to changes in brain development and behavior. This proposed model moved the autism-immune association from food allergy alone to food-induced autoimmunity—a situation in which a "confused" immune system mounts a damaging response against its host. As preliminary evidence for this "horror autotoxicus"[51] Vojdani et al. demonstrated, for the first time, that in some children with autism and predisposing immune response genes, the dietary peptides (molecule consisting of two or more amino acids) gliadin and casein bound to enzymes on the host cell surface. These children produced antibodies against gliadin, casein, and the cell's own molecules, resulting in an autoimmune reaction.[52]

They subsequently compared this food-induced autoimmune reaction in patients with autism with that seen in patients with established autoimmune disease ("mixed connective tissue disease"). In both groups, antigliadin antibodies were present and cross-reacted with human cell surface proteins—on this occasion, peptidase enzymes. The authors proposed that these autoantibodies might cause membrane enzyme dysfunction and immune dysregulation affecting the nervous system.[53] Vojdani et al. also showed that some children with autism have antibodies against a milk protein (butyrophilin); these antibodies cross-reacted with certain important brain proteins such as myelin basic protein (MBP)—a constituent of the insulation that surrounds nerves—suggesting a mechanism by which, in autism, milk antigens may contribute to autoimmune responses to nerve tissues.[54]

FROM MOLECULES TO INFLAMMATION

An autoimmune *reaction*, for example, the binding of antibodies that are cross-reactive with foods and host antigens, does not on its own constitute an autoimmune *disease*. It is also necessary to have inflammatory pathology and/or disturbance of cell function arising as a consequence of this immunologic interaction. On a potentially convergent track to Vojdani and colleagues, Ashwood et al.[55] reported the novel observation of marked disturbances in immune cell (lymphocyte) numbers and function in the intestines of children with autistic regression and GI symptoms. Lymphocytes isolated from the intestinal lining of such children exhibited a striking increase in the level of the potent proinflammatory molecule tumor necrosis factor-alpha (TNF-α) and a decrease in the level of interleukin-10 (IL-10), a counter-regulatory cytokine that acts to downgrade the immune response and limit inflammation. The findings of microscopic inflammation and a marked proinflammatory immune cell activation in the intestinal mucosa are reminiscent of other inflammatory bowel diseases and put the gut front and center stage in some forms of ASD.

Independently, Dr. Harumi Jyonouchi, an immunologist from the University of Medicine & Dentistry of New Jersey, and her colleagues reported an association between immune reactivity to common dietary proteins and excessive proinflammatory cytokine production in a subset of ASD children when their blood lymphocytes were exposed to endotoxin, a component of bacteria that is highly prevalent in the gut, is better known for causing fever during infections, and is a major stimulant of innate (natural) immunity in the gut mucosa.[56]

Jyonouchi and her colleagues then sought to resolve whether such abnormal immune responses were just part of these children's innate immune constitution or whether they were the result of chronic GI disease secondary to allergic reactivity to food.[57] To do so, they studied cytokine responses of immune cells from the blood that were exposed to bacterial endotoxin. Responses in children with ASD, with and without GI symptoms, including those on unrestricted and elimination diets, were compared with neurotypical children with non-IgE-mediated food allergy on similar diets and healthy children.

The first observation was that, regardless of dietary interventions, endotoxin-exposed immune cells from the blood of children with ASD and those with non-IgE-mediated food allergy produced higher levels of TNF-α than did healthy children. In support of the original findings of Ashwood et al., ASD children with GI symptoms on an unrestricted diet produced more of the proinflammatory cytokine IL-12 and less anti-inflammatory IL-10 than other groups. Those children with ASD, GI symptoms, and an unrestricted diet had the most marked immune imbalance.

Overall, their findings indicated intrinsic defects of innate immune responses in ASD children with GI symptoms, supporting the probability of a gut-immune-brain axis operating in these children to produce the manifestations of autism.[58] An interesting observation that set the ASD children apart from more common forms of non-IgE-mediated food allergy is their apparent failure to generate IL-10—the anti-inflammatory cytokine—in an effort to limit the inflammatory response. This observation clearly requires further study.

In order to determine which common foods might be driving the inflammatory responses in ASD children with GI symptoms, the authors measured cytokine production in response to whole cow's milk protein (CMP) and its major components[59] as well as to gliadin and soy. Exposed to milk proteins, ASD children with GI symptoms produced more proinflammatory cytokines than did control subjects. They also produced more TNF-α with gliadin. Even in those ASD children with no GI symptoms, cow's milk protein stimulated lymphocytes to produce more proinflammatory cytokines than did control subjects. The findings provided clear evidence of a link between food allergy and GI symptoms in children with ASD.[60]

As the evidence continues to mount for a gut-immune-brain interaction in some children with ASD—perhaps a majority of the current epidemic wave—a pathogenic mechanism is consolidating around food allergy, intestinal inflammation, autoimmune responses in neural tissue, and symptomatic disease. As with celiac disease, the proof of the pudding is in *not* eating; do diets that exclude potentially allergenic foods lead to resolution of the behavioral symptoms of ASD?

SELECTIVE FOOD EXCLUSION IN THE TREATMENT OF AUTISM

For autism, the mainstay of dietary intervention has been the gluten- and casein-free diet. In 2010, the results of two randomized controlled clinical trials were available that confirmed the benefit of this approach in ameliorating the behavioral symptoms of autism.

Anne-Marie Knivsberg and her colleagues in Norway performed a single-blind, controlled study to evaluate the effect of a gluten- and casein-free diet for children with autism. Twenty children with autism were randomly assigned to either the diet or the control group and underwent developmental and behavioral testing. The experimental period was one year, after which observations and tests were repeated. A significant reduction in autistic behaviors was found for participants in the diet group but not for those in the control group.[61]

Replication is a key to scientific validation; in the recent study titled "The ScanBrit Randomised Controlled Study of Gluten- and Casein-free Dietary Intervention for Children With Autism Spectrum Disorders," Whiteley et al. undertook a two-stage, twenty-four-month controlled trial in which seventy-two Danish children aged four to ten years were randomly assigned to either diet or non-diet groups.[62] In stage one, all children were tested at baseline, eight, and twelve months with respect to any behavioral changes. After twelve months, seventeen children in the non-diet group were switched to the diet, and eighteen already on the diet were asked to continue. Inter- and intra-group comparison of symptoms revealed evidence of sustained clinical improvements for those children on the diet. This effect eventually plateaued at a higher level of functioning.

The authors concluded that ". . . the data provided evidence of sustained clinical improvements in groups receiving the dietary intervention compared to controls . . . dietary intervention may possibly affect developmental outcome for ASD children."[63]

For autism, by 2010, the threads of a compelling pathological axis of gut-immune-brain interaction in ASD were coming together. Key aspects of the gut-immune-brain axis in ASD were consistent in many respects with the prototypic model of celiac disease. Jyonouchi and colleagues were to add a further piece to the jigsaw puzzle by linking the beneficial clinical and immunological responses to dietary intervention in a preliminary study. In their patients with ASD, the elimination diet helped to resolve GI symptoms and autistic behaviors while at the same time normalizing cytokine responses in these patients' immune cells. The authors concluded that "Dysregulated production of inflammatory and counter-regulatory cytokines may be associated with non-IgE-mediated adverse reaction to common dietary proteins in some ASD children, indicating therapeutic significance of dietary interventions. . . ."[64]

Jyonouchi and her colleagues had succeeded in linking non-IgE-mediated food allergy, GI symptoms, and elevated inflammatory cytokine production in a substantial number of ASD children in response to clinically suspect foods like cow's milk protein, soy, and gliadin. They had also linked normalization of these parameters to dietary intervention, at least in preliminary studies.[65] But many questions remain unanswered. For example, in children with cow's milk protein–associated non-IgE-mediated food allergy, dietary exclusion leads to sustained improvement in GI symptoms. In contrast, for some children with ASD and this same allergy, GI symptoms recur despite a strict exclusion diet. Jyonouchi et al. found that after having started the appropriate diet, these children's immune reactivity to milk and wheat proteins declined over three months but rebounded by six months, despite their having continued with the diet.[66] This was not seen in food-allergic children who did not have ASD. While GI symptoms also improved initially, they returned in these children with ASD. On the other hand, behavioral symptoms including irritability, hyperactivity, and lethargy improved on diet and did not relapse. There is something different about the ASD group that distinguishes their response from more typical non-IgE-mediated food allergy; Jyonouchi believes that they have a continued problem with innate immunity that might lead them to react to a succession of foods—not just those initially eliminated from the diet. I believe that this effect may be linked to their apparent difficulty in producing adequate counter-regulatory or anti-inflammatory cytokines like IL-10 that restore and maintain immune tolerance in the intestine. Whatever the basis of this anomaly, it requires continued vigilance and reassessment of these children, based at the very least on the status of their GI symptoms, in order to manage their continuing dietary issues and intestinal disease.

CONCLUSION

In 2010—at the time of the Arizona MSBP hearing—there was good evidence of immunological intolerances to common foodstuffs in a significant proportion of patients with ASD. It was also evident that these intolerances may be mediated through a variety of immunologic and inflammatory mechanisms and may directly or indirectly impact behavior.

In a detailed review of the relevant medical literature, published the year before the Arizona hearing, Dr. Jyonouchi concluded: "In summary, convincing data support the presence of chronic GI inflammation in ASD children, but the etiology of this GI inflammation is not well understood and is likely affected by multiple genetic and environmental factors. [Non-IgE-mediated food allergy] can partially explain the GI symptoms and apparent beneficial effects of dietary interventions in some ASD children, especially young ASD children."[67]

As will become evident, these matters received no consideration whatsoever in the prosecution of the parents of the Arizona 5.

PART II

Chapter 5

MÜNCHAUSEN SYNDROME BY PROXY: A CHECKERED HISTORY AND AN UNCERTAIN FUTURE

Münchausen syndrome by proxy (MSBP) was first proposed as a disorder in 1977 by Dr. Roy Meadow, an English pediatrician. His proposition was based upon two distinct cases of illness falsification. The first involved tampering with the child's urine samples to elicit false test results, and the second involved an administration of toxic doses of salt leading to the child's death.[1]

William (Bill) Long, professor of law, who was until 2006, a visiting professor of law at Willamette University College of Law in Salem, Oregon,[2] has written a detailed, critical review of MSBP,[3] including its origins, its shifting definitions rooted in many uncertainties, and its challenged standing, particularly following misuse of the diagnosis in the case of Sally Clark[4] by its originator, Dr. Meadow, in perpetrating serious and extremely damaging injustices against parents. Sally Clark lost two children to sudden infant death syndrome (SIDS). In the absence of any obvious risk factors for SIDS, the chance of one such death was estimated at 1 in 8453 live births.[5] Meadow squared the denominator to provide a risk of 1 in 73 million for two siblings dying in this way. In his expert statement at Sally Clark's successful appeal, Professor Dawid of University College, London, described Meadow's figure as "highly misleading and prejudicial."[6] Her children's deaths and her imprisonment effectively killed Sally Clark.

Thirty-three years after it was first proposed, MSBP is still about abuse; however, the role of *abuser* has, in my opinion, ominously shifted in many cases to healthcare professionals—doctors, psychologists, and Child Protective Services

(CPS)—and by proxy, prosecution lawyers and the courts. Inevitably, the victims in such cases are the families.

This section seeks to focus on the criteria for determining MSBP in order to identify possible and actual sources of error in the setting of ASD. For the purpose of this report, the first important reference is to Dr. Donna Rosenberg's classic case review of 1987[7] from the University of Colorado.

Rosenberg's initial definition comprised four components of the syndrome cluster, including:

1. Illness in a child which is simulated (faked) and/or produced by a parent or someone who is in *loco parentis*;
2. Presentation of the child for medical assessment and medical procedures;
3. Denial of knowledge by the perpetrator as to the etiology (cause) of the child's illness; and
4. Acute symptoms and signs of the child abate when the child is separated from the perpetrator.

Rosenberg's report is based upon 117 cases garnered from the medical literature. Coupled with her paper's dramatic title—"Web of Deceit"—and her willingness to infer a diagnosis of MSBP in the absence of requisite evidence, her report gives little or no heed to the false-positive cases (and inevitable harm) that inadequate and non-systematic case ascertainment would inevitably incur. First Meadow himself and later Long were to point out the glaring errors in her analysis with, for example, double-counting cases and the failure of the majority of cases to meet her own criteria for diagnosis of the syndrome. One can see just how problematic Rosenberg's original criteria—relying largely as they do on circumstantial rather than objective evidence—would be in the setting of ASD and just how vulnerable the parents of a child with ASD would be, particularly if one or other of these criteria could be omitted at will (as Rosenberg has done) in the formulation of a diagnosis of MSBP. For example, in the context of Rosenberg's criteria 1–4:

1. It is the position of certain pediatricians that since some parents have their children on a "strange diet" GI symptoms are to be expected.[8] In other words, the parents are responsible for these symptoms.
2. In addition to their autism, ASD children have often been seen by doctors for allergies, ear infections, asthma, seizures, and GI symptoms as well as by nutritionists, physical therapists, occupational therapists, acupuncturists, chiropractors, and behavioral therapists.

3. For the majority of ASD cases, no one knows the cause. Not only do the parents not know what caused their child's symptoms, but with possible MSBP in mind, the healthcare professional may have considered that their "feigned" ignorance of autism's causes is compounded by the audacity to have suggested that a vaccine might have been responsible.
4. Since children with ASD have good days and bad days, the coincidence of apparent symptomatic improvement and the absence of parents may occur by chance and should be interpreted with the utmost caution.

DSM-IV AND DSM-IV-TR (1994 AND 2000; APPENDIX B) RESEARCH CRITERIA

Thirteen years after Rosenberg's paper and still uncertain as to whether MSBP[9] represented a new category of mental disorder, the psychiatric community placed it in the Appendix (B) of the DSM-IV with other disorders deserving further research. The research criteria for the determination of the disorder comprised:

•   Intentional production or feigning of physical or psychological signs or symptoms in another person who is in the individual's care.
•   The motivation of the perpetrator's behavior is to assume the sick role by proxy.
•   External incentives for the behavior (such as economic gain) are absent.
•   The behavior is not better accounted for by another **mental**[10] disorder.

The confusion that has bedeviled the field is exemplified by the substantial discordance between the DSM-IV and Rosenberg's criteria. Rosenberg, like Meadow, saw MSBP as an "Illness **in a** child[11] which is simulated . . . ," whereas DSM-IV requires the "Intentional production or feigning of physical or psychological signs or symptoms **in another person**[12] . . . " thereby attaching the diagnosis to the perpetrator. Moreover, the DSM-IV criteria focus upon the motive of the perpetrator, whereas Rosenberg does not. But how does one establish the motive "to assume the sick role by proxy" in the absence of a frank confession? And the absence of any external incentives for the behavior might simply (and likely) reflect the parents' desire to have their child well again. As Eric Mart, PhD,[13] psychologist and defense expert in the Arizona case explained in court, the measurement of secondary gain on the part of the parent(s) is "generally inferential and speculative."

This is not a sound basis for taking away anyone's children and destroying lives. Most importantly, however, neither the DSM-IV nor Rosenberg's criteria contain the essential exclusory requirement that "**the behaviors of the parent/ guardian and the child are not better accounted for by objective evidence of relevant physical illness in the child.**" The selective reference to an alternative mental disorder in the DSM-IV criteria is entirely inadequate, particularly in the setting of ASD.

ROSENBERG REVISED

In 2003, seemingly concerned that confusion might hinder the diagnosis of MSBP, Rosenberg presented a major and important revision of her original criteria,[14] criteria that had, up to this point, "served to convince courts and others of the prevalence, insidiousness and need for early intervention where MSBP was suspected."[15] Professor Long pointed out that Rosenberg's revised definition, set out below, is so narrow that it would require a complete rewriting of all the MSBP literature to date and would also call into question the importance of the diagnosis. Her revised criteria for a definitive diagnosis consist of the following:

1. Child has repeatedly presented for medical care.
2. Test/event is positive for tampering with child or child's medical situation.
3. Positivity of test/event is not credibly the result of test error or misinterpretation or specimen mishandling.
4. No explanation for the positive test/event other than illness falsification is medically possible.
5. No findings credibly exclude illness falsification.

These criteria have a far more forensic feel to them. Criterion number two requires positive evidence of wrongdoing. In this respect, it goes further that the DSM criterion of the "intentional production or feigning of physical or psychological signs or symptoms in another person," which provides no indication of how solid the evidence for this "feigning" should be; in case reports, the diagnosis of MSBP has relied upon circumstantial evidence and no more.

For the first time—and long overdue—was the requirement that an MSBP diagnosis has to happen "*at the end* of a rigorous clinical differential diagnosis (professional process of elimination)."[16] This is a strikingly different emphasis from the way the MSBP label had been used up to that time. Rosenberg correctly observes that rather than increasing the weight of medical evidence in support of a diagnosis of MSBP, accumulating data ". . . may sometimes instead diminish its likelihood."[17]

In other words, diagnostic due diligence would reduce the likelihood of making a false-positive diagnosis with its attendant heartaches for families. This could only be a good thing.

MSBP IN ASD

In the setting of ASD, abuse does occur, but it needs to be clearly distinguished from MSBP. For example, aversion shock therapy, the delivery of moderate electric shocks by caregivers to condition the behavior of children with ASD as was, until very recently, used by the Judge Rotenberg Educational Center in Massachusetts,[18] was one such state-endorsed abomination. Tragically, parents can reach such levels of despair that they take their children's lives and often, in such cases, their own as well. Neither of these are MSBP.

What of the published cases in which the diagnosis of MSBP has been presented as fact and GI symptoms form part of the allegedly factitious clinical presentation? One example, presented by Dr. Patrick Ip, illustrates that practice is a long way from perfect.[19] It involved a twelve-year-old boy with clear features of a pervasive developmental disorder (PDD), including speech delay, moderate mental retardation, behavioral problems including self-giggling (presumably spontaneous, apparently senseless laughter), temper tantrums, biting people, and playing with feces. These symptoms will be all too familiar to parents with children on the autism spectrum. The diagnosis of speech delay and mental retardation were made at a child assessment center, and his additional behavioral problems were sufficiently severe to have required extended hospitalization. He was managed as a psychiatric inpatient over a period of nine months; despite this, his symptoms appear to have persisted.

With respect to his multiple symptoms of low-grade fever, recurrent colds, allergy, spontaneous bruises, abdominal distention, chronic constipation, and blood in his stool, his only medical investigations appear to have been blood tests, a chest X-ray, and a lymph node biopsy. Specific GI investigations were neither mentioned nor do they appear to have been performed.

The mother in this case had clear psychiatric problems of her own, having been diagnosed with Briquet's syndrome.[20] The presence of this disorder—characterized by multiple symptoms for which no cause can be found—will clearly have impacted not only the physician's perception of likely MSBP but the objective risk of such a disorder. Whether, in this case, the label of MSBP is attached to mother or child—since both had a mental disorder that would better account for the behavior—thus the diagnosis of MSBP foundered on the DSM criteria. In addition, the absence of an adequate GI evaluation in this case means that it should have been inadmissible as MSBP and most certainly would now be, based upon our current understanding.

TRAGEDY: DIAGNOSTIC ERROR AND INEXPERT MEDICAL OPINION

And then there are those cases that turn the diagnosis of MSBP inside out. Two such cases are used to describe the consequences arising out of diagnostic error and inexpert medical opinion, situations that are relevant to the experiences of the Arizona 5 reported below.

In the first case, a five-month-old boy was admitted to the hospital with abdominal pains and a metabolic acidosis which, based upon laboratory testing, was diagnosed as deliberate poisoning with ethylene glycol (antifreeze).[21] Poisoning was suggested, CPS became involved, and the child was removed from his parents. While in foster care he suffered a further severe episode of acidosis and later died in the hospital.

Based upon the discovery of a half-empty container of antifreeze at her home, the mother—five months pregnant with her second son—was arrested, charged with murder, and imprisoned. Two months after the second son's birth, in a repetition of his brother's illness, he developed a metabolic acidosis that was correctly diagnosed at a different hospital from the one that investigated his late brother as a rare metabolic error called methylmalonic acidemia (the body cannot break down certain proteins and fats, resulting in a build up of methylmalonic acid in the blood).

Despite this, the mother was found guilty of murdering her first son, and she was sentenced to life imprisonment as a result. It was only after her dead son's samples were retested and correctly diagnosed as having the same rare disorder as his younger brother that the conviction was overturned.

The second case arose out of a parental custody dispute over a daughter. Psychological profiling was undertaken on the parents and child, during which the daughter's guardian ad litem reported to the psychologist that the mother was causing illnesses in her daughter in order to maintain the position of caregiver. The appointed psychologist had no prior experience of MSBP. Based upon what she subsequently read in some Internet and medical articles, and despite warnings given her by the experts that she should not try to make such a diagnosis if she lacked adequate training or experience, she reported that there was a "reasonable case to suspect that [mother] suffered from MSBP." Over six months later, realizing her error, the psychologist filed a second report, concluding that her allegations of MSBP were unsubstantiated. Citing precedent,[22] the courts gave the psychologist absolute immunity from prosecution.

In his essay Professor Long cited these cases as illustrations of how ". . . laws that were originally meant to protect children went horribly awry when allegations of MSBP were thrown into the mix."[23]

As will become abundantly clear in the following case of the Arizona 5, when allegations of MSBP were thrown into the mix at an early stage, the issue of confirmatory bias rapidly and rabidly set its teeth into the collective medical perception of the family's "disorder." As Dr. Eric Mart explained to the court, "Confirmatory bias is a natural human tendency, when you're investigating something, to come to an immediate theory about something. That this guy robbed this bank [sic]. That child seeks abuse by her stepfather and then what happens is that people—and it's an unconscious process—look for everything that supports their hypothesis and neglect the information that cuts against it. The police call it tunnel vision."[24]

I disagree with Dr. Mart as to the level of conscious processing that drives the need to validate this bias, certainly in the context of the Arizona 5. I am also concerned about its contagious potential, one that insidiously transmutes confirmatory bias to groupthink and ultimately into mob behavior that threatens and intimidates the accused. Dr. Mart summed up the status of what some call MSBP and others factitious disorder by proxy on the basis of the empirical evidence that supports it—"think pieces"[25] rather than science—as he described them in the Arizona court: "So it's kind of garbage in, garbage out."[26]

And for now, it is sufficient to add that Dr. Mart, like Professor Long, has called for the diagnosis of MSBP to be abandoned. With that I can agree.

Every medical specialty has its high-risk clinical situation: during my surgical training in the UK my special interest—an interest that has grown with time—was inflammatory bowel disease. One complication of Crohn's disease is a rectal fistula, a septic tract from the inside of the bowel onto the skin of the perineum. Badly managed by an inexperienced surgical trainee (registrar[27]), the surgical exploration of these tracts, starting with a fistula probe, can lead to catastrophic problems for the patient—incontinence, for example. It was said by my surgical professors that a registrar with a fistula probe is more dangerous than a monkey with a spanner (wrench). Similarly, in the hands of some wayward pediatric specialists, MSBP is to autism what this probe, wielded by a registrar, is to a rectal fistula: more dangerous than a monkey with a spanner.

PART III

Chapter 6

THE ARIZONA 5

Against this broader evidential and historical backdrop, I now turn to the specific case of the Arizona 5—five children who were taken from their parents on suspicion of MSBP. As Christmas 2010 approached, the children remained in foster care, separated from one another and with highly restricted parental visitation rights. So, when this chapter was written, the judge had yet to rule on the charge of MSBP. In contrast with the legal maxim of innocent until proven guilty, the parents are deemed to be of sufficient risk to their children that their guilt must be disproven before the court while they endure the pain and grief of separation, a separation that may be permanent.

As is standard in such cases, the judge imposed a gag order stating that disclosure of anything heard in his proceedings that leads, or might tend to lead, to the identification of these children will be considered as contempt of court. Any perpetrator is liable to imprisonment. Such a ruling, while intended ostensibly to protect the children, serves in fact to protect the accusers. CPS, its informers, and its expert witnesses seem able to operate behind a cloak of secrecy, delay, obfuscation, and legal immunity,[1] facts that become self-evident from an analysis of the Arizona 5. At the same time, the defense must race for the finish line already one lap down, hamstrung by lack of documentary evidence (that is at the disposal of the accusers), with defendant-parents, emotionally distraught, facing the prospect of never seeing their children again. So it is that this story—with the parent's approval—is being made known. The judge will no doubt have something to say about it.

Certain facts have emerged during the course of this analysis that may, from medical, legal, and humanitarian standpoints, perplex the reader. There is no simple answer except to say that the system is broken—irreparably damaged—and needs to be recognized as such, and entered into history as a lesson learned. The analysis is based upon the documents supplied to the defendants' lawyers by Phoenix Children's Hospital (PCH, where the allegations of MSBP originated) and from other medical practitioners involved in the children's care; interviews with parents, family members, friends, and caregivers; and a thorough review of the relevant medical literature. The documents supplied by PCH were incomplete, delivered to the defendants' lawyers piecemeal and in disarray, with different children's records mixed in together. Even worse, by the time the defendants' lawyers received the documents they were apparently left with little more than one week to prepare their defense. Dr. Mart, a psychologist and expert witness retained on behalf of the parents described in court how he had inadequate time to review the records, which were just crammed together in boxes, providing him with ". . . the most challenging record review I have ever been involved in."[2]

Witnesses appearing on behalf of the prosecution did not seem to feel it necessary to voice the same complaints.

In my analysis I will seek to rely on the objective evidence. Matters of opinion will be dealt with in the context of this objective evidence as to the evidential weight that they should carry. In the end, however, this analysis is my opinion. What will become evident to readers is how the narratives of the Arizona 5 stand in marked contrast with those cases of MSBP originally described by Professor Roy Meadow. Beyond this observation, I will not seek to preempt the analysis. Where I have abstracted from records and transcripts, I have made every effort to conserve what I have taken to be the original context and meaning.

THE PARENTS

Notwithstanding their current crisis, the parents remain happily married after fourteen and a half years. After four years in the Air Force, the father went back to school to train as a special education teacher, working mainly in group homes. Already disabled after having the wrong knee operated on by surgeons at Walter Reed Army Medical Center in Washington, D.C., at forty-six he sustained a second injury and retired on disability.

When she was seventeen, the mother broke her neck in a car accident. After three years of nursing school, she had to drop out because of the residual effects of this injury[3] coupled with the physical demands of nursing. She ultimately earned a degree as a licensed practical nurse (LPN). She also retired at the age of thirty on disability as a result of continuing problems with her earlier neck injury. Since retirement, their lives have been dedicated exclusively to raising and caring for their children. They are a religious family and have been sustained throughout their present ordeal by their Christian faith and the strength of their bond as a family. As the mother said in interview, smiling at her husband, "I am married to my best friend."

The mother had achieved some notoriety through a clash with Child Protective Services (CPS) many years before. When she was twenty-five in Syracuse, she had a daughter, Cherilyn, by a previous relationship. Now twenty-three years old, Cherilyn works as a missionary on the Caribbean island of St. Croix. I had the pleasure of interviewing Cherilyn when she returned to Arizona to support her mother through the court ordeal.[4] When she was two, she was taken from her mother into foster care as a victim of alleged sexual abuse. In fact the mother, a naïve single parent, was referred to CPS after calling a local community helpline with questions on breastfeeding her daughter. During the conversation she asked whether it was normal to feel sexually aroused during nursing. I will return to this later but, in short, Cherilyn was removed by CPS, the mother was arrested and imprisoned, the allegation was thrown out of court, and the mother filed a claim against CPS and won damages. Despite this, mother and daughter were separated for one year. Cherilyn, now twenty-three, still suffers nightmares about " . . . the white car that stole her from her mother."

Before moving to Arizona, the family lived in Syracuse, New York. It was there on July 29, 2003, that their third child (Child 3) was assessed at the Margaret L. Williams Developmental Evaluation Center at the Upstate University Hospital for severe developmental and behavioral problems. These are discussed in some detail below. Although the parents were aware of slow development in at least one other of their children, they had no additional concerns about the possibility of ASD at this stage. This is an important point that will be revisited later in the context of the first appearance of the specter of MSBP.

New York State routinely tests all small children for lead exposure, and the child tested positive. The paintwork in their 1895 house was the likely source. In fact, both Child 2 and Child 3 had high blood levels on routine testing reflecting their current exposure in 2002–3. The mother, looking for effective treatments, learned about the biomedical approach to the treatment of childhood developmental disorders at a Defeat Autism Now! (DAN!)[5] conference in Syracuse, New York, in October 2003. Because of adverse effects of New York's climate on Child 3's asthma, the family acquired some land in Arizona, planning to move and build there. On the lookout for a local autism expert, the mother heard about Dr. Cindy Schneider, a physician in Phoenix with extensive experience in the medical treatment of autism. This doctor, previously an OB/GYN, is the mother of a son and a daughter with autism.

The mother chose well. Dr. Schneider has published on autism science in some of the world's leading journals.[6] She was the founding president and medical director of the Southwest Autism Research & Resource Center (SARRC) and is currently the medical director of the Center for Autism Research and

Education (CARE) in Arizona. She sat on the Research Committee of the Medical Investigation of Neurological Disease (MIND) Institute at the University of California, Davis, from 2001 to 2005.

The mother made a call to Dr. Schneider's office that was answered by Cynthia Macluskie, who was working at that time with Dr. Schneider. Ms. Macluskie, a tour-de-force mom and autism advocate, described her personal experience with the benefits of biomedical interventions. Ms. Macluskie is the mother of a boy who, once profoundly autistic following an adverse vaccine reaction, has made remarkable progress on intensive biomedical intervention to the extent that he no longer has a diagnosis of autism,[7] a fact that is central to the ensuing narrative. In fact, he is enrolled in a current research project funded by the National Institutes of Health that is studying "recovered" children.[8] Ms. Macluskie was later to testify in court on behalf of the parents; under oath she confirmed the history of the Child 3's referral to Dr. Schneider on the basis of a developmental disorder associated with possible lead poisoning.[9]

Dr. Schneider agreed to take over Child 3's care, so the mother made her first visit to Arizona with Child 3 in April 2004. During a follow-up visit at her medical office on February 14, 2005, attended by all the family, Dr. Schneider recognized developmental problems in the remaining children and raised her concerns with the parents. Suspecting that they might have some shared environmental exposure causing or contributing to their developmental problems, Dr. Schneider conducted extensive testing on all the children for, among other things, heavy metal poisoning, in accordance with official guidelines.[10] This testing confirmed that lead toxicity was a potential problem in all of the children.

All five children were later referred to a developmental pediatrician, Dr. Sidney Rice, for formal assessment of their behavioral and developmental problems. The process was not straightforward, since the State of Arizona wanted them evaluated instead at a "behavioral health clinic." At a subsequent administrative hearing of the Health Department, the parents argued that, based upon the abnormal results of the heavy metal testing, the children's developmental problems were likely to be medical in origin. The hearing examiner agreed, and the children were approved to see Dr. Rice. What follows are the narratives of the children, numbered 1 to 5 according to their birth order.

Chapter 7

CHILD 1

hild 1 is a boy born on December 30, 1997. His cognitive developmental trajectory was, according to his parents, entirely normal up to the age of three. He was a very happy, engaging child whom his mother described in a recent interview as being "perpetual sunshine; just happy, happy, happy."

At three and a half, he received a nitrous oxide anesthetic (a possible mitochondrial toxin) during a dental procedure. Although not proof of cause and effect, his cognitive and behavioral problems started at this point. His mother describes how he became more difficult and moody and stopped smiling. His organizational skills evaporated so that he could no longer clean up the toys in his room. Tasks that he had mastered now confused him and his frustration led to problem behaviors.

Over the years, delays in Child 1's gross and fine motor skills emerged and he experienced problems with balance and coordination. Eventually he stopped smiling altogether. The engaging, gregarious child was gone; the perpetual sun had set.

Dr. Schneider recalled the first time she met Child 1 when he was seven years old and he came with the entire family to her office on July 5, 2005, for a follow-up visit for Child 3. She described her first impressions of the children as they stood in her office:

> They really worried me; they were skeletal, dark circles under their eyes, white like ghosts. They had no muscle tone—they had no muscle. Their bellies were bloated and swollen. Just like the children you and I see all the time.

I have never met these children, but I feel that I know them well. In her records Dr. Schneider described Child 1 as "thin, pale, and introverted."

His affect was flat, and he responded reluctantly to questions. While his vocabulary was adequate, she noted that his use of language and conversational skills were not age appropriate. On physical examination she confirmed that his balance and coordination were poor and that his fine motor skills were likely delayed. She considered his presentation to be consistent with pervasive developmental disorder—not otherwise specified (PDD-NOS), which she thought might have occurred as a consequence of lead toxicity, given the test results in his younger brother.

Based upon Dr. Schneider's concerns and findings, including an elevated lead level,[1] Child 1 was referred after some delay for further evaluation by Dr. Rice, the developmental pediatrician, to assess his requirement for remedial services. On July 24, 2006, when he was eight, Dr. Rice did a diagnostic assessment. In a follow-up letter dated August 22, 2006, to Dr. Spies, Child 1's primary care physician—a letter whose opening statement is pivotal to an analysis of events that followed—Dr. Rice declared that her assessment of Child 1 had been based upon "neurodevelopmental history, physical and neurological examination, and developmental assessment. . . . performed at this visit."[2]

Her letter to Dr. Sipes included the following diagnoses: Asperger's syndrome [in the absence of speech delay],[3] hypotonia [low muscle tone], non-verbal learning disability with a significant discrepancy between verbal skills, and his visual perceptual skills and written expression. Finally, she added, ". . . toxic exposures with elevated lead levels."[4]

It was not until he was about eleven and into an early puberty, however, that Child 1's behavior regressed markedly with loss of self-regulation involving anger, aggression, and physical violence against objects, himself, and other people; in short, he was out of control. When seen by a child psychiatrist, Dr. Gayle Gregory, at the West Yavapai Guidance Center, on January 28, 2008, it was determined that a diagnosis of childhood disintegrative disorder (CDD)[5] was most appropriate. (This is a historically rare condition, grouped under ASD, that usually involves late-onset, severe autistic regression.) However, it appears that, in light of his earlier problems and in the absence of attendant mental retardation, which usually accompanies CDD, a formal diagnosis of autism was given to Child 1. It is true to say that the parents expressed a preference for a diagnosis of autism which, although less severe than CDD, entitled their son to remedial services.

The mother contacted Dr. Rice by e-mail on March 4, 2009, naturally concerned about the deterioration in his condition. Reminding her that she was the mother of five of Dr. Rice's patients with ASD, she asked Dr. Rice, for children on the spectrum, "Is this normal? Do boys usually get worse at this age? What can we expect? Should we come back to see you? Behavioral health doesn't want him. They [Dr. Gayle Gregory] diagnosed him but have no plans for follow up care."[6]

Dr. Rice responded the following day, confirming that "I absolutely remember you. . . . Many kids get worse with puberty. It is probably a combination of hormones and increased social awareness that causes anxiety and stress. I would be happy to see him again."

Not only did Dr. Rice remember this family with five ASD children, but characterized Child 1's deterioration as something that is seen in many such children.

Child 1's physical health took a dramatic turn for the worse when in December 2008, shortly after recurrent low-grade fevers, leg pains, and a rash on his lower body, he developed severe abdominal pains and started vomiting blood (hematemesis). On December 12, 2008, he went to the emergency room at PCH, where, following an enema, he passed altered blood in his stool (melena). Melena is black and tarry, the color and texture resulting from alteration of the blood by stomach acid; it is indicative of bleeding from high up in the GI tract, usually the stomach or duodenum. On examination, Child 1 had abdominal tenderness and a coalescent purpuric (area of bleeding within the skin) rash[7] and swelling (edema) of his lower extremities. Investigations found thickened bowel loops on abdominal imaging, indicative of inflammation, and blood in his urine (hematuria). The diagnosis was Henoch-Schönlein purpura (HSP).[8] Despite Child 1's evident intestinal problems, the attending pediatric gastroenterologist, Dr. Pasternak, apparently did not seem to feel that diagnostic endoscopy was indicated at this stage. Child 1 was prescribed analgesia and discharged home where his problems continued.

And for this unfortunate family, sorrows were to come "not as single spies, but in battalions."[9]

While the father was dealing with a very sick Child 1 at home, the mother was back at PCH with one of the younger boys, Child 4, who had been admitted as an emergency, having perforated his inflamed appendix.

Child 1's discharge from PCH was premature; after just two days he required readmission to the hospital. On December 14, 2008, the father took him to the local ER for continuing symptoms, principally severe abdominal pain and dehydration. Lacking pediatric inpatient facilities but recognizing his serious condition, the local ER doctor sent Child 1 back to PCH with clear instructions to admit him. At PCH Child 1 was readmitted by Dr. Cooper, the resident, and Dr. Carter, the attending physician. Dr. Cooper noted that he was "doubled over in pain. . . ."[10]

His pain was not even relieved by morphine. He was managed with various painkillers, rehydration, and bed rest. Nevertheless, his abdominal and joint pains continued despite multiple medications, necessitating a review by the pain management team. The mother later described how, at this stage, Child 1's condition had been reported to Dr. Bradstreet, an autism specialist, and Dr. Hellmers, an allergist-immunologist, both of whom were involved in this child's care. Both indicated that he should be on steroids—powerful immune suppressant and anti-inflammatory drugs—to control his HSP. The father went to The Emily Center, a reference library in PCH specifically provided for parents to research their children's problems, where the recommendation of the two doctors was confirmed. He subsequently discussed this treatment option with Dr. Carter, who apparently dismissed it. Dr. Carter's opinion was not shared by Dr. Shishov, a rheumatologist who was brought in to consult on Child 1's HSP-related joint pains. In fact, according to the father, who described Dr. Shishov as an excellent clinician with an unusual bedside manner, he said Dr. Carter's opinion was "nuts . . ." and he walked out of the room. Dr. Shishov started Child 1 on steroids to control his inflammation. At this point, Child 1 had already been in the hospital for seven days.

During this hospital admission, Child 1 developed a marked and progressive anemia (hemoglobin 8.3 g/dl[11]; normal >11.5 g/dl), almost certainly due to intestinal blood loss. On day eight, he was started on intravenous feeding because he could not tolerate oral nutrition due to pain and nausea. In light of his continuing severe GI condition and in the absence of any definitive diagnostic tests, the parents requested that their son's care be transferred to Dr. Ursea, a second PCH pediatric gastroenterologist who had some experience with children with ASD.

After eleven days, on Christmas Eve, despite not having been definitely investigated for his abdominal distress and the source of his blood loss and having yet to see gastroenterologist Dr. Ursea, Child 1 was sent home again. The mother recalls that he spent the next two days at home lying on the floor outside the bathroom, writhing in pain and crawling frequently to the toilet to throw up. Mother described how he had screamed in pain like a woman in labor, adding that "it's one of the most distressing things I have ever had to witness."

Increasingly concerned, the father spoke by phone to an ER triage nurse at PCH about his son's condition. He was asked to describe his son's vomit and was told that it sounded like blood. It has since been alleged that, rather than being a nurse's interpretation of the father's description, it was the father who claimed that his son was "vomiting blood"; this is denied.

HSP can be complicated by damage to the kidneys, intestine, skin, and joints, and associated with pain, swelling, bleeding, and general debilitation. Child 1 had all of these. In fact he had severe, protracted inflammation of the small blood vessels throughout his body leading to chronic multi-organ disease. His initial, belated steroid therapy failed and needed to be intensified in light of his continuing "profound" symptoms.[12] These symptoms included principally abdominal, joint, and muscle pains, for which he was followed by Dr. Ursea and the rheumatology practice of Dr. Shishov and Dr. Ede through January and February 2009. On January 8, 2009, Dr. Ursea wrote to Dr. Sipes reporting that he was still testing positive for blood in his stool and urine. She replied, "I discussed this case with Dr. Shishov and we both agree that his symptoms are 100% due to severe HSP."[13]

Dr. Ede reviewed Child 1 on a monthly basis. On January 31, 2009, concerned with the adverse effects of long-term steroid therapy, he started Child 1 on methotrexate.[14] Better known as an anti-cancer drug, methotrexate is also a powerful immune suppressant that has been useful as a "steroid-sparing" therapy in prior case reports of HSP.[15]

Both Dr. Ursea and Dr. Ede noted, independently, that Child 1 was refluxing repeatedly during his clinic visits. This was associated with halitosis and burping. Dr. Ursea was concerned that this may have been related to intestinal yeast (*Candida albicans*) overgrowth as a consequence of the immunosuppressive treatment. At that time, he also had a severe herpes simplex virus–associated cold sore, a lesion that characteristically breaks out during periods of immune depression. On February 14, 2009, Dr. Ede reviewed Child 1 in the rheumatology clinic. His white blood cell count had risen to 16.3×10^6 per ml—nearly twice the upper limit of normal—a finding that strongly suggested a flare of his HSP. Child 1 was far from out of the woods.

As far as Dr. Ursea's management of Child 1 was concerned, it was his reflux symptoms, combined with continued abdominal pain and blood loss that led her to admit him for endoscopy in February of 2009.

But Child 1's condition deteriorated further, preempting his planned admission. On February 24, 2009, he was readmitted to PCH with persistent abdominal pain, vomiting blood (hematemesis), and the passage of maroon-colored blood in his stool (hematochezia). In the ER he was seen by three people: Dr. Hazelhurt, a resident; Dr. Weiss, the attending physician; and a medical student, Jason Samuels. That he was unwell was not in doubt. In addition to his continuing symptoms of intestinal blood loss and abdominal pain, he had objective measures of continuing illness including a raised inflammatory marker in his blood[16] and positive tests for blood in both his stool and urine. All of these were consistent with ongoing severe HSP. At this stage, he was clinically dehydrated with a critically low blood pressure (80/50 mm/Hg compared with the normal value of 120/80 mm/Hg).

It was later claimed that no healthcare professional had ever witnessed Child 1's intestinal blood loss,[17] implying that this alleged symptom was parental confabulation. This is inconsistent with Dr. Weiss's clinical record of

February 24, 2009, that documented "chronic black tarry stools (that always test + for blood)."[18]

Dr. Weiss's record clearly implies that these abnormal stools had been specifically tested and were consistently positive for blood. The record review of Dr. Krigsman, pediatric gastroenterologist and expert witness on behalf of the parents, disclosed also that Child 1 had only passed these bloody stools after being given an enema at PCH, where this was documented.[19] The fact was that this child was in serious trouble and the medical team at PCH was a long way from having the matter under control. Somewhat incongruously and completely at odds with the clinical situation, Dr. Weiss, in summarizing Child 1's condition wrote, "**Reportedly all 4 sibs have autism and father was an autism specialist in NY**[20]—**quite a coincidence!?**"[21]

He went on to speculate about the possibility of "**?? M by P,**" and below that entry he added, "**Behavioral referral.**"[22]

It is here that we find the first reference to MSBP ("M by P"). Dr Weiss's speculation on this "diagnosis" appears to have rested, irrespective of the child's obvious physical illness, solely upon the coincidence that all five siblings suffered autism while father "was an autism specialist."[23]

The following day, February 25, 2009, Child 1 was reviewed by two further doctors, resident Dr. Longhurst, and once again by Dr. Carter as the attending physician. It will be remembered that, during Child 1's previous admission, Dr. Carter had declined to prescribe steroids for Child 1, a decision that was deemed to be "nuts" and was overruled by the rheumatologist Dr. Shishov.

Dr. Longhurst documented the father's frustration that his son had not been seen by a gastroenterologist the previous night. According to Dr. Longhurst, he was threatening to leave PCH and take his child to another hospital because no treatment had been given. Dr. Longhurst sought to reassure him that the gastroenterologist had been informed and that rehydration was the first important step in his child's management. Unknown to the father, she had also documented that she was aware of the concern over possible MSBP and that she planned to call the social work department with respect to this. She offered no explanation.

As the senior of the two doctors, Dr. Carter reviewed Dr. Longhurst's assessment and added her own note to the record. Among other things, she documented that the father had reported his child's "functional immune deficiency," a diagnosis made by a local immunologist, Dr. Hellmers, on the basis of an inadequate level of antibody immunity to tetanus and *Streptococcus pneumoniae* (Prevnar) vaccines. Notably, Child 1's tetanus antibody level (titer), measured at PCH in December 2008, was not protective.[24] This immune deficiency was due to be treated by Dr. Hellmers with intravenous immunoglobulin (IVIG).[25] IVIG is a donated blood product made up of the concentrated antibody fraction of the blood that contains a broad spectrum of protective antibodies. It is used to reduce the risk and severity of infections in patients with antibody deficiencies.

Dr. Carter was suspicious of the father's claim. She called Dr. Hellmers for clarification and subsequently wrote that she did not accept his anti-tetanus titer as evidence of immunodeficiency, since he was not fully vaccinated. Furthermore, since Child 1 was born in 1997 and Prevnar was introduced in 2000, he would have been unlikely to have received it. In addition, she claimed that Dr. Hellmers had said that he made the diagnosis of immunodeficiency solely on Child 1's low *S. pneumoniae* titers. She added, " . . . of note, some schools of thought hold that IVIG helps with autistic behavior."[26]

Dr. Carter specifically took issue with Dr. Hellmers's diagnosis of a functional immune deficiency and, on that basis, refused to prescribe IVIG, informing the father of her position. At the end of her note she added, "**Psych/Social— complex sit'n [situation] social work involved.**"[27]

That same day, Child 1 was also seen by the pediatric gastroenterology team. The gastroenterologist documented the child's abnormal blood tests at this time, including a raised marker of inflammation and evidence of dehydration,[28] the latter almost certainly a result of vomiting and poor fluid intake. Child 1 was already booked to have GI investigations on the following day, February 26, 2009, under Dr. Ursea, including upper and lower GI endoscopy and capsule enteroscopy (a pill-sized camera that images the small intestine). Prior to his endoscopy, Child 1 was reviewed by Dr. Carter, who had tracked down his vaccination history and identified that he had not received Prevnar but had received a fourth dose of DTaP on December 28, 1998. On this basis, she continued to take issue with Dr Hellmer's diagnosis of immunodeficiency and the use of IVIG. However, she now switched tack from immunodeficiency, stating that ". . . present research shows question of benefit for autism spectrum disorder with IVIG."[29]

She continued, " . . . at present IVIG is not FDA approved for autism symp[tom]s,"[30] and once again informed Child 1's father of her decision not to prescribe it and her reasons why. It is notable that Dr. Hellmers had prescribed IVIG to treat Child 1's immunodeficiency and *not* his autism symptoms, a point that was reinforced later in court by Dr. Hellmers himself. Nonetheless, there is a medical literature that indicates substantial benefit from IVIG in the amelioration of autism symptoms in some children,[31] and an awareness of this may have been the source of Dr. Carter's confusion.

On top of everything else, father apparently became "angry" at Dr. Carter's intransigence and requested that another pediatrician take over his child's care.

At the conclusion of her record and her involvement in Child 1's care, she wrote under the heading "Social":

> Family "fired" me. In past [they] have also fired one of my hospitalist partners. Discussed with administration [the] best course of action. Plan made to t'fer [transfer] case to [pediatrician Dr. Ijaola]—will call them to discuss pt [patient]. Concern for fictitious d/o [disorder] + Munchausen by Proxy. [Social Work] involved + aware of concern.[32]

From this sequence of events, one is inclined to assume that Dr. Carter called PCH administration because she had been fired from the case. This is understandable; it is a difficult and unusual situation and not unreasonably, she needed advice on how to proceed. Had MSBP been Dr. Carter's primary concern, the proper course of action would have been to contact the social services department or Child Protective Services (CPS) specifically; both are departments within the Arizona Department of Economic Security. It appears that during the course of the exchange between Dr. Carter and PCH Administration, possibly fearing legal repercussions from the parents, it was determined that attack was the best form of defense. Unfortunately, no record of Dr. Carter's conversation is available.

Later, in expert testimony, and based upon his forensic analysis of approximately one hundred cases of alleged MSBP, the psychologist Dr. Mart emphasized that the origin of an MSBP allegation in the vast majority of cases followed a falling out with the reporting doctor, on which he opined, "I'm not sure that it's always a good reason."[33]

I would go further and suggest that in circumstances of parent-caregiver conflict, the professional must consciously avoid this diagnosis for fear that any antipathy toward the parents might interfere with an objective view of the child's medical problems.

In addition, it is not certain how the discordance between Dr. Weiss's concern for MSBP (the coincidence of multiple siblings with autism and father an autism specialist) and that of Dr. Carter (diagnosis and treatment of immunodeficiency) was reconciled, if indeed it ever was. Nor is it evident how either of these doctors' respective positions fulfilled any of the criteria for MSBP advanced by the American Psychiatric Association[34] or Dr. Rosenberg,[35] as discussed in Part 2.

Returning now to the objective medical narrative, the following day, February 26, 2009, Child 1 underwent endoscopy that revealed gastric and duodenal erosions (ulcers). Even after several weeks on powerful medication, microscopic examination of intestinal biopsy tissues still showed an acute inflammation (duodenitis). This pathology—part of his HSP—was very likely the source of his intestinal blood loss.

So it was that, by the end of February 2009, Child 1 had received a diagnosis of autism and was suffering from "severe" HSP with potentially life-threatening intestinal hemorrhage from erosions of his stomach and duodenal lining. Other clinical findings of note were blood tests on September 10, 2010, showing an elevated IgE antibody (consistent with allergy) and deficient diphtheria and tetanus antibodies, markers of a possible functional immune deficiency. Not content with this as an explanation for his problems, the possibility of MSBP had been raised and reported to social services.

The source of Dr. Carter's conflict was, in fact, a professional disagreement between her and the immunologist, Dr. Hellmers, as to the significance of Child 1's antibody titers, the validity of a diagnosis of functional immunodeficiency, and the merits of treatment with IVIG. While Dr. Hellmers had prescribed IVIG for the treatment of an immunodeficiency, Dr. Carter had refused to order it for the treatment of autism. It is no wonder that the parents were confused. The family had endured their oldest son's suffering in the face of a somewhat tentative medical approach to his severe illness. Finally, based upon the perceived benefits of IVIG in his child and Dr. Carter's intransigence, the father had asked for another pediatrician to take over Child 1's care and in her own words, Dr. Carter had been "fired."

Dr. Mart noted in testimony that the case actually boiled down to " . . . a disagreement between medical doctors . . . "[36] of which functional antibody deficiency was just one issue. Having made this observation, he indicated that further consideration of an MSBP diagnosis was somewhat redundant.

This hospital admission concluded for Child 1 with a review by Dr. Iajola, a pediatric internist to whom the patient had been referred by Dr. Carter as her replacement. Dr. Iajola made no mention of MSBP in the patient's chart and recommended discharge home.

In an interview with the parents in early 2011, they were adamant that the course of their child's severe HSP was altered initially by steroids and latterly by IVIG that was instituted by Dr. Hellmers. After just two infusions of IVIG, they said, his abdominal and joint pain, his purpuric rash, and his intestinal bleeding all improved. Attempts to reduce the steroid dose led to a return of the HSP symptoms. The parents maintain that the IVIG allowed them to finally stop the steroids once and for all. This may have been coincidental, but the parents thought not, and Dr. Ursea certainly remarked on it. As a possible treatment for HSP, it may be worth bearing in mind.

IVIG was not the parents' only bone of contention with Dr. Carter. During the early days of his HSP, the father had referred Dr. Carter to literature that he had found in the hospital's reference library describing the potential benefits of steroids in alleviating HSP. Dr. Carter had resisted, and it was the rheumatologist, Dr. Shishov, who started this treatment. He was right to have done so; a review of the medical literature in 2007 with a meta-analysis of data from all valid clinical trials indicated that steroids were beneficial, particularly for HSP-associated abdominal pain,[37] which was Child 1's most troublesome complaint.

The parents were emphatic that for the four children in this family that received IVIG, it "changed their lives." Nonetheless, the parents had become, by proxy, victims of a divergence of opinion between two doctors on the rationale for and merits of a seemingly beneficial treatment.

Despite the question of MSBP having been referred to the social services department, this was not pursued. At the time of writing, no documents are available to report on how the matter was handled and why it was not pursued. The parents had no knowledge that the question of abuse had ever been raised until their children were taken from them and charges were filed sixteen months later. This referral to social services—despite having been made without any opportunity on the part of the parents to respond—was to play a supporting role later on, re-emerging with a pejorative spin in the matter of Child 2, and was no doubt instrumental in shaping the drastic actions of CPS.

Eventually, with the help of heavy-duty, and arguably belated, medication including corticosteroids, methotrexate (a potent immunosuppressive drug), and IVIG, Child 1's life-threatening disorder eventually settled. Later, in court, as evidence of parental abuse, the prosecuting counsel returned repeatedly to the fact that Child 1 had had over sixty medical appointments in an eighteen-month period.[38] Given his severe multisystem disorder, this is hardly surprising. Ironically, had Child 1's initial treatment been more proactive and aggressive, the number of appointments might have been substantially fewer.

Sadly, Child 1 has developed cataracts as a likely consequence of his steroid treatment. Medicine sometimes harms as well as helps. His eye disease will require medical follow-up and possible surgery: in other words more doctors' visits. Will the treatment of this iatrogenic disease, a disease caused by the physician, also be labeled as abusive?

Chapter 8

CHILD 2

Child 2 is a girl who was born on November 5, 1998. Her early development appears to have been normal. Contemporaneous documents are not available to me to confirm this. However, in October 2010 during the course of the legal proceedings, such documents were apparently available to Dr. Sharon McDonough-Means, a developmental pediatrician who reviewed Child 2's case, along with those of her siblings. She wrote, "12 months: very vocal, walking with wide-based toddler gait. 15 months—babble a lot, 2 word phrases (likely by history)."[1]

The parents report that when she was two and a half years old, she became quiet and withdrawn, and her mother initially attributed this to the birth of her third child. However, as Dr. McDonough-Means observed, at three years there was "stranger anxiety"[2] and that by four years there were, "articulation concerns."[3] Child 2 was seen on July 5, 2005, by Dr. Schneider, who described her as having become:

> Very shy and withdrawn at age 4 for unclear reasons . . . She has difficulty comprehending events coming in the future and other concepts of time. . . . She has a few chores around the house such as setting the table, but cannot remember what items need to be placed there . . . Delayed echolalia occurs, often involving phrases from videos. She is a thin, pale and extremely introverted child with an unusually fearful affect.[4]

Dr. Schneider noted that Child 2 had recently been seen by a neurologist who thought that she was "depressed." Although Dr. Schneider had no report to refer to, she was told that this specialist in diseases of the nervous system had found no neurological deficits in Child 2. In contrast with the specialist, on neurological examination of Child 2 Dr. Schneider noted:

> . . . deep tendon reflexes were markedly reduced throughout all extremities. Increased sympathetic activity was noted in the left upper extremity. . . . Her

left pupil fatigued rapidly with light and a right palatal paresis was evident. Finger to nose testing was poor bilaterally, but particularly on the left, indicating involvement of the left cerebellum.[5] Disdiadokokinesis[6] on the left was also observed.[7]

As a testament to her clinical acumen, Dr. Schneider had elicited signs of focal neurological injury affecting Child 2's cerebellum, in particular. These symptoms cannot be faked, particularly by children. Readers may remember from Part 1, Chapter 3 that the cerebellum appears to be particularly vulnerable to damage from the downstream effects of an allergic intolerance to wheat gliadin. It is also a part of the brain that is very susceptible to lead poisoning[8] and important in autism.[9] Dr. Schneider's diagnosis in Child 2 was PDD-NOS with considerable deficits in social and motor skills with autistic features.

In light of the family history of lead exposure, Dr. Schneider recommended that Child 2 undergo a chelation challenge: giving an infusion of a substance that binds heavy metals in the body, facilitating their excretion in an effort to reduce the metals' toxicity. The lead in Child 2's red blood cells was high, and the amount excreted in her urine after chelation was extremely high.[10]

Child 2, when she was six, was seen by Dr. Schneider on October 12, 2005, who wrote:

[Child 2] has responded very positively to treatment with [chelation], glutathione, zinc, probiotics, [folic acid] and [vitamin B12]. Her concentration has improved, she is making more rapid progress academically, and she has begun to speak to children outside her immediate family. While these gains are very encouraging, her challenges remain great.[11]

To assess her eligibility for special needs services, Child 2 was subsequently referred to Dr. Rice, the developmental pediatrician, by her primary care physician, Dr. Sipes. When reporting back to Dr. Sipes after the consultation on August 2, 2006, Dr. Rice once again introduced her report with a standard qualification of her assessment: "Neurodevelopmental history, physical and neurological examination and developmental assessment were performed at this visit."

Her diagnosis of Child 2 consisted of autism, hypotonia, and toxic exposure associated with elevated lead levels. She made recommendations for physical, occupational, and education therapies.

Dr. McDonough-Means cited one further record from Dr. Rice, when Child 2 was seven and a half years old, that described "hypotonia, poor balance, definite neuromotor integration difficulties; poor eye contact, facial tics when stressed; patterned, constrained behavior; perseverative on topic. Impression was Autistic Disorder, mild."[12]

So, the formal developmental assessment by Dr. Rice put Child 2 somewhere on the mild end of the autistic spectrum. While her early development appeared to have been normal, she became withdrawn in her third year, and clear behavioral abnormalities and motor problems emerged at around three to four years of age. Dr. Schneider's intervention had produced evident benefits for this child.

The problems with CPS really started in earnest for this family when on March 16, 2010, Child 2, then eleven years old, was seen by Dr. Carter—the same Dr. Carter who had been "fired" by the father one year earlier. The encounter took place in the ER at PCH. Child 2 was suffering with right shoulder pain, a pain that radiated to the right hand and forearm,[13] following an injury while on a recent family trip to Mexico. A clinical examination and X-ray at a medical center in San Diego shortly after the injury had apparently shown subluxation (partial dislocation) of the right acromio-clavicular (AC) joint. After returning to Arizona, Child 2 had her right AC joint "realigned" in four or five sessions with a chiropractor. He had subsequently ordered an MRI, which showed narrowing of the right subacromial space. However, his manipulation did not alleviate the problem, and it was the continuing pain that took them to the ER at PCH on March 16, 2010.

In an interview, the mother[14] described to me how she had been accompanied in the ER by a witness. This witness, Ms. Teri Holloway, was a family support program manager, there at the mother's request for support from Mentally Ill Kids In Distress (MIKID), a local organization. The mother and Ms. Holloway met for the first time at that ER visit. Ms. Holloway later described Dr. Carter's behavior as odd.[15] Apparently she came and went several times, questioning the mother and/or daughter on each occasion but spending no more than five to ten minutes with them in total. According to the mother, no examination of Child 2's shoulder was undertaken by Dr. Carter in the presence of either her or Ms. Holloway, both of whom remained with the child throughout. In fact, according to the mother, Dr. Carter undertook no physical examination of Child 2 at all. The mother recalled that Dr. Carter's note of this consultation was confined to " . . . less than one page of writing, in pencil, that ended with the single word 'Münchausen'."

Here we encounter a major discrepancy between the mother's report of events and the attendance note written by Dr. Carter. Following the MSBP charges, the parents were sent Dr. Carter's one-page summary with the allegation of "Münchausen." The hospital records obtained by the parents' lawyers did not include this important document, and having come from the parents rather than the hospital records, by virtue of chain of custody rules, it was apparently not admissible as evidence and was not considered further.[16] What was provided, instead, was a detailed report—apparently written by Dr. Carter on the same evening of March 16, 2010—that describes not only the medical history that she had obtained from the mother, but also her findings on examination of Child 2 on that occasion.

Dr. Carter's report is disproportionately detailed for a five-to-ten-minute consultation, running as it does to five single-spaced, handwritten pages. On closer inspection, her report confirms that Child 2 was seen by her at 6 PM on March 16, 2010. Toward the bottom of her report she wrote, "Time 60 mins," and below this, a record that she concluded her report at 8:30 PM on the same day. It appears that, since this annotation is likely to have been made for billing purposes, "60 mins" reflects the total time spent on this patient including her write-up.

It is usual practice for a doctor to make handwritten notes of the patient's history as he or she goes along and write up the examination findings at the conclusion of the physical examination. Although this is not invariable, it is not clear why Dr. Carter's interview with the mother and daughter, having started at 6 PM, should have finally been written up two and a half hours later when the time spent on this patient was apparently only "60 mins." Whatever the case, it does not explain the discrepancy between the mother's claim that Dr. Carter did not undertake an examination of her child and Dr. Carter's written report of her examination findings.

The discrepancy is thrown into considerably sharper relief by the observations of two of the witnesses: Ms. Holloway and Child 2 herself. First, Child 2 was interviewed by Heather Williams of CPS at the family home on March 20, 2010. At that time, according to the mother, she told Ms. Williams that she had not been examined by Dr. Carter in the ER. This was confirmed by Ms. Holloway who had been with Child 2 throughout the time that Dr. Carter had dealt with this child in the ER. There was, apparently, no other opportunity for Dr. Carter to have undertaken an examination as she had claimed. In a larger meeting that took place at the family home in May 2010, with representatives from CPS, including Ms. Williams, and an additional representative of the family, Ms. Holloway endorsed the claims of both mother and daughter in her account of events.

The record of Dr. Carter's physical examination of Child 2 is quite extensive, involving the nervous system, the abdomen, the respiratory and cardiovascular systems, and of course, the right shoulder. Her record of her examination of Child 2 is set out below in some detail for the purpose of forensic analysis. Her examination findings, largely written in the form of medical acronyms and shorthand, are found on page two of her five-page report. She opened by describing Child 2 as a "well appearing 11yr female. [No abnormalities detected]. Makes good eye contact. Answers [questions] appropriately."[17]

An examination of Child 2's eyes and associated nervous system integrity followed with "pupils [left and right] equal and reacting to light and accommodation. Extraoccular muscles intact. Sclera white, conjunctiva pink." Next, Dr. Carter examined Child 2's ears. She described her tympanic membranes [left and right] as clear, her nose and oro-pharynx as clear, and her tonsils as not red or enlarged, with no exudate.

Examination of the tympanic membranes, which separate the external and middle ears, would have required the use of an otoscope, an instrument that virtually all mothers and children recognize. Ms. Holloway confirmed to me that at no stage did Dr. Carter examine Child 2 with this medical instrument.

She described Child 2's head size as normal [normocephalic] with no evidence of trauma [atraumatic]. There was no evidence of swollen lymph glands [lymphadenopathy], and her neck was supple.

Turning next to Child 2's respiratory system, Dr. Carter described this as "normal, left and right. Clear to auscultation [listening with a stethoscope] bilaterally." She examined Child 2's heart, which she described as "heart sounds [S_1S_2] normal. No murmurs, rubs or gallops [MRG; also requiring use of a stethoscope]."

Next she examined Child 2's abdomen, which she reported as being "soft, not tender with no distention, no enlargement of the liver or spleen [hepatosplenomegaly; HSM] and no masses." Examination of Child 2's genitalia was "deferred," and she found no evidence of lymph gland swelling.

Finally, she reported on her examination of Child 2's injured shoulder: "Right upper extremity [no] swelling or redness. No blue discoloration appreciated even p [sic] [Right upper extremity] held with down and side for 2–3 mins. Free range of movement of right hand, wrist, elbow, shoulder. Patient winced with arm supine and right shoulder abducted."

What is very odd is the fact that, according to the mother and Ms. Holloway, they were in a hospital corridor throughout their time in the ER. At no time were they admitted to an examination room. It seems unlikely that such an extensive examination, particularly of a child—and one the mother described as being extremely shy—would have taken place in public in a busy ER.

In an interview with Teri Holloway on January 26, 2011, I asked her to confirm whether or not Dr. Carter had actually examined Child 2 as she had claimed in her record. Ms. Holloway replied, "Absolutely not."

According to this witness there had been no examination of Child 2 that involved the nervous, respiratory, and cardiovascular systems or the abdomen as documented by Dr. Carter. Ms. Holloway could not even recall Dr. Carter examining the child's injured shoulder. In fact, she vividly remembered that Child 2 and her mother were seated side by side on the hospital gurney throughout. "Mother would have had to move for any examination to have taken place," Ms. Holloway said. Ms. Holloway was present throughout the examination and to the point Child 2 was admitted to the hospital ward. This point of admission was also Dr. Carter's last clinical contact with Child 2.

This issue clearly needs to be resolved. Both versions of the events of March 16, 2010, cannot be correct. It is either the case that the mother, her daughter, and their witness are wrong, or Dr. Carter is guilty of fraud and, as a consequence, gross professional misconduct. The case against this family—the allegation of MSBP—has been framed around Dr. Carter's successive reports to social services, and if she has intentionally misled them, then whatever the consequences for Dr. Carter, the case against the parents must be summarily dismissed and any adverse findings overturned.

Toward the end of Dr. Carter's five-page ER note, a degree of hostility is evident on several levels. As in the case of Child 1, she appears to have taken exception to the diagnosis of functional antibody deficiency in Child 2. This had been identified and treated, as in the case of her brother, by immunologist Dr. Hellmers, on the basis of "low antibody titer." Dr. Carter also commented that "the patient does not exhibit obvious signs of autism to me." She continued, "When asked if the patient is still meeting criteria for [a] diagnosis of autism mom said, 'I refuse to answer that question.' When asked why mom said, '. . . because it might make her lose services.'"[18]

The mother reported that she actually said, "I do not wish to answer that question because it's not in her best interests."

The mother's version of events is supported by Ms. Holloway. The mother's immediate concern had been for her daughter's pain, not her autism. Nonetheless, it is worth noting that Child 2 had, according to several observers, responded to treatment including chelation, exclusion diet, nutritional support, and IVIG. In the process, her autistic traits had receded. The mother may have been reasonably concerned that her daughter's recovery might be used to justify removal of beneficial services such as occupational and educational therapy. Not unreasonably, she may not have wanted to advance an unqualified opinion on her daughter's diagnosis and risk the removal of any of these beneficial therapies, a situation that might have led to reversal of her daughter's improved well-being.

Dr. Carter decided to admit Child 2 for further assessment. This came as a complete surprise to both the mother and Ms. Holloway;[19] no one had expected or asked for admission to the hospital. Ms. Holloway wrote later, "This action for a hurt shoulder seemed very odd. Typically X-rays or other tests would have been performed and families are asked to follow up with their primary care doctor or specialist."

Dr. Carter's skepticism about the mother's story beyond the matter of Child 2's shoulder is indicated by the fact that her admission plan involved placing Child 2 on a normal diet. She had already noted two pages earlier in her medical notes that the child was on a restriction diet that excluded casein, gluten, various oils, and soy. Ignoring these dietary exclusions was at best cavalier and at worst downright dangerous.

The final item in Dr. Carter's admission plan was an intention to consult with the social worker out of her concern for "**Munchausen by proxy and/or vulnerable child syndrome**[20] for this child and her siblings." She also added that she was "concerned about inappropriate use of medical resources for unproven diagnoses; in particular IVIG [every] 3 weeks."

The basis for her concern about MSBP is not clear and will be discussed below in the context of the criteria for this diagnosis. Whatever her current developmental status, Child 2 had received a professional diagnosis of autism. The mother had been informed by medical professionals that her daughter had a likely MTHFR gene mutation (the MTHFR gene provides instructions for making an enzyme called methylenetetrahydrofolate reductase, which is important to folate metabolism, methylation, and detoxification), a functional antibody deficiency, GERD (gastroesophageal reflux disease), high blood lead levels, and a damaged right acromioclavicular joint.[21] As in the case of Child 1, Dr. Carter's principal issues appear to have been with Dr. Hellmer's diagnosis and treatment of the immune problems and, in addition, the fact that Child 2 "did not look autistic" to her. Neither of these issues had any direct bearing on the child's presenting complaint, shoulder pain, for which Dr. Carter had been consulted but had apparently failed to properly assess. Nonetheless, Dr. Carter took it upon herself to stop Child 2's exclusion diet and involve CPS on behalf of all five children.

Child 2's time in the hospital is notable for the report of physical therapist Alison Perkins, whose job it was to help with the assessment and treatment of the shoulder injury. Three days after Dr. Carter's examination, Ms. Perkins reported, on March 19, 2010:

> Area 1. Pocket of swelling over the [right] AC joint that was notably boggy.
> Area 2. Multiple muscle spasms noted along the medial border of the right scapula and into the right trapezius.

These findings, made three days after Dr. Carter's examination and, therefore, a further three days for the shoulder to have healed, found no mention in Dr. Carter's clinical record from the ER.

The social work department record from March 17, 2010, is, at least for the first several entries, relatively innocuous. Other than noting the need to get Child 2 up to date with her immunizations, it documents the parental concern over their child's continuing shoulder pain, the family history of chronic illness, their limited finances/resources, the stress of hospitalization on the family, and the parents' willingness to cooperate. Anica Herren, a child life specialist— someone who apparently assists with the activities of daily living—spoke with Dr. Carter, presumably in order to understand better the nature of her concerns over possible MSBP. The note refers to a "multiple, chronic complex history." Crucially, the note referred to the fact that Dr. Carter was attempting to make contact with Dr. Hellmers, but, at that point, had failed to do so. This point is critical since it was Dr. Carter's conflict with Dr. Hellmer's diagnosis of functional antibody deficiency and his decision to treat with IVIG that had triggered her allegations against the parents in the first instance. For Child 2, Dr. Carter had intended to resolve this crucial issue with Dr. Hellmers—an issue central to the merits of her allegation of MSBP—but, in fact, filed her allegation before having done so. In fact, there is no record of any contact with Dr. Hellmers ever having been made by Dr. Carter in respect of this child. In other words, the issue at the heart of the allegation of MSBP was never resolved by Dr. Carter.

The next significant encounter was between Child 2's father and a social worker at his daughter's hospital bedside. Both parents were becoming increasingly frustrated that they could not get IVIG for their daughter according to her prescribed three-weekly schedule while she was in the hospital—a hospital admission that the parents had not anticipated, requested, nor felt was necessary. The father then requested that the issue of pain relief and IVIG be resolved by a treatment team and a representative of the PCH administration, stressing that he wanted "to get effective pain relief and IVIG and get [his daughter] out of hospital as soon as possible."

The social worker noted that later during this same interview, he apologized for his negative attitude, which, according to the father, arose out of frustration and concern for his child.

Child 2's mother was later interviewed by a social worker who noted the mother's report of her daughter's obvious pain despite her normally having a "high tolerance to pain." Conflict followed when she told the mother that it was unlikely that IVIG would be given to her daughter during that admission. Mother told the social worker that she did not have the authority to make that decision. Later in the same interview, the mother apologized to the social worker, her frustration apparently arising out of the failure to control her child's pain. The pain physician subsequently made further recommendations concerning suitable analgesia for Child 2, and she was discharged home on March 19, 2010.

In an interview with the parents,[22] it seems that their angst over IVIG had arisen because Child 2 was due for her prescribed IVIG as an outpatient while she was an inpatient in the same hospital. The outpatient nurse, who scheduled and administered the IVIG, had been encouraging the mother to arrange for IVIG to be given by the inpatient staff, and the inpatient staff was, in turn, reluctant to oblige. The parents, caught in the middle, were at a loss to understand why two departments of the same hospital could not communicate and coordinate this process between them.

None of what had happened to this point could reasonably be construed as evidence of abuse, let alone MSBP. The parents' behavior was a reasonable reflection of their justified concern, including their wish to comply with Dr. Hellmer's treatment orders for IVIG. Dr. Carter had blocked Dr. Hellmer's recommended treatment for immunodeficiency on the mistaken basis that it was being used for the treatment of autism, but she had failed in her stated intention of contacting Dr. Hellmers in order to justify why she had done so. This was particularly important since, unlike Dr. Hellmers, she was not, by her own admission, an expert in immunology.[23] While Dr. Carter had also questioned Child 2's current autism diagnosis, this was not her field of expertise either.[24] Neither did she take any steps at that time to contact the diagnosing physician to seek the opinion of the relevant expert. The final entry in the social work record flagged the fact that Childs 2's brother had been referred to CPS in 2008, but that entry failed to mention that no grounds for action were ever established. Instead, the entry read "Heather [Williams, SW] is hoping to collaborate with the medical team at PCH, the [primary care physician] and DDD to begin building a case that might warrant an investigation for CPS."[25] The entry was signed by social worker Nicole Ordway on March 18, 2010, just two days after the social work department had become involved with Child 2's case.

Several additional observations are merited. On March 17, 2010, under the request, "State reason for suspicion of abuse and describe extent of injury or neglect," PCH social worker Jennifer Slatteri, in her CPS report, wrote, "possible/suspected emotional and physical abuse re patient stated/reported chronic, complex multiple medical diagnosis." Below this, under the request for "other information which might be helpful in establishing case," she added, "autism, mitochondrial disorder, functional immunodeficiency, asthma, hypotonic, MTHFR[26] deficiency reported by parents with no mitochondrial document [sic] of diagnosis."[27]

The basis of Ms. Slatteri's suspicion of MSBP was that the "[patient] stated/ reported chronic, complex multiple medical diagnosis." Thus, in the eyes of Ms. Slatteri, Child 2's mother had already become a "patient"—someone suffering a disorder—and the evidence for this preemptive and baseless status was the mother's description of her child's "chronic, complex multiple medical diagnosis."

Notwithstanding Ms. Slatteri's presumption of the mother's pathology, this report reflects a clear lack of understanding: in 2010 it was documented in the peer-reviewed medical literature that autism, mitochondrial disorder, MTHFR deficiency, and hypotonia could well be part of a single, integrated disease process with a plausible and coherent chain of cause and effect.[28] In her defense, Ms. Slatteri might argue that she was not qualified to recognize this coherence to Child 2's medical disorders. Since this is undoubtedly the case, she should never have been in position to take the factitious leap that turned a concerned mother into a suspected abusive psychiatric patient.

From the GI perspective, Child 2 was first referred to Dr. Ursea and seen on March 27, 2009, with a history of chronic regurgitation that was worse at night, waking her from sleep. This is classical in gastroesophageal reflux, where more frequent and severe symptoms occur characteristically when lying down. She underwent endoscopy on June 6, 2009. The microscopic findings of mild esophagitis in biopsies obtained in this procedure were described by Dr. Ursea in a letter of June 24, 2009. Child 2 was treated with acid-reducing drugs and her symptoms improved, although they never quite went away.

Chapter 9

CHILD 3

Child 3, a boy born in Syracuse, New York, on July 7, 2001, was, in fact, the first of the siblings to be diagnosed with autism. He developed normally to eighteen months of age and, according to the mother, was advanced in his motor skills. On December 16, 2002, he received his primary MMR and pneumococcal (Prevnar) vaccines plus his fourth round of *Haemophilus influenzae* type b and DTaP vaccines. Eight vaccines were given at once, a medical procedure for which no prospective safety study has ever been conducted. Just over one week later on Christmas Eve, he returned, unwell, to Dr. McCarthy's office. She wrote, "Child seems uncomfortable even in sleep since shots. Loose BMs [bowel movements]."[1]

The link between his novel symptoms and his shots had been made contemporaneously by the parents and documented accordingly by Dr. McCarthy. On the basis of a red left eardrum, Dr. McCarthy prescribed antibiotics. Child 3 was seen again by the office nurse on January 2, 2003, with vomiting, and again on January 6, 2003, with continued vomiting and diarrhea "pouring out of diaper." The antibiotics were stopped in light of these symptoms. By January 13, 2003, he had developed a severe diaper rash suggestive of secondary infection. On January 28, 2003, just over one month since his previous eight shots, while still unwell, he received injections of his third polio and second Prevnar vaccines.

Following the second set of shots, he had to be carried from the doctor's office screaming. In an interview with Cherilyn, the mother's eldest child who helped to raise her younger half-brothers and half-sister, she recounted that " . . . the day after he got vaccinated it was a different child. You know, it was like we took the wrong child home from the doctor's office."

Within forty-eight hours of receiving these vaccines, he stopped walking and he started waking up in distress as his sleep pattern deteriorated further. Over the ensuing weeks his disturbed sleep continued to get worse. At a pediatrics acute care visit on March 15, 2003, the nurse recorded, "Cranky. [Decreased] sleep and won't lie down. Screaming in sleep last night."

Similar entries continued over the following months with repeated reference to his sleep and GI disturbances, and in addition, a tendency to severe acute upper respiratory infections. On June 3, 2003, Dr. McCarthy recorded the ominous hallmark signs of his emergent developmental disorder: "Repetitive behaviors—not ritualistic. 18 mo shots given late—screamed nights. Then sore throats."[2]

In this entry, the link between his symptoms and his eighteen-month vaccines was reinforced. Under "chief complaint," Dr. McCarthy wrote, "Almost 2 year old [with] parents for trouble sleeping . . . waking up in middle of night screaming . . . does not want to be touched." Below that, she wrote, "Not speaking. Active . . . all over room." And under "assessment," she wrote, "Behaviors that parents concerned about and night terrors."[3]

By June 30, 2003, he had developed a left lower lobe pneumonia, confirmed by X-ray, and was admitted to the hospital on July 1, 2003, for intravenous antibiotics. The admitting doctor considered the pneumonia to be due to probable *Streptococcus pneumoniae*, which would have been ironic in light of his recent Prevnar vaccination. It was also evident that by this stage Child 3 had restricted his diet, a common feature in children with ASD, and was "refusing most foods." Here we find one of the first references to food allergies, made by a Loretta Caffey (possibly a dietician although who was responsible for the use of the term "food allergies" is not clear). Beyond this point, Child 3 suffered recurrent wheezing consistent with a diagnosis of non-atopic asthma that required long-term asthma medication. This diagnosis was subsequently confirmed by Dr. Hellmers, the allergist and immunologist.

On September 11, 2003, Dr. McCarthy documented that "parents want to hold vaccines." Not only did the parents make a positive decision at this stage to stop further vaccination, but Dr. McCarthy had, according to her own records, offered no resistance to the parents' wishes.

Thereafter, Child 3 developed a constellation of increasingly severe problems, including seizures, language regression, aggression, hand flapping, toe walking, and echolalia. In addition to these more typical features of autism, he became hypotonic with associated motor delays. As referred to earlier, a very high pain tolerance was a feature of this child's disorder. Consistent with his general deterioration was the fact that his linear growth and weight gain fell in his third year. Between November 17, 2003, and November 15, 2004, his weight fell from the ninety-fifth percentile to around the sixtieth. In light of his training in special education, the father wondered whether he was suffering from a pervasive developmental disorder such as autism. The mother doubted this since she felt that his lack of social aloofness was inconsistent with what she had heard of this disorder.

Child 3 underwent extensive developmental testing on at least four occasions. After concerns were first raised by Onondaga (New York) County Early Intervention Program, he was referred for formal developmental assessment. This initially consisted of an evaluation at the Margaret L. Williams Developmental Evaluation Center in Syracuse, New York, on July 29, 2003, when he was two years old. The diagnostic team, a school psychologist and an occupational therapist, noted that "the family would like help with [Child 3]. They feel his development is not 'typical.'" They also noted that "[Child 3] is a beautiful blond-haired little boy who came to his assessment dressed in neat, clean, age appropriate clothes. . . ." This was to be reiterated later in their report: "[Child 3] is a beautiful little boy who has the benefit of a devoted family."

In New York he was diagnosed with multiple developmental delays, a disorder of sensory regulation, and motor delays. His use of joint attention—drawing the attention of others to something he considered to be of mutual interest— meant that in the assessors' opinion he did not merit a diagnosis of PDD. One of the most significant aspects of this evaluation is that it took place two weeks after Child 2 had been started on a gluten- and casein-free diet. The assessors commented:

> Two weeks ago they started him on a gluten and casein-free diet and they have seen remarkable changes for the better. They were pleased to report that he was able to participate for as much and as long as he did during this assessment, and report that he would not have been able to do as much as he did two weeks ago before starting the diet.

In the light of medical concerns—diarrhea up to twelve times per day and raised lead level—he was seen at the same center one month later, on September 3, 2003, by Dr. John Friedman. Dr. Friedman's observations are instructive.[4] He noted that Child 3 had suffered longstanding diarrhea, but that since the institution of the gluten- and casein-free diet over six weeks previously, Child 3's stooling pattern had improved. Later on in his report, Dr. Friedman offered his own observations on the parent's choice of diet for modifying aberrant behaviors, " . . . I mentioned that anecdotally, elimination diets may be helpful, but specific allergy testing [likely a reference to testing for IgE allergy in 2003] may not be diagnostic." In an addendum to his report, Dr. Friedman noted that the parents wished to pursue both an allergy consultation and heavy metal testing.

The salient points of this initial series of assessments are that Child 3 had major developmental issues, he was medically unwell, and both his behavior and his GI issues had responded symptomatically to a gluten- and casein-free diet. As will become relevant to matters arising later in allegations from agents of CPS, the parents are described as "devoted" and they took no issue whatsoever with the developmental diagnosis that their child was given at that time.

Pursuing the possibility of lead toxicity had led the family to the office of Dr. Schneider at her autism treatment clinic in Phoenix on April 19, 2004. The mother and Child 3 attended this appointment with the child's maternal grandfather. Dr. Schneider's record described the reason for this clinical consultation to be Child 3's "developmental delays and associated medical concerns."

This was an accurate representation of Child 3's prior assessment in New York and no other behavioral diagnoses—autism included—were claimed for this boy by the parents. Dr. Schneider went on to document Child 3's chronic diarrhea and hospitalization on three occasions for asthma. She noted that his bowel symptoms had improved dramatically on the gluten- and casein-free diet. She also noted that temporary fasting during an episode in the hospital with pneumonia led to him becoming more alert and focused. At the Royal Free Hospital in London, we had noticed and reported the exact same clinical improvements with fasting ASD children during bowel preparation prior to colonoscopy.[5] This kind of novel, idiosyncratic symptom, reported by independent sources, goes a long, long way in my book in mitigating any claim of the parents feigning illness in their children.

In a detailed history of Child 3's problems, Dr. Schneider recorded significant impairments in language, social skills, and a range of activities and interests. She noted that even though he was comforted by the presence of his mother or grandfather, his interaction with them did not include any shared expressions of joy or pleasure, referencing for reassurance or approval, or showing objects of interest. In addition, he was not observed to point or follow a point. In the light of these features, she concluded that "[Child 3's] presentation is consistent with autistic disorder."[6]

Child 3's lack of joint attention was a crucial discriminating factor between the diagnosis of multiple developmental delays in New York and Dr. Schneider's view in Arizona that he had an autistic disorder. Here one becomes aware of how symptomatic presentation on a given day may substantially influence the diagnostic label. She determined that, in order to achieve meaningful progress, Child 3 required a much higher level of intervention than the weekly speech and occupational therapy and the one hour per week of individual tutoring that had been prescribed in New York. She also considered that further medical testing was required and ordered a Sage Complement Antigen Test for food allergy (see Part 1, Chapter 3). She later communicated Child 3's results[7] on this test to his parents so that they might act on them appropriately.

On April 29, 2004, in Syracuse, New York, at a follow-up visit at the Margaret L. Williams Developmental Evaluation Center, Child 3 was reviewed by a different team of assessors. He had now been on an apparently beneficial exclusion diet for approximately nine months. Notably, referencing the parents, the assessment team reported, "[Child 3] demonstrated attachment to both parents. [The mother] was in the evaluation room for most of the evaluation process. She calmly supported her son and redirected him, as appropriate. [Child 3] was obviously attached to both of his parents who appear dedicated to his well-being."

The assessors' conclusion, at least in part because Child 3 exhibited joint attention on this occasion, concurred with that of the earlier assessment at the same New York center, i.e., "global developmental delay" and not an ASD. In an addendum to the report, Dr. Friedman of the assessment team noted the parents' concern about a possible ASD diagnosis and the inadequate level of services but did not mention their previous consultation with Dr. Schneider. He noted, "They did not agree with our impressions and recommendations."

Dr. Friedman appeared to have made no effort to contact Dr. Schneider to discuss the basis for their different diagnoses for and consequent treatment of Child 3. New York, where the family was still living at this stage, was not prepared to invest in an increased level of services for this child.

The Sage test came back positive for food allergy. Three months later, following a phone consultation with the mother on July 17, 2004, Dr. Schneider recorded Child 3's continued progress after all allergenic foods identified in this test had been excluded from Child 3's diet. She wrote, "His language has increased to utterances of up to 5 words in length, he is making spontaneous comments, and he is noticing things in his environment as never before. His concentration is better and he does not become frustrated as easily as in the past." It should be noted that the results of randomized controlled clinical trials of gluten- and casein-free diet[8] validate such clinical experiences. His stools were still loose but had reduced from 8–10 per day down to 3–4 per day. Dr. Schneider also recommended nutritional supplementation and the exclusion of soy from his diet.

As further validation of the mother's original concerns, his red blood cell lead level was very high.[9] The option of chelation following correction of his mineral imbalances was considered by Dr. Schneider. Mother also reported that Child 3 had been diagnosed with very brittle teeth with virtually no enamel. Many children with ASD suffer with gastroesophageal reflux (GERD) whereby stomach acid erodes their teeth, necessitating multiple fillings and extractions, yet another reason for prompt and proper treatment of GI disorders in this group of patients.

In light of his seizure symptoms, Child 3 also underwent electroencephalography (electrical recordings of brain wave patterns) on November 18, 2004, at age three. The report read, "Abnormal recording due to pronounced run of independent focal spike discharges originating in the occipital area.[10] Left more than right. In addition, the background was mildly diffusely slow and disorganized. Suggestive of seizure disorder originating in the occipital area, left greater than right, and also mild diffuse bilateral cerebral dysfunction." The report was signed by a Dr. Hector Santana. One *further* concern of the parents' for their son had been entirely justified.

Following the family's move to Arizona, Child 3 was evaluated by Dr. Rice on August 2, 2006, who, having characteristically described her evaluation as being based upon "neurodevelopmental history, physical and neurological examination, and developmental assessment," diagnosed Child 3 with " . . . autism with language and motor regression, hypotonia, and sensory integration [problems]."

She also noted his toxic environmental exposure with high lead levels, and she made recommendations for speech and occupational therapy and educational intervention.

Child 3 was seen again by Dr. Schneider on February 26, 2007. By this stage he was passing 1–2 normal stools per day and had gained weight and developed some muscle mass. Academically, he was attending full-day kindergarten with an aide and was progressing very well. Thus it seemed from the perspectives of the parents, Dr. Schneider, and Dr. Rice, Child 3 was making demonstrable progress. Further, objective evidence of improvement was a normal brain recording (EEG) performed at the request of Dr. Kara Lewis, a neurologist from the local St. Joseph's Hospital. It is quite possible that this improvement may have been as a direct consequence of his gluten-free diet since gluten can provoke seizures,[11] and it may be that disappearance of the epileptic focus in his brain, seen on an earlier EEG, was a result of his restriction diet.

The ever-diligent Dr. Schneider identified in Child 3 another clue to possible vulnerability to environmental toxins in the form of a genetic deficiency in a certain enzyme called methylenetetrahydrofolate reductase (MTHFR), which made it difficult for him to use vitamin B12 and folic acid. This deficiency limits the ability of the body to efficiently detoxify and deal with the metabolic consequences of infection and inflammation. By her methodical approach, Dr. Schneider was able to modify his treatment further to compensate for this deficiency.

Child 3 was also followed by Dr. Kara Lewis, the pediatric neurologist at PCH, because of his continuing seizures and the emergence of tics. Records of these consultations were not available at the time of writing.

Child 3 was seen again by Dr. Rice on April 24, 2010, due to parental concerns about his profound learning difficulties and his highly variable behavior. By this stage, the parents had decided to homeschool all of their children because Child 3 and his siblings were not getting the help they needed, apparently due to budgetary restrictions on special education services in Yavapai County public schools. During this consultation, Dr. Rice conducted a further neurodevelopmental assessment involving, as before, a neurological examination, testing of gross and fine motor skills, language and problem-solving skills, and observations of social and other behavioral patterns. She described Child 3 as having a past history of a Landau-Kleffner variant. Landau-Kleffner syndrome (LKS) is an autism-like disorder associated with epilepsy and abnormal electrical recordings of the brain (EEG).[12] LKS variant is a term that has been coined for children with autistic regression with an epileptic pattern on their EEG.[13] On this occasion, she concluded her assessment, not with a diagnosis of autism, but with the diagnosis of severe visual/spatial learning disability and auditory/visual learning disability. Clearly, his clinical presentation had changed. She made treatment recommendations including further expert referral.

Child 3's developmental trajectory can be summarized at this stage as falling into three broad phases: the first, normal development to around eighteen months of age; the second, regressive encephalopathy, or brain disorder, causing cognitive, developmental, sensory, and motor dysfunctions associated with focal brain injury and associated GI distress. This phase was presaged by a documented adverse reaction to immunization. Biomedical interventions during the second phase appear to have heralded a third developmental phase associated with progressive, incremental recovery.

The distinction between his first diagnostic assessment of global developmental delay in New York and subsequent diagnoses of ASD by Dr. Schneider and Dr. Rice in Arizona appear to have rested, at least in part, on the symptom of his lack of shared attention. Child 3's recovery was, in my opinion, largely a function of interventions initiated by his parents, Dr. Schneider, and Dr. Hellmers (see Part 3, Chapter 4).[14] His recovery is documented by Dr. Schneider and is evident in the sequential assessments of Dr. Rice. These record the more recent loss of his autism diagnosis, a finding that is consistent with the assessment of Dr. Blitz-Wetterland on behalf of CPS (see below).

It is said that if you ask ten lawyers for an opinion, you will get ten different opinions. It should not surprise anyone familiar with childhood developmental disorders that, similarly, different views are regularly expressed by different professionals. These views for Child 3 will have been impacted inevitably by treatment, maturation, and factors as mundane as whether he is having a good or a bad day. The respective professional perception of his condition and the recommended treatment inevitably influenced the parents, who wanted only the best—that is, the most intensive—services, for their child. They relied upon the opinions of professionals. This is not illness falsification by any stretch of the imagination. But later in this sorry tale, that is exactly how this discordance between professional opinions was to be construed.

From the GI perspective, Child 3 was initially investigated for symptoms of gastroesophageal reflux on November 15, 2004, when he was three, at Crouse Hospital in Syracuse, New York. He had a series of X-rays taken after drinking a radio-opaque contrast medium so that the passage of this medium could be monitored as it passed from his esophagus into his stomach and beyond. The official report, which confirmed his doctor's clinical suspicion, read, "Mild-to-moderate-intermittent gastroesophogeal reflux disease."

Child 3 was later seen in Phoenix by Dr. Ursea on December 26, 2007, at age six, for evaluation of weight loss and diarrhea. As noted above, she documented that developmental regression and explosive diarrhea started at eighteen months of age and that his parents had associated these events with his eighteen-month immunizations. His behaviors included manifestations of GI distress referred to in Part 1, Chapter 1, such as screaming, self-injury, and biting and scratching of others. He suffered diarrhea for eighteen months, three times per day, with runny, malodorous stool containing undigested food. His stool was positive for blood and fecal eosinophil protein, a marker of immune activation in the intestinal lining. Finally, as described above, testing for non-IgE-mediated food allergy had revealed an intolerance of multiple foods.

In a detailed letter to Dr. Sipes, the children's primary care physician, that was written prior to Dr. Ursea's investigation of Child 3's GI symptoms, she wrote:

> I appreciated the opportunity to participate in the care of this lovely family. It does seem that there is a psychological component to some of his symptoms as he tends to do much better when he is at home and being fed at home. I advised the family that they should probably keep that as a stable variable at this point until we know more about the possibility of presence of organic reason for his symptoms.

Notably, this history of improvement at home is at odds with MSBP for which, according to Dr. Sanders, children characteristically improve when removed from the abusive parent(s). On the other hand, compliance with diet, and therefore any associated benefit, is more likely in a home environment.

Dr. Ursea's speculation about a psychological component to his GI symptoms was premature and later dispelled—as she had predicted—by the findings on upper and lower GI endoscopy, undertaken on January 30, 2008. Histopathology confirmed GERD and eosinophilic inflammation of the small intestine and entire colon. Analysis of his duodenal biopsy for digestive enzyme activity revealed a severe deficiency of disaccharidases, consistent with the histologic diagnosis of eosinophilic gastroenteritis. Dr. Ursea recommended a referral to Dr. Rose, an allergist, on the basis that his intestinal disease was a clear manifestation of an allergic response to foods. She stressed in her report that the only way to control Child 3's disorder was "dietary restrictions that exclude foods that trigger an allergic response."

In her extensive correspondence about Child 3 with Dr. Sipes, Dr. Ursea referred to his food allergies on a number of occasions, drawing attention to the fact that significant behavioral problems accompanied dietary infractions. She also documented the fact that his symptoms of reflux were improved on Nexium (a drug that blocks the production of stomach acid) and that IVIG[15] had contributed to reversing his failure to thrive and reduced his acute infectious illnesses.

So it was that the sentinel child in this stoic but unfortunate family—the first child to have received an ASD diagnosis, complicated early in its course by epilepsy; a child with clear evidence of systemic pathology in the form of a food-allergic gastroenteritis, GERD, and possible lead poisoning; and a child whose problems appear to have been triggered by immunizations—had arrived at this diagnostic determination following multiple expert assessments. Crucially, these assessments involved not only the parents' narrative but also direct, objective examination and testing of Child 3.

Treatment had led to clinical improvement; a combination of Nexium for his reflux, an exclusion diet for his allergic gastroenteritis, IVIG for his immunodeficiency, and nutritional supplements for his general well-being, had led to significant improvement in symptoms. One example of this was weight gain while on an exclusion diet, a clear indication that the diagnosis of food intolerance resulting in failure to thrive was in fact correct.

However, a very different complexion was put on Child 3's circumstances once he had been taken from his parents and placed in foster care. Apparently at the request of a CPS-appointed general pediatrician, Dr. Jacobsen from PCH, an assessment was undertaken in the Department of Neurology on August 31, 2010, by Dr. Blitz-Wetterland, a developmental pediatrician. In her report,

Dr. Blitz-Wetterland reviewed Child 3's history. Like so much of what was to follow in this case, the factual omissions, the unwillingness to consider alternative explanations, and a raw bias permeate her report. As an opening example, notable— even extraordinary—by its omission was any mention of the fact that Child 3 had been professionally diagnosed with an ASD on several occasions in the past.

Of particular concern is that in an interview with the foster mother, Dr. Blitz-Wetterland was apparently informed that "[Child 3] was tested for food and environmental allergies and that he was negative for any allergies."

The basis for this statement is false and potentially dangerous [See Part 1, Chapter 3]. It seems that not only had Child 3's Nexium been stopped, since his foster mother reported that "he was taking no medications," but also that his exclusion diet had been abandoned for a "normal diet," thereby exposing him to potentially harmful food allergens. There is reference to the fact that "he had mild diarrhea after a visit with parents on Saturday, but it did not persist." It is difficult not to infer a pejorative—even accusatory—tone here in light of the general tenor of Dr Blitz-Wetterland's report.

A formal evaluation was performed on Child 3 using the Childhood Autism Rating Scale (CARS), a diagnostic instrument on which he did not score in the range for autism. Instead, he was determined by Dr. Blitz-Wetterland to have learning difficulties, a significant articulation disorder, and a coordination disorder with delayed fine and gross motor skills. This diagnosis accorded with that of Dr. Rice. At several points in her report, she drew attention to the fact that Child 3 appeared "overly friendly." She followed this with a reference to her "vast experience in treating children in foster care due to abuse and/or neglect," adding, "It is common to see children from those types of situations who are either overly friendly or significantly withdrawn."

Dr. Blitz-Wetterland allowed herself considerable latitude in the symptomatic presentation of abuse and neglect. In contrast, nowhere did she describe his previous ASD diagnoses or draw attention to the fact that, for example, articulation/ coordination disorders and a history of EEG-confirmed seizures are hard neurological features of an organic neurological condition and not some hallmark of parental psychopathology.

The issue of affection in children with autistic regression is dealt with in my book *Callous Disregard: Autism and Vaccines: The Truth behind a Tragedy.*[16] The historical view of the child with autism is that of an aloof loner who shuns physical and emotional engagement. This may be the case when autism results from an injury in utero when there has been no opportunity for normal emotional interactions to shape an infant's development. However, in those children like Child 3, who regress into autism after a period of normal or near-normal development, the reciprocal benefits of mother-baby and other interactions become established during that early period of normality. Thereafter, in spite of the child's ensuing developmental challenges, affection may remain, albeit that, in the setting of strangers, it may not be regulated in a normal way. But Dr. Blitz-Wetterland, with her "vast experience," saw it somewhat differently. Her prejudice becomes manifestly obvious when reviewing her recommendations for Child 3's continuing care. She wrote:

> **I am concerned about the multiple weekly visits with the parents.** The children currently have 4 supervised visits per week with the parents. Per [foster mother's] report, between visits, school, and homework, the children have very little time to just relax and play. None of the children have had the opportunity to learn how to ride a bike. **I would like CPS to consider reducing the number of visits to a longer visit on the weekend and one visit during the school week.**[17]

No case had ever been proven; no case had ever been so much as reasonably articulated, and yet for this family the thumbscrews were to be turned a little tighter. Finally Dr. Blitz-Wetterland stated, " . . . **I am concerned that all of the children have some atypical behaviors that are commonly seen in children who have lived in neglectful or inappropriate parenting environments.**"[18] But Dr. Blitz-Wetterland had only assessed Child 3. How in the world was she able to pull this diagnosis on children numbers 1, 2, 4, and 5 out of thin air? Not even her "vast experience" permitted this considerable and totally inappropriate leap of faith, having only assessed one of the children.

There was to be one further professional report on the Arizona 5, an analysis undertaken by Dr. Sharon McDonough-Means, a developmental pediatrician instructed by the parents' lawyers in October 2010.

Seeking from the outset to confine her assessment to the objective findings, in order to eliminate any question of parental bias or deception, Dr. McDonough-Means wrote, "The objective findings . . . were the historical material used [and] NOT the reported history which most often came from one or both parents."

After reviewing Child 3's history she wrote, "Final impressions: Autistic Disorder, very likely based on early *objective* history. **Positive response to interventions and treatments with significant improvement in general behavioral functioning. . . .**"

She continued, "The evaluator during the 4 & 8/2010 evaluations questioned or refuted the diagnosis of Autistic Disorder. This is compatible with the **positive therapeutic response expected from the biomedical, educational and**

therapeutic treatments, i.e. improvement in all regulatory control skills . . . and in social interaction."[19]

In other words, Child 3's apparent loss of his autism diagnosis over time could reasonably be attributed to his positive symptomatic response to therapy: therapy such as diet and supplementation with which his parents had so diligently complied. His progress from autism to developmental delay could be attributed to biomedical intervention, not just as a matter of opinion, but in line with the peer-reviewed published medical science[20] that was available at that time to anyone who cared to read it.

Chapter 10

CHILD 4

Child 4 is a boy born on December 12, 2002, in Syracuse, New York. His developmental problems were first identified by Dr. Schneider at the family visit on April 19, 2004. She assessed him again at the age of two years and eight months on August 2, 2005, after testing for lead toxicity. She recorded that his parents had first become concerned about their third son's development after a high fever in response to his two-month vaccines, after which he became more difficult to engage. Dr. Schneider wrote, "He never cooed or babbled and did not speak his first true word until 18 months of age. Most language is now echolalia."

There was also a history of delayed motor milestones: Child 4 did not sit independently until thirteen months of age, never crawled, and did not walk until eighteen months. He had been assessed in New York by a speech therapist who diagnosed him with delays for which he received speech therapy. At thirty months, his receptive and expressive languages were delayed at a level of eighteen months and eighteen to twenty-four months respectively. When seen by Dr. Schneider at thirty-two months, she noted that his gait was immature. As with his siblings, his balance and coordination were poor and he had delayed fine and gross motor skills. In addition, she noted that he had no functional language, poor eye contact, echolalia, and blank staring spells.

Child 4 was evaluated by Dr. Rice on August 6, 2006, at forty-two months, to determine his need for remedial services. As with the other children, Dr. Rice's evaluation was based upon "neurodevelopmental history, physical and neurological examination, and developmental assessment." Dr. Rice noted that he had hand flapping, repetitive behaviors and poor regulatory control of mood, emotions, and behavior. He was apparently preoccupied with wheels and was bothered by changes in routine.

Her diagnoses for Child 4 were consistent with those of other family members and included autism, hypotonia, and toxic exposure associated with high lead levels. Dr. Rice reviewed Child 4 two years later when she confirmed her earlier diagnoses of autism and hyotonia, this time with valgus deformity (outward angulation) of the ankles.[1] Child 4 was also assessed by Dr. Gregory, the child psychiatrist, who apparently confirmed the diagnosis of autistic disorder.[2]

Finally, Dr. McDonough-Means, the developmental pediatrician, reviewed Child 4's records, focusing on the objective developmental and behavioral assessments for the purpose of providing an expert opinion to the family court. She too, concluded that he had an autistic disorder.

From the GI perspective, he had never tolerated dairy products, which produced loose, foul-smelling stools and excessive gas. Elimination diet and probiotics had produced some symptomatic improvement. Dr. Schneider noted Child 4 to be thin and pale, with poor muscle tone and very poor eye contact. She witnessed and documented his echolalia and the fact that he did not appear to have any functional language. A blood test performed on this occasion indicated poor function of his mitochondria, the batteries of the body's cells. Urine testing, as with his siblings, showed a provoked[3] lead level in the very high range,[4] for which he underwent chelation therapy to bind and remove the lead from his tissues.

He was seen by Dr. Ursea on August 1, 2008, when he was five for a GI assessment. Between the ages of ten months and two years, he suffered vomiting, bloating, and diarrhea associated with poor weight gain. At two, he was started on a gluten- and casein-free diet, whereupon his weight gain improved and his diarrhea and bloating stopped. His vomiting remained a problem, however, recurring on a cyclical basis, with three–four nights of vomiting every three–four months. Physical examination revealed no obvious abnormality. However, his stool tested positive for blood.

Upper GI endoscopy performed on March 19, 2009, showed friable, erythematous (reddened) mucosa in the stomach and duodenum. Microscopic analysis of his biopsies revealed mild esophagitis extending over at least nine centimeters of his lower esophagus, eosinophilic gastritis, and mild duodenitis. He underwent a sigmoidoscopy and biopsy on the same occasion, the results of which were normal. Gastric emptying studies on April 21, 2009, and April 23, 2009, identified multiple episodes of GERD and a persistent hiatus hernia. He was treated with Nexium. On January 26, 2010, Dr. Uresa notes that his GI symptoms had resolved, and the Nexium was stopped.

Chapter 11

CHILD 5

Child 5 is a boy who was born on August 23, 2004, in Syracuse, New York. Having passed his initial developmental screening, his parents reported that he underwent language regression and loss of eye contact at around nine to ten months. He was seen by a speech therapist who requested that he get fully evaluated. He was subsequently referred for assessment at the Northern Arizona University Institute for Human Development for developmental concerns. He was seen on July 14, 2005, age nine months, for developmental assessment, including observation of play and movement, and review of his medical records. He was described as having "moderate delays in the acquisition of gross motor skills and of cognitive skills in specific areas of attention and memory. He is also demonstrating significant delays in the area of self-concept and social roles and his expressive communication."

He was seen by Dr. Tim Jordan, a developmental pediatrician, on February 21, 2006, at eighteen months. Using a range of observational tests including at least part of the Autism Diagnostic Observation Schedule (ADOS), Dr. Jordan diagnosed him with having either PDD-NOS or an expressive language disorder.

He was seen by Dr. Saunder Bernes, a pediatric neurologist at PCH on March 15, 2006, who described him as "having some behaviors that certainly would suggest a pervasive developmental syndrome and possibly childhood autism."

Following his initial encounter with Dr. Schneider in May 2006, a lead level performed on a first-morning urine sample (unprovoked by chelation challenge) was elevated.[1] He was then evaluated further on June 21, 2006, by Dr. Mary McLellan, a psychologist with the Arizona Early Intervention Program. She conducted psychometric testing, including the Caregiver Interview, Bayley Scales of Infant Development, the Cognitive, Socioemotional and Adaptive Behavior Scale, and the Autism Diagnostic Observational Schedule (ADOS). She reported that according to his ADOS score " . . . his ability to communicate and relate to others shows indications similar to other children who have been diagnosed on the autistic spectrum."

Despite evident developmental problems, at this time she did not think that a diagnosis of autism was appropriate although she considered him to be a significant risk for developing this condition. As with his siblings, he also underwent a review by Dr. Rice on July 25, 2006. Once again, at the risk of my appearing pedantic, her assessment was based upon "neurodevelopmental history, physical and neurological examination, and developmental assessment." Her diagnoses in Child 5 included autism, hypotonia, and elevated lead levels.

He returned for a full evaluation with Dr. Schneider on September 8, 2006. She confirmed the history of developmental regression at around eleven months, consisting of loss of receptive language, the use of gestures, and social withdrawal. Delayed motor development, including poor coordination and poor gross and fine motor skills were also noted. On examination he was pale and thin, with marked periorbital edema (swelling around the eyes caused by fluid in the tissues). His gait was immature and his eye contact was poor. As is typical of such children with developmental disorder and GI distress, his abdomen was distended, and his weight (sixty-fifth percentile) for height (ninetieth percentile) was low.

Following the institution of a strict exclusion diet and nutritional supplementation, by the time he was reviewed by Dr. Schneider nine months later on July 27, 2007, he had made obvious cognitive gains and put on weight.

At age five, Child 5 was assessed by Dr. Gregory, who noted his blunted affect and the fact that he looked quietly at the same car for thirty minutes during his assessment. She noted possible articulation difficulties and hypotonia. Her diagnosis was of autistic disorder.

Finally, Dr. McDonagh-Means rendered her expert opinion to the family court that included "Hypotonia; early, generalized developmental delay with communication more delayed than motor. Autistic Disorder with all of the underlying specific developmental skill delays. Regression at 10 months may have occurred; unable to objectively document that."

From the GI perspective, Child 5 was seen by Dr. Ursea on December 29, 2008, at the age of four months, with a history of hoarse voice and halitosis. He suffered from recurrent respiratory symptoms and choking when drinking fluids and was thought by Dr. Ursea to have GERD. He also suffered occasional abdominal pains, nausea, and constipation but was otherwise physically well. Unlike his siblings, he did not have a diagnosis of functional antibody deficiency and consequently did not receive IVIG. In light of the fact that he was unvaccinated, his tetanus and S. Pneumoniae antibodies would have been irrelevant. Dr. Ursea treated his tentative diagnosis of reflux with Nexium and his symptoms of GERD settled.

In summary, this family consists of five children with developmental disorders, who have all, at some stage (and for some, on several occasions), been diagnosed by a qualified professional(s) as being on the autistic continuum.

It will be recalled that it was largely Dr. Schneider's clinical acumen that identified developmental problems in Child 3's siblings. The other children had not been brought to Dr. Schneider because the parents were seeking a diagnosis of autism; they were not even aware of the possibility of an ASD diagnosis at that stage. Recognition of this fact is vital in any objective deconstruction of the case made against the parents. Readers will recall that in the case of Child 1, in the ER of PCH on February 24, 2009, the attending physician Dr. Weiss had proffered the seemingly random speculation that: "Reportedly all 4 sibs have autism and father was an autism specialist in NY[2]—quite a coincidence!?" followed by "?? M by P."[3]

Rendering that dangerously factitious speculation unsustainable is Dr. Schneider's observations on the developmental problems in the four previously undiagnosed children. It was she—not the parents craving medical attention by proxy—who first brought attention to their possible autistic disorder that was subsequently confirmed by Dr. Rice and others.

All of the children have GI issues, including gastroesophageal reflux disease, that have, except in the case of Child 5, been formally diagnosed as inflammatory in nature by clinical and laboratory testing by qualified medical experts. Children numbers 1, 3, and 4 have more extensive GI pathology in addition to their reflux disease. In the case of Child 5, a pediatric gastroenterologist made a provisional diagnosis of reflux based upon symptoms and treated the patient accordingly, leading to symptom resolution. A medical expert in pediatric immunology diagnosed children 1–4 as suffering from a functional antibody deficiency and treated this with IVIG, something to which another pediatrician—not an immunologist—took exception. This immunological conundrum—central to the plot—is dealt with below.

PART IV

Chapter 12

BUILDING A CASE: INTRODUCTION

I am stuck for a collective noun, one that captures the congruence of motive, the unity of purpose and mutual encouragement, and the guiding beliefs—the ethos—that characterize the community of women who now join with Dr. Jodi Carter—the informant—center stage. These include Dr. Susan Stephens, MD, medical director of the Comprehensive Medical and Dental Program of the Arizona Department of Economic Security (ADES), Ms. Heather Williams of CPS, also part of ADES, and Dr. Mary Sanders, a psychologist from northern California and prosecution expert on MSBP. At the risk of causing offense, I will refer to them as the Sorority, not because they have anything in common with Gamma Phi Beta and its derivative university societies but because I cannot erase from my mind's eye the image of Shakespeare's three weird sisters.

Were these sisters simply blessed with a supernatural wisdom that foretold, act by act, Macbeth's royal ascent, his troubles, and ultimately his death at the hand of one who was not "of woman born?" Or were they essential—catalytic—to the story; did they foment in Macbeth's latent ambition and his wife's rabid sense of social entitlement, a tragedy that, had they never appeared through the filthy air, would have been avoided—end of story? Aware of the dangers of pursuing too far Macbeth as an allegory for the Arizona 5, I will leave it there and to you, the reader, to form your own opinion of who did what and why. . . . Who made this story?

BUILDING A CASE

Dr. Stephens testified that this family had fooled over 30 doctors in two different states . . . She also talks about the family having fooled the Division of Developmental Disabilities, various state and federal agencies, and two separate advocacy groups.

Jennifer Kupiszewski, attorney for the father.
November 1, 2010.[1]

On March 20, 2010, the sky did not fall, but it certainly slipped. The evening prior, Child 2 and her mother were on the road north, making the three-hour journey home from Phoenix Children's Hospital (PCH), when they were rear-ended. The impact gave Child 2 a sharp reminder of her shoulder injury, hurt her low back, and left her feeling miserable for the rest of the journey home. Unbeknown to the family, four days earlier, on March 16, Dr. Jodi Carter had referred the case of Child 2 to the social work department, and the previous day Heather Williams of CPS had expressed her intention of "building a case" against the parents for possible abuse.

On that day, March 20, 2010, two CPS workers knocked, unannounced, at the family's front door. Shocked and completely unprepared for this intrusion, the parents agreed to meet with them on the front porch, where they presented their children to CPS officials so that they could see for themselves that the children were all well. One CPS official, Heather Williams, questioned Child 2 about her shoulder and her experience in the emergency room at PCH. The mother later explained to me that this was when Child 2 confirmed that she had not actually been examined by Dr. Carter while in the ER, despite Dr. Carter's record to the contrary. At one stage the parents, justifiably fearing the motive behind CPS's visit and their questions, indicated that they wanted to call an attorney. Apparently, they were told by Ms. Williams that they were being uncooperative, and the option of simply calling the police and having the children removed was suggested as a way of discouraging the parents. In the event, no attorney was called.

In a later e-mail exchange with Dr. Carter and others, Ms. Williams wrote, "When I initially went to the home the parents would not let me see the kids."[2] According to the parents' narrative—a detailed account of the children's interactions with Ms. Williams—this statement is completely untrue. Clearly, both versions cannot be correct.

In response to CPS's questions about the extent and variety of the children's diagnoses, the parents responded that they had documentary proof of these medical conditions from doctors. According to the mother, Ms. Williams stated that if they could provide proof of this, then the matter could be closed. The mother promptly went indoors, photocopied the relevant medical documents, and handed them to Ms. Williams. But closing the case was not her intention.

On April 9, CPS officials came again. The children were not present, but the parents had arranged for various witnesses to be there either in person or on a conference call. These witnesses included Teri Holloway, who had accompanied mother and daughter (Child 2) to PCH during their encounter with Dr. Carter. It was during this second meeting with CPS that Teri Holloway confirmed Child 2's description of events in the ER and the fact that Dr. Carter had not examined this child's shoulder at any stage. Unhappy with the presence of witnesses and the absence of the children, Heather Williams apparently described them as " . . . the hardest parents she had ever had to work with."

Sometime between late April and early June, the mother received a call from an unspecified "agency." The caller said that she had been asked to contact the family to see what they needed. The mother asked what service they provided, only to be asked the question, "What service is it that you need?"

This exchange went back and forth for several minutes ending up with neither the mother nor the caller being any the wiser. Apparently, the agency had been asked to make contact by social services, but beyond that no one knew quite why or what for. No service had been requested by the family and none had been specifically offered. The mother recalled that, on the basis of this conversation, she was later accused by CPS of refusing services. The provenance and the purpose of the call remain a mystery.

The parents and Ms. Williams arranged that the children would be interviewed on May 7 at West Yavapai Guidance Center. Although this was agreed to by both parties, CPS was later to claim that its officials had been refused access to the children; the mother denies this, and certainly the Yavapai interviews took place. In the presence of a witness, there, once again, at the behest of the parents, Child 3 asked Ms. Williams if she was there to take them—the children—away. Ms. Williams denied this, replying, "No one is going to take you away."

On June 15, the sky came crashing down. The family was just back from a trip and the mother was unpacking. The father and children were leaving the house to go fishing, getting them out from under their mother's feet. The parents remember Child 4 running back through the front door shouting, "Daddy, there's men with guns and badges."

In a few breathless moments it was all over. Two armed deputies and at least three CPS employees had removed all five children, bewildered and distraught, and taken them into protective custody.

During the raid, the mother recalls desperately trying to give instructions to CPS workers on the children's dietary needs and which children should be placed together in foster care in an effort to reduce their trauma, while frantically trying to pack their favorite toys. And all this in the face of an assault team whose only interest seemed to be getting the children out the door and away as fast as possible.

The parents do not know where their children stayed that night. In fact, they were not allowed to see their children at all for two weeks. The children were later housed in Phoenix, where the parents would travel three hours by car and three back for a two-hour visit three times per week. They were later moved closer to the family home, but the strict limit on visitation rights remained.

Behind the scenes, there was considerable activity, and small mountains of paperwork were generated. Much of this paperwork was not made available to the parents and their lawyers until the week before the hearing. Therefore, their ability to defend themselves against the allegations was constrained accordingly.

Here, I will consider in detail several key documents provided by the prosecution—reports from CPS, doctors, and psychologists—culminating with the prosecution's expert psychologist, Dr. Mary Sanders, that led to charges and the court hearing.

The relevant documentary evidence starts with a string of e-mails exchanged among the Sorority: Ms. Williams, Dr. Carter, and Dr. Stephens. The first knot in this string was titled "[Family Name] Summary" and was sent from Ms. Williams on March 23, 2010. She started by assuming ownership of the problem: "I have a family [name] that lives in the middle of Ash Fork where there are no neighbors that claim to have 5 autistic children."[3]

While the reference to having no neighbors is odd, it is nonetheless an allegation that would return to haunt the family later. Ms. Williams continued, "They have the documentation to support autism in all 5 children. The first problem is that all of the children are also diagnosed with mitochondrial disorder, functional antibody deficiency, asthma, GERD [gastroesophageal reflux disease], hypotonia [low muscle tone], and MTHFR [methylenetetrahydrofolate reductase] deficiency. The second problem is that some of the providers do not feel that the children have autism or that the parents are giving symptoms of things that are not really happening."[4]

Ms. William's referred to Dr. Carter's interactions with Child 1 and Child 2, the latter's concern for factitious disorder by proxy, and quoted Dr. Carter as having admitted, somewhat tortuously, " . . . these parents have never been caught in the act of doing anything to the children [but] they continue to elaborate the symptoms of things that they can find no medical explanation for."[5]

Ms. Williams then quoted Dr. Sipes, the children's primary care physician, as reporting how "very aggressive," "hostile," and "pushy" the parents were and that they " . . . will not listen to the direction of the doctor, [and] they will basically tell her what they need when they come in and won't leave until they get it."[6]

As we have already seen, a review of Dr. Sipes' medical records on the family over an extended period reveals no evidence in support of this allegation, nor has Dr. Sipes ever provided testimony or documentary evidence to this effect, with one exception. Child 2 received a low back injury in the car accident on March 19. When the parents called Dr. Sipes (the child's longtime doctor) in some distress asking for her help with this injury, she declined to give it, apparently on the basis that insurance reimbursement on such injuries is not paid out until the patient no longer requires treatment, thereby incurring significant delays in payment. On the one hand, Dr. Sipes had a professional obligation to provide care for Child 2, but on the other, she did not wish to do so. The parents had called Dr. Sipes, as the mother put it, "Advocating on behalf of their daughter with a doctor we had been with for a long time."

Dr. Sipes declined her request; her unofficial reason was, apparently, the issue of insurance reimbursement. But in order to dismiss the family from her practice, this reason was neither valid nor defensible. The parents subsequently received a letter from Dr. Sipes stating that they had been " . . . rude and disrespectful."

Apparently this was a valid reason for their dismissal. Another general practitioner, Dr. Polstein, said that she would certainly take a look at Child 2's back, which, following her examination, she described to the father as being "beat up."

Returning to Ms. William's record of her conversation with Dr. Carter, in characterizing the latter's description of Child 1, she wrote, "He had [Henoch Schönlein Purpura] which is an autoimmune condition that was self-limiting [sic]."

As a matter of fact, Child 1's HSP had been anything but self-limiting, having required powerful and highly toxic immunosuppressive treatment, including high-dose corticosteroids and methotrexate, to bring it under control. After falsely representing the significance and severity of this HSP diagnosis, Ms. Williams continued, "The thing that got [Dr. Carter's] attention is autism and other 1000 rare diagnosis [sic] that are attached to this child."[7]

In a gratuitous aside, and in marked contrast with her dismissal of HSP, Ms. Williams had greatly exaggerated Child 1's diagnostic status out of all proportion to any parental claims. With reference to Child 1's HSP, Ms. Williams— once again, summarizing her conversation with Dr. Carter—stated, "He [Child 1] needed to be there at that time but he kept coming back."[8]

I am compelled to interpret the fact that "he kept coming back" as having been intended to imply the parents' craving unnecessary medical attention. It will be recalled that the second occasion that Child 1 was admitted to PCH was on December 14, 2008, on the instructions of a local ER doctor because of severe abdominal pain and dehydration. He was started on steroids for his joint pain, an integral part of HSP's symptom complex, and both the rheumatologist, Dr. Shishov, and the gastroenterologist, Dr. Ursea, agreed "that his symptoms are 100% due to severe HSP." However, Child 1's joint pains were also turned in to something sinister as Ms. Williams continued by stating that according to Dr. Carter, "Dad had done some reading on [HSP] and came back with vague conditions such as joint pains."

What an extraordinarily low opinion Dr. Carter must have had of her colleagues in the Rheumatology Department at PCH who continued to follow and treat Child 1 on the basis of the arthritis associated with his severe inflammatory disease for many months all, apparently, because "dad had done some reading" and come up with a new complaint as a consequence.

Notwithstanding the fact that the father had "fired her" in February 2009, the majority of Dr. Carter's complaints against the family centered upon the diagnosis and treatment of functional antibody deficiency.

Ms. Williams moved on to Child 2: " . . . they showed up with [Child 2] with a bogus arm thing which is nothing by the way."[9]

Later in the same e-mail, Ms. Williams noted that an MRI of Child 2's shoulder, when read by a radiologist, had shown inflammation. She went on to state that, in most cases " . . . ice, IBU [probably ibuprofen], and stretching should cure."[10]

In fact, a simple perusal of the hospital record of Child 2's admission with the shoulder injury would have also identified the detailed note of the physical therapist, Alison Perkins, made on March 19, 2010: "Area 1. Pocket of swelling over the [right] AC joint that was notably boggy. Area 2. Multiple muscle spasms noted along the medial border of the right scapula and into the right trapezius."

These clinical findings plus inflammation on MRI and the treatment regimen that Ms. Williams quotes as being curative are incompatible with a "bogus arm thing." Ms. Williams continued, "Mom said that the child was diagnosed [with autism] in Tucson but the year she was [sic] stated she was living in New York."

Implicit in Ms. Williams' tortured grammatical conjunction is that mother was lying. In fact, Child 2 was diagnosed with an autistic disorder in Tucson by Dr. Rice on August 8, 2006. The year the mother stated that Child 2 had received her initial autism diagnosis, she was not, as Ms. Williams wrongly asserted, living in New York, but in Arizona.

In the penultimate knot in this e-mail string, Dr. Susan Stephens of ADES provided some challenging melodrama, accusing the father of " . . . forcing ER doctors to put IVs into his children despite the doctors totally disagreeing with this, demanding skin biopsies, and reporting too many infections to count on each child which are not supported by the primary care physician."[11]

The problem is that few if any of these instances were referenced in any way that allows them to be identified in the children's medical records. Yet Ms. Williams concluded, "I think there is plenty of evidence that this family has factitious disorder by proxy (Munchenhausen [sic] by Proxy), however the complicating factor is that they have engaged multiple doctors in crazy therapies with them!"

In breathing new life into the dark legacy of psychiatrist Leo Kanner's "refrigerator mother"[12] and Bruno Bettleheim's[13] infanticidal psychopath, the blame for this scam—the deception of successive guileless physicians—lay fully on the shoulders of the parents: "This has all been based upon what the parents reports [sic], re: symptoms or what other doctors have allegedly stated or recommended."[14]

I have been unable to identify where, other than in the records of Dr. Carter, reports of symptoms and doctors' recommendations have differed from the clinical records. Dr. Stephens formalized her own allegations in two reports. In the first, written on June 10, 2010, she described it as her role " . . . to assist CPS in the assessment of complex cases of alleged abuse and/or neglect."[15]

She had been asked to review the medical records of the five children because of "Concerns raised by Dr. Jodi Carter, a staff pediatrician from Phoenix Children's Hospital (PCH) who has cared for these children on multiple inpatient hospitalizations."

In fact, Dr. Carter had seen only two of the children in this context: Child 1 on two occasions, and Child 2 on a single occasion. Dr. Stephens went on to document the records of the various doctors she had relied upon. She claimed, "I was told that these five children all have autism, the same metabolic disorder, and functional antibody disorder. There were concerns raised about the types of treatments, supplements, and diet these children were receiving because of their autism. What I found when I reviewed the records surprised me."[16]

What surprised *me* is the extent to which what Dr. Stephens was told and what she wrote do not accord with the documentary record—but more of that later. It appears to be the case, however, that the concerns that had been brought to her attention were, at least at this stage, confined to "crazy treatments" given specifically because of the children's autism, including supplements and diet. But as she ventured further into the records, things took upon a far more sinister complexion. She continued, "Based upon my review of the medical records, the **parents report conflicting information**[17] to every pediatric healthcare provider they see."[18]

She went on to list some of the multitude of issues that concerned her including, "previous diagnoses, immunization history, medical treatments, home therapies, in-home interventions, which pets, if any, the family had in the home, what the medical issues were for each child, what the previous consultant said or recommended, and results of laboratory tests."[19] Her list of concerns, notable for lack of any specific examples, was not, she indicated, exhaustive.

She continued, "The parents report many signs and symptoms of illness for each child that appear undetectable to the medical specialists. There are **MANY VERY CONCERNING** aspects of these cases and most of the medical interventions, treatments, and work-ups center around what the parents are reporting and not what the pediatric specialists are finding."

Having reviewed the children's medical records, I can find little to support Dr. Stephen's myriad, grave, and wide-ranging allegations. There is no question that the parents' reports of behavioral symptoms reflected real developmental disorders in their children. Their reports of GI symptoms lead to the identification of bona fide GI pathology. So what precisely were these illnesses that were "undetectable to medical specialists"; where are these illusory ills to be found?

The problem with Dr. Stephens' report to this point is that, despite her litany of claims and allegations, she cites not one specific incident by reference to the relevant medical records. Despite having described the cases' "many very concerning aspects," she provided no reference to an actual event. Her report, which continued in this vein, described a conference call—effectively a turning point in the case—that took place on June 9, 2010, among Drs. Carter, Weiss, Sipes, Rice, and Lewis. The stated purpose of the call was " . . . to share observations and concerns about the children and parents, the medical issues, which diagnoses are real (documented) vs. factitious, and to trace the source of the diagnostic testing and previous diagnoses that these children have been previously labeled with. . . ."[20]

These were diagnoses, including MTHFR deficiency, mitochondrial disorder, functional antibody deficiency, asthma, and gastroesophageal reflux, that had, according to Dr. Stephens, "been dispelled when the facts were shared by these doctors."

Dr. Stephens appeared to draw a line between those diagnoses that were real by virtue of having been documented, presumably by the diagnosing physicians, and those that were factitious, presumably because they had not been diagnosed and documented but instead had been contrived by the parents.

During the actual dependency hearing in Family Court, Dr. Stephens was asked to explain the purpose of the June 9 conference call in more detail. She replied, "I was trying to do what I call primary source investigation. I was trying to get to the original diagnosis."[21]

In her further response, Dr. Stephens was unable to provide a coherent explanation for why Dr. Hellmers, Dr. Schneider, and Dr. Ursea had been excluded from this conference. Given that these specialist medical practitioners were the primary sources for the documented diagnoses of MTHFR deficiency, functional antibody deficiency, asthma, and gastroesophageal reflux (as well as lead toxicity, food allergy, and ASD), they should, for Dr. Stephens' purposes, have been on the call.

As for asthma, this had been diagnosed and documented specifically in children numbers 2 and 3 in New York, prior to the family's move to Arizona, and in Child 4 by Dr. Hellmers in 2010. More recently, all three children had been under the care of Dr. Hellmers for their asthma.

Gastroesophageal reflux disease (GERD) had been diagnosed and documented by Dr. Ursea by endoscopy and histology in Child 2 (June 18, 2009), Child 3 (January 21, 2008), and Child 4 (March 19, 2009). Based upon their symptoms and Dr. Ursea's and Dr. Ede's clinical observations, Child 1 and Child 5 were diagnosed with and treated for GERD by Dr. Ursea on October 14, 2009 and December 29, 2008, respectively.

In her report of May 10, 2010, Dr. Stephens went on to describe the views of those who had participated in the teleconference. First up, MTHFR deficiency and mitochondrial disorder were considered under a single heading by Dr. Lewis.

MTHFR (previously defined in this chapter as methylenetetrahydrofolate reductase) is an enzyme that in humans is encoded by the MTHFR gene. MTHFR catalyzes the production of active folic acid which then operates in what is called the methylation cycle to reduce levels of the potentially toxic amino acid homocysteine. Genetic variation in this gene may lead to the production of less active forms of MTHFR and inefficient synthesis of the active form of folic acid. MTHFR gene mutations are associated with an increased risk of miscarriage, congenital neurological defects, heart disease, and some cancers.

Dr. Lewis, the pediatric neurologist, described briefly what the MTHFR enzyme does, just how common genetic mutations are in the Caucasian population, and how MTHFR deficiency should not be considered a dramatic metabolic disorder but a common and treatable disorder. In fact, the treatment of this condition is nutritional supplementation with the active forms of folic acid and vitamin B12.

It is not certain what relevance this exposition had to the matter at hand or in affirming the parents as abusers. No one had ever suggested that it was a dramatic metabolic disorder, certainly not in anything I have read. Most reassuring, however, was Dr. Lewis' observation that MTHFR disorders are treatable. One must ask, therefore, whether it was abusive of the parents to treat a perceived MTHFR deficiency in their children. Genetic testing of Child 3 had found him to have this defect. The parents were told by Dr. Schneider that their other children were likely to have the same issue. It was not unreasonable, therefore, for them to have reported this when relating their children's respective histories. However, they acknowledged on several occasional that, for other than Child 3, no formal diagnosis of MTHFR deficiency had been made.

Mitochondrial disorders in autism, first investigated in an ill-fated cohort of twelve children reported in the *Lancet* in 1998,[22] refers to a malfunction in the batteries, the energy reserves, of the body's cells (see Part 1, Chapter 2). It is here that oxygen and sugar get turned into useful energy. Malfunction of mitochondria is characterized by oxidative stress, an abnormal metabolic state that was documented in four of the five children.[23] Despite this, the mother had clarified to Dr. Carter that mitochondrial disorder had never been proven in her children.[24]

Later, in court, both Dr. Jacobsen and Dr. Stephens were to confuse MTHFR defects and mitochondrial disorders. Dr. Jacobsen was to claim, "MTHFR deficiency which is actually a mitochondrial disorder that is present in 30% of the population . . . It is not of any major significance at all."[25]

Dr. Stephens claimed wrongly that mitochondrial disorders are very, very rare,[26] followed closely by the claim that they affect 30% of the population, so common in fact that they are " . . . a normal variant and not something that you would treat."[27]

When asked whether he thought that any of the children had this disorder, Dr. Jacobsen replied, "No, other than the very benign type that I mentioned."[28]

I take that as a "yes."

The next item of concern was the alleged functional antibody deficiency. In her earlier claims, Dr. Stephens wrote of being told that all five children had this disorder. If this was the case, she was misled, but not by the parents. Child 5 did not receive this diagnosis from Dr. Hellmers or from anyone else and, accordingly, was not treated with IVIG. This would have been easy for Dr. Stephens to check before making her allegations.

The likely source of this disinformation was Dr. Carter herself, who had documented in Child 2's admission summary of March 16, 2010, "All sibs have autism, MTHFR deficiency, functional antibody deficiency."[29]

Moreover, and a point that I have belabored previously, it was Dr. Hellmers who diagnosed the children with this disorder based upon laboratory testing. How Dr. Hellmers did that testing and whether the children did or did not have this immune disorder is not the point. The parents were explicitly told by a medical expert that their first four children did have a functional antibody deficiency and that it was on this basis that they were being treated. These diagnoses were documented and were, according to Dr. Stephens' criteria, therefore real.

It would have been factitious for the parents to have denied this diagnosis in their children after explicitly receiving it from Dr. Hellmers.

Dr. Carter waded in on the possible side effects of IVIG, its cost, its limited supply, and the fact that while some studies have shown benefit in treating autistic symptoms, IVIG " . . . is NOT considered part of the standard of care and is not FDA approved for use in the treatment of autism."[30]

These facts are entirely irrelevant given that IVIG was not being given to treat autism but rather to treat a functional antibody deficiency. With respect to their autism, Dr. Stephens stated, "It was doubtful that any of the children even currently met the diagnostic criteria for autism."[31]

From her confusion of tenses, it is not clear whether she meant that Dr. Rice and others had got the diagnoses of autism wrong in the past or whether, if tested currently, the children would not meet the criteria for autism. I take it from the use of the word "currently" that she means at the time of writing her report. The difference is crucial since one is contrary to the historical documentary evidence whereas the latter is consistent with Child 3's documented clinical improvement in response to biomedical and behavioral treatments. Either way, except in the case of Child 3, who was reevaluated in early 2010 (see below), Dr. Stephens' position amounts to little more than conjecture.

Dr. Stephens concluded with the opinion of the above medical professionals that:

- These children have histories of unexplained illnesses, resulting in too-numerous-to-count doctor visits, hospitalizations and invasive medical procedures.
- The children in this family have illnesses that extend beyond the normally expected frequency or degree of seriousness.
- It appeared on many occasions that the parents may have exaggerated or induced illness in the child.
- The children have had unnecessary laboratories/tests/invasive procedures done because of reported symptoms from parents that appear to have been fabricated or greatly exaggerated.

These are extremely serious allegations. This analysis moved the goalposts from the original concerns of Dr. Weiss (the coincidence of multiple siblings with autism and the father an autism specialist) and Dr. Carter (diagnosis and treatment of immunodeficiency) to the proposition that not only had the parents deliberately induced illness in their children but they had done so on many occasions.

It is singularly difficult to deal with allegations that are so nonspecific in that they were not linked back to actual cited events. For example, which of the children's illnesses were unexplained and which of those unexplained illnesses would lead to "too-numerous-to-count doctor visits, hospitalizations and invasive medical procedures"? Let me deal first with the specific clinical presentations that brought these children to the attention of Drs. Weiss and Carter at PCH and thereby, into the hands of CPS. These clinical encounters involved Child 1 and Child 2.

First, in the case of Child 1 and his illness of December 2008, HSP was an "unexplained"[32] but real and serious condition. Over the course of his protracted illness, he required numerous (although countable) doctors' visits and medical procedures, some of them potentially life-saving. Despite his obvious illness, Dr. Carter and others appeared to have insinuated falsification, having alleged that no healthcare professional had witnessed the blood in Child 1's stool. This allegation must be offset against the repeated positive testing of his stool for blood and his gastric and duodenal ulceration that could certainly have produced melena (black, altered blood in stool) and bloody vomiting, entirely in accordance with the parents' story.

More to the point, Dr. Carter's version of events is not consistent with Dr. Weiss's clinical record of February 24, 2009, that documented "Chronic black tarry stools (that always test + for blood)."[33] As set out in Part 3, Chapter 2, the clear implication was that these abnormal stools had been specifically recovered for testing and were consistently positive for blood.

Arguably, if Child 1 had received more appropriate medical care and been managed in the hospital during the initial phases of his HSP rather than discharged prematurely only to require readmission a short time later, the passage of blood just might have been evident to other doctors as well. His illness was protracted and, by its nature, of a fluctuating course, itself influenced by the treatment he received. Any part of this could have been anticipated from clinical experience with HSP. There is no evidence, none whatsoever, that the parents exaggerated or *induced* this illness in their child. Finally, Dr. Stephens does not provide a single substantive instance whereby laboratories/tests/invasive procedures were performed on Child 1 because of fabricated or greatly exaggerated symptoms reported by the parents.

In the case of Child 2, it was a shoulder injury that caused her presentation to Dr. Carter. She was in pain and, notwithstanding the fact that perception of and response to pain in children with an ASD may be altered in comparison with neurotypical children,[34] adequate pain relief was what the parents sought for their child. Instead, using Child 2's shoulder injury as a pretext, in my opinion, the parents were set up by Dr. Carter in an elaborate sting operation (see Part 3, Chapter 3). Beyond this, Dr. Stephens' summary falls by the wayside.

Exaggeration of illness is part of the elusive syndrome of MSBP; but where does the guilt lie in this case? Observe, for example, Dr. Stephens' exaggeration of the history of illness in these children. This falsification appears to have been contagious. Having started with Ms. Williams' claim of "1000 rare diagnosis [*sic*]"[35] attached to Child 1, falsification infected her colleagues. For her part, Dr. Stephens starts in with the claim that Dr. Carter had cared for these children on multiple occasions. One can only infer that "these children" refers to all five siblings that she had referred to earlier in the same sentence. As a matter of fact, and as stated above, Dr. Carter had only seen two of the children during inpatient hospitalizations: Child 1 on two occasions and Child 2 on one occasion.

Second, her review of the medical records had led her to the position, stated in paragraph four of her report, that the parents had reported conflicting information to *every* pediatric healthcare provider they saw.

Third, she talks of a "multitude of issues," the "many signs and symptoms of illness for each child that appear undetectable to the medical specialists," and the "**Many very concerning**[36] aspects."

Fourth is her conclusion that the children have had " . . . too-numerous-to-count doctor visits, hospitalizations and invasive medical procedures."

Fifth, and far and away most seriously in my opinion, she refers to the "many occasions" on which the parents may have induced illness in the child, that is, deliberately caused their children harm.

Finally (at least for the report under consideration), and with an irony that is reserved for the righteous she referred to symptoms in the children that the parents had "greatly exaggerated."

Dr. Stephens' facility with exaggeration carried over to her testimony when she claimed that Child 1 had had "multiple colonoscopies" for "alleged bleeding."[37] In her book, these colonoscopies were an example of abuse, presumably indicting Dr. Ursea by proxy.[38] Countering Dr. Stephen's fictional tale, Dr. Krigsman, pediatric gastroenterologist and expert witness, was able to confirm that Child 1 had undergone only one colonoscopy and that it had been essential for diagnosing the source of his pain and intestinal bleeding.[39]

Dr. Stephens was, of course, entitled to her opinion; however, in a matter of this importance, that opinion should have been supported by the documented facts: facts that are not vulnerable to being disturbed or frankly refuted on any reasonable and objective reading of the evidence. Dr. Stephens' report, littered with hyperbole, error, and speculation—and lacking any specifics—was highly vulnerable.

On October 7, 2010, Dr. Stephens produced a second report, ostensibly on the basis of concerns raised not just by Dr. Carter, but also by a second doctor, presumably Dr. Weiss, who had seen Child 1 in the ER at PCH in 2008. After the referral of the case of Child 1 to social services at that time, beyond an internal review, it was apparently not considered worthy of investigation. For some reason, presumably Dr. Carter's latest allegation, it surfaced once more.

In this second report, Dr. Stephens described herself as having a " . . . great deal of expertise in the screening and identification of children with autism spectrum disorders,"[40] having worked at an autism center for almost seven years. Her review of the records led her to the opening conclusion that " . . . it did not appear that any of the children actually had a diagnosis of autism."[41]

She then listed—and this is the first time these are presented in any formal articulation—the reasons why the children were taken into foster care. They read, "**Suspected Factitious Disorder by Proxy** (formally called Münchausen Disorder by Proxy), **Suspected child abuse** in that the children were being subject to potentially harmful therapies to treat their supposed autism that they may not actually have. This included use of **chelation therapy** and monthly **intravenous infusions** of IVIG . . . a **human blood product**."[42]

Dr. Stephens went on to describe some of the serious side effects of these treatments. She identified the fact that chelation therapy is used to remove heavy metals from the body, citing lead, arsenic, and mercury specifically. In an effort to highlight the dangers of chelation, she drew attention, in bold type, to the fact that in August 2005 a five-year-old boy with autism had died from chelation while receiving this therapy intravenously in a physician's office in Pennsylvania. In this, as in other matters, she was wrong. In fact, there had been a prescribing error, and this child had received the wrong drug,[43] resulting in fatal depletion of his blood calcium and cardiac arrest. The fact that a drug error and not chelation therapy had caused this child's death was later confirmed by Dr. Mary Jean Brown, chief of the Lead Poisoning Prevention Branch of the Atlanta-based Centers for Disease Control and Prevention (CDC).[44]

On the following page, Dr. Stephens started into her findings, based upon assessments by various pediatric specialists. But before doing so, she delivered her verdict: "This is a case of Factitious Disorder by Proxy."

In her mind there was no room for doubt: why should there have been? She had been affirmed in her belief by the report of psychologist and expert witness for the prosecution Dr. Mary Sanders (see below). Dr. Stephens seemed to scream from the page: "This is a case of child abuse . . . These children have been subject to unnecessary procedures, tests, therapies, and evaluations. As stated above, many of the 'therapies' that the parents have pursued have significant potential associated risks. In addition, the children have been placed on restrictive diets for their 'autism,' have not been fully immunized (protected) and have not been allowed to socialize with age-appropriate peers or regularly attend school and prove academic success."[45]

In building a case against the parents, two further elements had been introduced to bolster the allegations of systematic abuse of these children: lack of immunization and social deprivation. While the matter of social deprivation is dealt with below, immunization deserves a chapter of its very own.

Under her next heading—emboldened and underlined—Dr. Stephens wrote, **"None of the children have autism."**[46]

She continued with a summary of a consultation, apparently with a CPS-appointed general pediatrician, Dr. Jacobsen, who had assessed the children two weeks previously, while they were in foster care and off their restricted diets. More will be said of this later, but for now it is sufficient to characterize the tone and balance of Dr. Stephens' report, factors that are evident, for example, in her review of Dr. Jacobsen's consult with three of the boys. He said, " . . . the three boys came in two weeks ago and everything was great. **They seemed much happier, well adjusted, and conversational. They all feel that the liberalization of both their diet and their hygiene regimens** (to be bathing more regularly) **was going very well."**[47]

In such cases, this statement amounts to an informal reference to the "separation test," a situation where the child improves in the absence of the abusive parent. The problem here is that Dr. Stephens provides no denominator, no qualification of her baseline, that is, from what point in time the boys had "seemed much happier." This could not have been a comparison with their status at home with their parents, prior to separation, since Dr. Jacobsen had not seen them at this stage. It must have been a comparison with their initial well-being in foster care when they were likely to have been their most disturbed. Nonetheless, the reader could easily be misled into thinking that they were now better off, being away from home, abuse, and deprivation.

Similarly, were they bathing more regularly than they had done at home (no mention of concerns about this had ever been raised before) or, alternatively, since their initial separation? Dr. Stephens' omissions—her failure to provide context for her claims of improvement in the boys—leaves only the insinuation that they were better off without their delinquent parents.

Later, in court, Dr. Mart picked up on this same issue in the face of repeated efforts by the prosecuting counsel to portray, to successive witnesses, the children as being in robust physical and mental health since separation from their parents,[48] their "recovery" having coincided with their removal. Specifically the prosecution suggested that, as evidence of parental fabrication " . . . the children becoming asymptomatic coinciding with removal from the parents' home is unlikely if not impossible."[49]

But where was their evidence of this coincidence, and more to the point, where was the support for the claim that they were fine or even better off in foster care? Dr. Mart was particularly critical of the absence of any baseline evaluations of the children by CPS prior to their removal as well as by the absence of any formal follow-up in all but the case of Child 3. How did anyone know they were better? All the court had heard was the word of those involved in prosecuting the case.

Dr. Krigsman also took exception to the prosecution's presumption of improvement coincident with separation, based upon what he perceived to be an inadequate clinical assessment by Dr. Jacobsen, the children's CPS-appointed pediatrician.[50]

The absence of objective baseline and follow-up data and the fact that, in reality, the children got progressively (rather than coincidentally) better because of the parents rather than in spite of them rendered the prosecution's baseless proposition nonsensical. CPS's failure to obtain baseline and follow-up data on the children, at home and in foster care respectively, was irresponsible, a failing compounded by their later baseless claims in court.

Returning once again to the report of Dr. Stephens, she commented next on the views of Dr. Rice, the developmental pediatrician who had seen and assessed all five children at the request of their primary care physician, Dr. Sipes. Dr. Rice's position on her developmental diagnoses in these children is central to the family's current predicament. Her apparent about face from her documented clinical assessments of these children to the meeting of professionals on June 9, 2010, as reported by Dr. Stephens, may ultimately be remembered as one of the greatest professional betrayals in this sorry and sordid affair.

In her second report on October 7, 2010, Dr. Stephens described Dr. Rice as " . . . a developmental and behavioral pediatrician considered to be an expert in the field of autism."[51] She continued, "Parents report to all providers that she allegedly made the diagnosis of autism in each of the children, except [Child 3]."[52]

As a matter of fact, Dr. Rice *did* make these diagnoses. In contrast with Dr. Stephens' assertion above, Dr. Rice first made and documented a diagnosis of autism in Child 3 on August 2, 2006. It appears that Dr. Rice sought to mitigate responsibility for her diagnoses after concerns over possible MSBP had coalesced into Dr. Stephens' frank allegations. For the purpose of her report, Dr. Stephens abstracted elements of a letter from Dr. Rice written on August 31, 2010, where she is alleged to have written, "During evaluations with the children, the primary information was provided by the parents. **Parents related that they both had an**

expertise in autism and that they described behavioral characteristics of severely impaired social interaction and odd repetitive behaviors. Parents described significant difficulties with eye contact (social skill), inability to interact with peers (social skill) and severe behavior issues that they related prompted them to homeschool the children."[53]

No problem so far, except to say that conflating the narratives of all five children, when some symptoms in each child were qualitatively and quantitatively different, was misleading. It is also worth clarifying that what had prompted the parents to homeschool was the lack of special educational facilities in Yavapai County's school system.

The second paragraph, abstracted from Dr. Rice's letter, takes on a subtly more pejorative character: "Evaluations with the [children] were challenging. Parents frequently interjected and were reluctant to have the children seen without their presence. This is a frequent concern for many parents because often parents are worried that their child will be either traumatized by being left or that something untoward might happen without their presence. Therefore I did not push to see the children without the parents. **During the evaluations parents would frequently interject for the children, so it was difficult to communicate with each child.** Several times parents described severe tantrums as children were coming to the clinic because of the change in routine or new place and although I did not see the tantrums myself, I did not feel I could discount their stories."[54]

There is nothing unusual, as Dr. Rice herself confirms, in parents wishing to accompany their children during visits to her office—quite the opposite. Although Dr. Stephens' report finds no mention in Dr. Rice's medical records, Dr. Stephens clearly seemed to feel that the parents' alleged tendency to interject on behalf of their children was significant since the bolded words are hers. This dynamic is relatively common in family consultations, particularly where children are reluctant or limited in their ability to communicate. Moreover, Dr. Rice appears never to have asked to see any of the children alone. So far, Dr. Rice had provided no grounds for concern whatsoever. Dr. Stephens then provided Dr. Rice's summary.

1. The diagnosis of autism is heavily dependent on parental history. **If the history is inaccurate, the diagnosis will also be inaccurate.**
2. As children develop, diagnoses become more clear over time. **Evaluations performed now would be more accurate than evaluations performed when the children were younger.**
3. **When I last saw [Child 3] in April of this year, I did not think he had characteristics of autism.** I spoke with the family briefly about this, but they wanted to discuss his learning issues rather than other diagnoses.[55]

The first two summary points, while entirely general in nature, are problematic. If the developmental/behavioral history is inaccurate, the diagnosis *may* be inaccurate. The diagnosis of a developmental disorder requires expert assessment of the child through observation and testing. If the results of this process are inconsistent with the parents' narrative, then the diagnosis may be in question.

At the beginning of each assessment (and my reason for belaboring this point), Dr. Rice had been very clear about the clinical parameters that guided her diagnostic process and documented this as "neurodevelopmental history, physical and neurological examination, and developmental assessment . . ."

In each case, Dr. Rice's conclusions as to her diagnosis are unambiguous and unqualified by concerns as to the parental history, inconsistencies between history and developmental assessment, lack of clarity due to the children's ages, or parental interjection. In fact, Dr. Rice diagnosed Children 2, 4, and 5 with autism and Child 1 with Asperger's syndrome at a range of ages from twenty-three months to nine years and four months. At that material time, she did not express any reservations about diagnosing these children, whatever their ages. She performed diagnostic assessments on Child 4 at the age of three years and seven months and again when he was five years and seven months of age. Her diagnosis of autism did not change with time.[56]

It is important to appreciate that, beyond fulfilling the criterion for starting before the age of three years, the diagnosis of autism is based upon the presentation of the child at that time: it is a diagnosis in the moment. For Child 3, Dr. Rice's diagnosis of autism was made when he was five years old. When she reassessed him at eight years and nine months, she diagnosed him not with autism but with severe visual/spatial learning disability and auditory/visual learning disability. She did not revise her previous diagnosis made "in the moment" over three years earlier, but reported on Child 3's current developmental status at that time. This later diagnostic status could reflect a number of factors including the beneficial effect of treatment that he had experienced. Child 1's diagnosis was *also* different at different ages, although on this occasion it was a reflection of his deterioration. He went from a diagnosis of Asperger's syndrome, a high-functioning ASD, to a much lower level of functioning following regression at around eleven years of age, befitting his provisional diagnosis of childhood disintegrative disorder/autism, made later by Dr. Gayle Gregory. Finally, nowhere in the records is there any mention of difficulties in assessing the children due to the presence of the parents or their interjections.

Dr. Rice's ASD diagnoses were key factors that, as they stood, undermined the case that CPS was building to the effect that these children never had autism. They were not diagnoses made by a rank amateur. Dr. Stephens herself had described Dr. Rice as an expert in the field of autism.

In court, Dr. McDonough-Means, a developmental pediatrician with thirty years' experience with autism was asked whether, in doing an evaluation for autism, she relied primarily on the parental report. She replied, "Absolutely not."[57]

Dr. Krigsman went further in his testimony. When asked what his opinion would be if Dr. Rice had made her autism diagnoses based solely on parental report, he responded, " . . . if, in fact, a physician gave a diagnosis of autism based solely on historical and parental reporting and because of that diagnosis entitles the child to tens of thousands of dollars and hundreds of thousands of dollars in services, that would be medical fraud."[58]

If Dr. Rice misdiagnosed these children, that is her responsibility; are all of her ASD diagnoses before and after the Arizona 5 similarly in doubt? Is she risking medical fraud by continuing to practice as she does? I doubt it. Dr. Rice's assessments appear to have been systematic and careful. She is an experienced professional and should not have depended, as she appeared to want her colleagues to believe, on the history provided by the parents but rather, as she herself stated repeatedly, on a "structured examination and assessment of each child." And nowhere in Dr. Stephens' report does she quote Dr. Rice as alleging that the parents gave an inaccurate history. But that was to change.

While Dr. Rice was not called upon to testify, she was alleged by Dr. Sanders or Dr. Stephens—prosecuting counsel was uncertain on this point—to have indicated that " . . . she no longer agreed with the diagnosis [of autism that she had made]"[59] and " . . . she did not believe any of the children had autism."[60]

In referring to Dr. Rice's alleged comments on the conference call of June 9, 2010, Dr. Stephens was diverging by the second from those contained in her report. Under oath, she was adamant that Dr. Rice had never given any of the children a diagnosis of autism[61] and that, in fact, "Dr. Rice made it very clear that she had not made the diagnosis of autism in any children."[62]

In later cross-examination she was pressed on this point by Tanya Imming, the mother's attorney: "But there were doctors who diagnosed the children and told the parents that their children had these diagnoses, correct?"[63]

To which she responded, " . . . no one told the parents the children had autism."

Dr. Stephens had started to unravel. She was headed down a road that no one, certainly not Dr. Rice,[64] had traveled before. There seemed to be only one way, and that was forward, headlong. She continued, "All the rest of the alleged diagnoses that Dr. Rice made were totally unfounded. She did not diagnose any of the children with autism. When you look carefully at her notes, she's very specifically clear about that."[65]

Dr. Stephens' claims appear to operate in a parallel universe to that of the case before us. I am unable to find where in the records Dr. Rice said any of these things. In contrast, I am able to find her clear and unambiguous diagnoses in the children. The only record of what she actually said to Dr. Stephens at that time was captured in the latter note above. It bears no resemblance to Dr. Stephens' claims on the witness stand. And why Dr. Stephens had not troubled to examine the independent autism diagnoses of Dr. Schneider and Dr. Gregory is yet another mystery.

Doctors—not patients—are responsible for their diagnoses. To seek to absolve oneself of this responsibility in the heat of the moment would be reprehensible. But with blood in the water and the Sorority[66] circling, it appears, according to Dr. Stephens at least, that this is exactly what Dr. Rice was attempting. Despite her central role in this case, she was not called upon to explain herself in court.

You may be wondering why Dr. Rice herself was not called upon to testify. A major dilemma for lawyers, both prosecuting and defending, is a hostile witness, one that does more harm than good to your case. In the case of Dr. Rice, both legal teams had likely assessed her alleged flip-flop professional opinion and decided not to call her on the basis that she could turn ugly.

So, had the parents sought a developmental diagnosis as part of a process of fabrication? Not according to the facts: Child 3 was healthy and developing normally until eighteen months of age. There was evidently no fabrication to this point. After an unusual series of vaccine exposures, untested in combination for safety, he exhibited a pattern of developmental regression and GI symptoms that are now tragically monotonous to many physicians who care for the medical needs of children with ASD. He was initially diagnosed with global developmental delay by an expert multidisciplinary team. His presentation some time later was consistent with an ASD according to two doctors, including Dr. Rice. He received intensive biomedical treatment under the care of doctors from different medical disciplines, and he improved. On reevaluation by Dr. Rice and Dr. Blitz-Wetterland, he still had problems but did not meet the criteria for autism. In other words, his clinical status had changed while he was on intensive biomedical and behavioral therapy. Dr. McDonough-Means captures this distinct possibility of cause-and-effect in her report on Child 3 of October 2010 when she stated that Child 3's loss of diagnosis " . . . is compatible with the positive therapeutic response expected from the biomedical, educational and therapeutic treatments."[67]

For their remaining children, the parents were not in the business of seeking out a developmental diagnosis at all. The likelihood that they were also affected came from the clinical observations of Dr. Schneider, and these observations were later confirmed by Dr. Rice and others. It's really as simple as that.

In court, Dr. Stephens testified on a number of other important issues where her opinion was also at odds with the facts. Asked whether children could grow out of a functional antibody disorder, she said, "No."[68]

In fact, children *can* outgrow a functional antibody disorder: the natural history of this disorder is that the *majority* of patients will normalize their antibody responses to bacterial polysaccharides by age five to six years, whereas only in a minority the defect may be permanent.[69]

She was to claim that IVIG therapy is " . . . a very risky procedure to perform"[70] that "did not help children with autism in any way."[71]

This statement is not reflected in the medical literature, as pointed out to the court by Dr. James Adams of Arizona State University.[72]

With respect to chelation for lead toxicity, a common finding in the Arizona 5, Dr. Stephens pronounced that at around a blood lead level of sixty micrograms per deciliter, the person starts having neurological problems.[73] In fact, neurological impairment is seen in children at levels below ten micrograms per deciliter.[74]

As evidence of parental falsification, she implied that the father had made up the claim that Child 1 was treated with methotrexate for his HSP.[75] "I reviewed his inpatient records and he absolutely did not receive that medication."[76]

In fact, he did receive that medication following its prescription by Dr. Ede, the PCH rheumatologist.[77]

She dismissed IVIG,[78] chelation,[79] and diet[80] as disproven or unproven and potentially dangerous treatments for autism. This is not the case, and while the findings are a matter of scientific debate, their status bears little resemblance to Dr. Stephens' claims. Use of diet, in particular, she characterized as "victimization."[81] "There is no research that supports its use . . . and unfortunately families of children with autism are easily victimized by a lot of people selling a lot of hopes and dreams . . . there is no medical reason for the children to be on it."[82] Part 1, Chapter 3, and a review of the children's medical records puts the lie to these claims.

Early in her testimony she disclosed her back-to-front strategy for the children, that is, first remove them from their abusive parents " . . . and then try to sort out what are the real medical issues."[83]

She later summarized what were, in her considered opinion, the real medical issues, " . . . the children don't have **any**[84] diagnoses and didn't need **any**[85] treatment . . . "[86]

Perhaps due to lack of the defense team's preparation time, the self-evident travesty of her testimony, or even the altitude of central Arizona—who knows—Dr. Stephens was let off very lightly in cross-examination. Quite why is something of a mystery since it allowed far more credence to her testimony than was deserved and permitted her behavior to continue. Reinforced further in this behavior by Judge Brutinel's finding against the parents, one anticipates that more such cases will be brought against parents of children with ASD by the Arizona Department of Economic Security, aided by Dr. Stephens. Somewhat paradoxically, she agreed that recovery from autism was possible.[87]

SOCIAL DEPRIVATION

In common with millions of other past and present citizens of the United States, the family lived in a rural setting. Strangely, Ms. Williams in her e-mail of May 23, 2010, seemed to feel it was significant that they had no neighbors. A vision of *Deliverance*, the sinister view of America's backcountry in James Dickey's 1972 screenplay, came to mind. Not only were they physically isolated, but, according to Ms. Williams, Dr. Stephens was of the opinion that ". . . [the children] have not been allowed to socialize with age-appropriate peers. . . ."

Dr. Stephens' allegation is best dealt with in the mother's words: "My children have never been kept isolated from others. Trisha [name] was our respite provider, and her children, [name] (12) and [name] (10), are close friends of my children. [Child 2] considers [name] her best friend. [Child 1] and [Child 2] spent overnights there, not for respite, but as friends. All of the children spent a decent amount of time there for respite, and Trisha has neighbor children that would come over and play with our children."

> [Child 1] has participated in Young Marines. That ended a few years ago when the group moved further away; it had been 45 minutes away and moved another half hour away. They met on a school night so the extra distance became problematic for homework and sleep. [Child 1] has played on a soccer team in the past, and participated in track and field and softball. He was on a swim team (the pool closed due to monetary problems). [Child 1] has been in youth groups in church. He participated in Awana, an international youth program, in the past. He has done other activities as well.
>
> In the 12 months before CPS stole him, [Child 1] attended dance camp near Tyler, TX (June 2009). In fact, all of the children participated. [Child 5] was too young, but he was able to hang out with [Child 4] and [Child 3] as those two needed extra support in the program. In September, he began attending school in Chico, California. We were staying on a base there, and all of the other students in the school were on base. The base has an Olympic-sized

swimming pool, hiking trails, basketball courts, etc. [Child 1] spent most of his free time with other kids, some his age, some older, some younger.

Then, in mid-November, we went to Fiji. [Child 1's] second night there he attended a youth group with Uate (he is our "adopted" son, he calls us Mum and Dad). We lived Fijian, so we were in the middle of Fijian people all of the time. [Child 1] spent time with other teens, and we were there with another family (they have three boys).

We came back to the States on Jan 12, spent a few days in Chico where he reconnected with his friends there, and then our family went on a bit of an explore. We traveled to Oregon, then down the Oregon and California coasts, coming home by way of Nevada (visited family). Then, home and we began to homeschool. [Child 1] went to church with us and we were hooking him up with the youth group there. In February, we spent a week in Mexico at an orphanage. [Child 1] spent time with the teen boys. They enjoyed marbles. (All of the children were there; [Child 2] preferred spending time with the younger children; it has been her dream for many years to work in an orphanage).

When we came home, life was tough for a little while because [Child 2] had hurt her shoulder in Mexico and she was in pain. We continued to home-school and attend church, the kids spent time at Trisha's. Then, two weeks later, CPS entered our lives (horribly, on March 20, [Child 1's] 13th birthday and ruined what should have been a big day for him). April and May we did family activities, he saw friends, went to church, but we concentrated a lot on school. We were trying to fit in a lot of school those months because the rest of our year would be very busy. Forgot to add for [Child 1] that he went to sum-mer camp two summers.

For this past year's plan, we were supposed to leave on June 17 to take [Child 1] to Texas for an SST, a camp of sorts that included time near Tyler, then a week in Chicago. This is designed for teens. Cherilyn (mother's twenty-two year old daughter) did this for several summers, and [Child 1] was so look-ing forward to going . . . he had been waiting to turn 13 for a couple of years because he so much wanted to be part of this. The rest of us, after dropping [Child 1] off in Texas, were headed to Wisconsin to see friends briefly before heading to New York for a friend's wedding and visiting family (the kids have cousins close in age). We were going to pick [Child 1] up and return home for a week or two before heading out to St. Croix for 5 weeks, where Cherilyn is. Cherilyn runs a summer camp, and two of the cousins attended. My kids were supposed to be there too. So we'd be there for camp, then spend a couple of weeks after that. We were to come home Sept 1. We were applying for a school in Ensenada, Mexico, that would run Sept 25 through December. My kids were to go to school right on the campus, with children from around the world. It is right on the ocean. Frank and I have been there; it is a lovely place.

This is not providing my children socialization?

[Child 2] did not have as many activities as [Child 1] by choice. We offered her many opportunities but she is more of a homebody and did not want to do as much. I think it is wrong to FORCE a child into activities if the child has no interest. [Child 2] sang in 3 talent shows, had time on the school radio station (that was in her IEP but we suggested to the super that it might help her, and he was in total agreement), played softball two seasons (would have last year if the shoulder injury and car accident hadn't gotten in the way). She did play soccer one year. She took swim lessons. She tried the swim team but did not enjoy it at all, so we did swim lessons and/or free swim while [Child 1] was in team. She went to summer camp two years, dance camp two years. We tried 4-H and she declined. Same with Girl Scouts. She did do AWANA [*sic*]. Last year in Chico she took ballet lessons. She had two very close friends in Chico and spent every available minute with the girls; these were her first "REAL" normal friendships of that nature, because it was the first time she was ABLE to relate (she had recovered enough, and Hannah was support- ive of her when [Child 2] pulled away because the group was too overwhelm- ing). [Child 2] learned to ride a bike last year, which was a big leap, and socially made life easier. Then, of course, she did the things I had listed for [Child 1] that the whole family did.

[Child 3] did not do as much for two reasons: age and ability. [Child 3] was 8 when he was removed. We tried soccer. He was not successful. We tried dance camp. It was not successful. We did a lot as a family, but [Child 3] was not in a place that he could succeed in outside activities. One thing our family did that I did not mention is summer SELF club, where special needs kids met once a week for games in the park, then a special at the library (music person, snake person, or other guest). [Child 3] struggled with even this; he found it over- whelming. He was more successful on our smaller family outings or at Trisha's.

[Child 4] was 7. He went to dance camp (which was not successful for him), but due to age, etc. had not been involved in many activities. He was too young for sleep-away camp (have to be 8). He did do swim lessons.

[Child 5] was 5. He hung out with his brothers' class at dance camp and had swim lessons. At 5, I don't know what activities away from the family would be expected . . . .

At least twice a month we would do a family activity, often more. We might go hiking (in May we went hiking to some small caves) or swimming. (We would go to a Motel 6 with a pool and the kids could swim that afternoon, evening, next morning. We did this fairly regularly, including the Sunday before the removal). The Saturday before the kids were taken, we went with friends to a children's home in northeastern Arizona. We frequently took the kids fishing; some would fish, others would throw rocks in the water, etc. We were a fairly active family. We have always had a trampoline and swing set, etc. We play ball with the kids. We went on picnics, went to parks and playgrounds. The week before the removal, we took the kids to the ballet! (Teri Holloway was there and saw us; we got the tickets through her. It was a special performance for children). We were members of zoos, and went to the zoo frequently. I tried to tell the CASA this stuff, but he only wanted to know what the kids did without us (they should have been in Scouts, etc.). Ash Fork is a very small place, and most of the kids here are not involved in a lot of activities. It also has a proportionately huge homeschooling population as many folks do not trust the school district. My children have had many more social experiences than the average Ash Fork child, so if my children are neglected for under-socialization, then the families of Ash Fork are in large part guilty of neglect by those standards (though not being part of groups is NOT actually considered neglect as far as I know, other than in the eyes of CPS).

As a father of four, I could have learned a lot from such parents.

The remainder of Dr. Stephens' concerns, including functional antibody deficiency, multiple environmental and food allergies, and their immunization status will be dealt with in separate chapters since they raise specific issues and introduce evidence from other doctors, whose contribution deserves to be considered in greater detail.

For Dr. Stephens, however, the case was absolutely clear cut, and with an almost tangible sense of rising hysteria she wrote, " . . . these children have been victimized and abused. I am concerned about the underlying pathology of the parents, their sophistication and ability to manipulate not only the medical community, but the advocacy communities. The parents have released their version of the children's healthcare information and engaged both MIKID (Mentally Ill Kids in Distress) and the Autism Society of America, in an attempt to keep these factitious disorders alive. In addition, they have successfully manipulated state and federal funding agencies [into] providing services and cash benefits intended for those who have a serious need. I would suspect that unless we are able to keep the family engaged in meaningful services within the state of Arizona, they will pick up and move on to another state where they can begin again."

The portent of harm hung heavy in the collective consciousness of the Sorority. Dr. Stephens thought she saw a dagger. "Come, let me clutch thee. I have thee not and yet I see thee still."[88]

And round about the cauldron these three went: drawing the ghastly visage of abusers from the confusion of smoke and steam; abstract, amorphous specters, frightening though formless, sick and sickening, if only they had been of any substance. The unraveling e-mail string needed only to end with, "When shall we three meet again?"[89]

Chapter 13

BUILDING A CASE: PART II

Today, January 7, 2011, I will write with a renewed sense of purpose, despite not having slept. For last night, the mother called me to explain, through breathless tears, that they—the family—had lost their case. In fact, in the words of one of the family's lawyers, their judge had "washed his hands of the case."

The mother explained that before recessing to celebrate the holiday season, the judge, the Hon. Robert M. Brutinel, had asked legal counsel from both sides why, in light of the evidence, he should not let the children return home for Christmas. According to the mother, the considered response of the senior lawyer from the District Attorney's office—the prosecution—threw her hands in the air like someone auditioning as a backup singer for Jellyroll Morton's *Red Hot Peppers* and exclaimed, " . . . because they might take the children to a doctor."[1]

Handed down, as it was, on the twelfth day of Christmas, Judge Brutinel's ruling, therefore, came as something of a shock. He ruled that "the children have been subjected to numerous invasive, painful and unnecessary medical tests because of the parents' reported history and insistence on treatment. Some of the treatments are potentially dangerous. The children have been treated as developmentally disabled due to autism, when they are not developmentally disabled."[2]

Over the Christmas break, Judge Brutinel was appointed to the Arizona Supreme Court, issued a finding of fact that, in his opinion, the children would not be safe with their parents, and handed off any further decisions to the incoming judge. Apparently in festive mood, he had given the defendants one working day to respond to his finding of fact. I spoke with the father's lawyer, who was able to confirm this. She was shaken, hurting both personally and professionally for the family and a case she knew should have been won. Something in the state of Arizona had changed for the worse; the Family Courts of Arizona are stacking up with autism cases, and it appears that parents who undertake a biomedical approach to the treatment of their affected children are being targeted. "Six months ago," the lawyer said, "I would have rejected a conspiracy." Now she's not so sure. Whatever the case, the system of justice to which she signed up lies bleeding.

FEIGNING FOOD ALLERGIES

In your practice over the last 30 years, have you identified a clinical association between autistic disorder and allergic reactions to certain food proteins?

Jennifer Kupiszewski, the father's attorney

Yes.

Sharon McDonough-Means, MD. Developmental Pediatrician[3]

No matter which way you look at it, whatever set of criteria you use to define MSBP, either faked,[4] feigned,[5] or falsified,[6] it comes down to the same thing: fabrication of illness in another lies at the heart of this diagnosis. One of the oft-repeated allegations against the parents was that they had claimed that all of their children suffered from multiple food allergies when, according to CPS and the prosecution, not only was there no objective evidence to support this claim but, in fact, testing of the children had positively excluded it.

In respect of food allergies, Judge Brutinel issued the finding that " . . . based, at least in part, on medical history provided by the parents, each of the children were diagnosed with multiple environmental and food allergies. Their parents had placed them on a restrictive casein free, gluten free diet. An evaluation after their removal concluded that none of the children suffered from allergies. The children have had a normal diet following removal without any negative effects."[7]

Notwithstanding Child 3's clinical history and diagnosis of a hallmark of food allergy, eosinophilic gastroenteritis, and the presence of eosinophilic pathology in other children, matters that will be discussed below, one of the first of very few references to food allergies that I could identify in the records was in a summary of allegations—unsigned and undated—provided by CPS.[8]

The document is titled "History of unexplained illnesses. Invasive medical procedures. Extended illnesses. Five pediatricians. Dispelled illnesses."

Included under the first subheading, "History of unexplained illnesses/ extended illnesses," is "Food allergies: As reported to multiple doctors, strawberries, tomato, pineapple, mushrooms, corn, milk, wheat, eggs, chicken, sweet potatoes, onions, peaches, peanuts, cashews, ginger, oregano, celery."

Later, under the heading of "Dispelled Illnesses," this document listed food allergies, along with autism, lead poisoning, and a number of other diagnoses. Finally, with respect to food allergies, under the subheading "Conflicting information to each of numerous doctors," it read, "The parents reported numerous food allergies to multiple doctors."[9]

It is not certain from the English usage whether conflicting information was given to each doctor, and many of them, or whether the author(s) meant something different altogether.

The next reference to food allergy is supplied by CPS-appointed general pediatrician Dr. Jacobsen, chief of ambulatory pediatrics at PCH, who was due to see all five children for review on July 15, 2010. It appears from his report that none of the children and their foster parents actually made the appointment as scheduled. Despite the absence of the children and their relevant medical records, and in advance of his intended testing for food allergies, Dr. Jacobsen seemed to feel able to take a significant risk and recommend the introduction of previously excluded foods. Not unreasonably, the foster parents went along with his recommendation.[10]

This further testing took place between the end of August and early September, when the children were evaluated for food allergy at the Arizona Asthma & Allergy Institute by a Ms. Susan Symington, a certified physician's assistant. As far as the testing went, the findings of food allergy were essentially negative for all children. An example of Ms. Symington's reports to Dr. Jacobsen on this testing is provided below for Child 3. Dated September 7, 2010, it read, "FOOD ALLERGY: ruled out today," and below this, "PLAN FOR THE POSSIBLE FOOD ALLERGY: ruled out today by allergy testing to 40 common foods and was negative . . ."[11]

There are several discrepancies and errors here that will be addressed below. At this point, however, what is somewhat concerning is that in light of the parents' alleged claims of multiple food allergies in their children and the potentially fatal consequences of reintroducing rogue foods in a random fashion prior to allergy testing, these actions bordered upon negligence. Had the parents done it, I have no doubt that it would have been listed as evidence of abuse.

References to food allergies were present in the records of Child 3. This child had clear evidence of a food allergic disorder. This evidence, which is referred to in Chapter Part 3, Chapter 4, came from at least five independent sources. Accordingly and appropriately, the parents *did* report this fact to doctors when asked about his history of allergies. The evidence came first from his medical history of diarrhea (containing undigested food) and weight loss, which was related to Dr. Jeff Bradstreet, a family physician based in Florida on December 13, 2007.

Dr. Bradstreet has extensive experience in the biomedical management of ASD and is a published author on this subject.[12]

The second piece of evidence came from a stool test, which was requested by Dr. Bradstreet on the same occasion, that showed elevated levels of *fecal eosinophil protein*, a marker of possible allergic inflammation of the intestinal lining.

The next piece of evidence came from a positive Sage blood test (Sage Complement Antigen Test) requested by Dr. Schneider that indicated Child 3's immunologic intolerance of certain foods. This testing has been discussed in Part 1, Chapter 3.

Child 3's medical history and test results, such as they were at that time, were related faithfully by the parents to Dr. Ursea in the gastroenterology clinic at PCH on December 26, 2007. A further piece of evidence of possible food allergy, obtained by Dr. Ursea at this time, was the demonstration of occult blood (blood that is not visibly apparent) in his stool.

The rational explanation for this constellation of medical history and abnormal test findings was the presence of intestinal inflammation, very likely food allergic in origin. On January 30, 2008, Dr. Ursea performed upper and lower GI endoscopy and definitively confirmed the presence of a combination of eosinophilic gastroenteritis and esophagitis—the latter being consistent with reflux in Child 3. Both of the pathological findings are characteristics of a food allergic disorder in children.

In order to determine the specific foods to which he was allergic, Dr. Ursea referred Child 3 to Dr. Hellmers, the immunologist, for patch testing.[13] This test, which at that time had been in clinical use for just three years, helps to identify non-IgE-mediated food allergies—the form suffered by Child 3. In court, he was asked what results were obtained in Child 3. "Well, the youngster came back with quite a bit of inflammation, as I recall, and so it was a little hard to identify specifically which one was—which test[s] were the major issues and I think that because of the amount of inflammation that the child had, Mrs. [name] didn't want to repeat the test."[14]

Dr. Hellmers confirmed that he had recommended that the positive test be repeated, but the mother had declined because of her child's obvious discomfort. Dr. Hellmers confirmed that with " . . . so many of the different foods being positive she just didn't want to put the youngster through that."[15]

It is hard to see how this could be interpreted as the mother craving medical investigation, either by proxy or otherwise. What it did confirm, however, beyond any shadow of a doubt, was a non-IgE-mediated food allergy in Child 3.

And he responded well to appropriate GI treatment. At the follow-up with Dr. Ursea on January 26, 2010, his acid relux had improved on Nexium. His main issue remained his food allergies; these provoked abdominal pain and reflux when he was exposed to offending foods and were managed appropriately by dietary exclusion until CPS came on the scene. The sequence of medical actions from Dr. Bradstreet through to Dr. Ursea was timely, appropriate, and undertaken according to standard of care. The careful diagnostic process enabled treatment that led to marked improvement in Child 3's overall clinical condition. Nowhere in the records is there any evidence that at any time the parents exaggerated or misrepresented the facts of Child 3's condition. In spite of his unambiguous and well-documented clinical findings, his foster parents and those responsible for his care pursuant to the intervention of CPS were either ignorant of or chose to ignore the facts and exposed him to foods that had a real potential to cause harm.

As for the remaining four children, I was unable to find a single doctor's record containing a parental claim of food allergies. Specifically, in Child 1, a routine enquiry for a history of allergies was sought by doctors on at least four occasions that I could identify, spanning the period of December 14, 2008, to February 24, 2009, when he was hospitalized with HSP. None were reported by the parents.

Child 2 had a history of asthma, diagnosed by a physician and treated with a steroid inhaler, but nowhere in the doctors' records available to me was there mention of food allergies, including the medical and nursing charts from her time at PCH with right shoulder pain, i.e., the records made by Dr. Carter. The same goes for Child 4 and Child 5. Notwithstanding the fact that there may be additional records to which I have not been privy, in their reports CPS, Dr. Stephens, and Dr. Jacobsen fail to identify or specify any factual evidence for parental claims of food allergies.[16] Nonetheless, Dr. Stephens, with the certainty and zeal that characterize her modus operandi, wrote in her report of October 7, 2010, *"None of the children have multiple environmental or food allergies."*[17]

She referred specifically to the results of Ms. Symington's testing: " . . . **allergy skin testing to the 40 common foods and all the results were negative for food allergies on each child**. Anaphylaxis due to adverse food reaction skin testing is negative and patient has been eating a regular diet for the past 8 months without any reactions."[18]

Having apparently been contrived by CPS and its agents, food allergies were subsequently listed in its damning category of "Dispelled illnesses." This reminds me of the primitive heads-I-win, tails-you-lose logic underlying the medieval process of diagnosing a witch; if throwing the accused in the village pond or dunking the unfortunate woman on the end of a pole caused her to drown, she was innocent. Alternatively, if she survived (obviously by invoking the "dark arts") she was guilty and put to death. CPS and Dr. Stephens had contrived an illness that they then had to be able to dispel. While this had the effect of further reducing the parents to frauds and pathological liars in the eyes of the court, in fact, it compounded Dr. Stephen's personal falsification of the children's disease status. Food allergy was confirmed and never dispelled in the case of Child 3 and does not appear to have been claimed to doctors—by the parents at least—for any other child.

Most significant of all the reports, however, was that of Dr. Mary Sanders, Berkeley psychologist and expert in the analysis of alleged cases of MSBP. In her report to the court of September 27, 2010—a defining document in the judge's determination on this case—she wrote, "The parents reported that all the children had . . . multiple environmental and food allergies."[19]

Later in her report she describes discussions that she had with some of the doctors and other healthcare professionals who had played a role in the children's care. These included: Dr. Katherine McCarthy (retired pediatrician, NY), Oryan Salberg (chiropractor), Dr. Robert Hellmers (immunologist), Dr. Albert Jacobsen (pediatrician), Dr. Kathryn Ballard (pediatrician), Dr. Sydney Rice (developmental pediatrician), Dr. Jeff Weiss (pediatrician), Dr. Kaleo Ede (rheumatologist), and Dr. Robin Blitz-Wetterland (developmental pediatrician). Notable for their absence from this list were Dr. Schneider and Dr. Ursea, key players in the issue of food allergy in this family.

In addition, Dr. Sanders supplied a table that ran for nineteen pages and contained relevant clinical details of each child—details that she had abstracted from the clinical records where she sought to compare and contrast the "Parental Reported Problems" with the "Findings." She described the contents of the table as being from those records that "seem pertinent."[20]

Among these documents there are three separate instances where food allergies receive mention. They are all for Child 3 and involve Dr. Schneider, who had ordered the Sage Complement Antigen Test that highlighted Child 3's specific non-IgE-mediated food allergies, and Dr. Ursea, who diagnosed his food allergic GI disease. Despite this, Dr. Sanders did not interview Dr. Schneider. From Dr. Sanders' review of the remainder of the "pertinent" medical records—presumably those upon which her allegations were based—and in her discussion with some relevant practitioners, there is not a single mention of food allergies in any other child.

But when examined by the prosecuting counsel on the opening day of the dependency hearing, in response to the question "Did the parents report that the children have multiple environmental and food allergies?" she responded, "Oh, yes. Absolutely." And then she continued, "Well—and I didn't see any testing for allergies . . . ."[21]

As outlined above, there was clear evidence of testing—positive testing—for allergies in the children's records, principally Child 3, ranging from the detection of eosinophil basic protein in his stool, through to the histological evidence of eosinophilic GI inflammation in Child 3 and Child 4. Dr. Mart, also a psychologist and expert witness on behalf of the parents, had the humility to demur in the face of questions about food allergy that clearly went beyond his expertise. But not Dr. Sanders—and she got it wrong.

But even if she had correctly identified the evidence of allergic disease, one wonders if it would have made any difference to her determination of the parents' guilt. Later in her testimony it was put to her by defense counsel, "If, in fact, hypothetically speaking medical diagnoses for these children are based upon objective diagnostic criteria and testing and not based on parent report, would that refute your diagnosis of Factitious Disorder by Proxy?" "Not necessarily," she responded, "it depends on if that explains all the falsifications."

So, according to Dr. Sanders, the falsifications exist and can be explained— but not mitigated—by objective evidence of disease. But where are these elusive parental claims that all their children had multiple food allergies? Is it possible that, in fact, the claims to such claims were, themselves, exaggerated? Or worse— were they fabricated in order that they could be later "dispelled," adding a new dimension to the legacy of Baron von Münchausen?

In a following chapter, Dr. Sanders' report will be scrutinized in some detail. At this stage it is sufficient to say that if her report were flawed, if it alleged parental claims for nonexistent illness(es) when there were none, and if rules of engagement for the investigation of alleged MSBP that she helped define have been broken, then she herself deserves an eponymous syndrome—one of her very own making.

FOOD ALLERGY

As discussed in Part 1, Chapter 3, food allergy comes in at least two major forms. The first is the one with which the public is more familiar, involving sudden and potentially life-threatening anaphylactic reactions ranging from hives to airway obstruction and cardiac arrest. Peanut allergy is a classical example of this problem. The second major form of food allergy, which may overlap in common parlance with food sensitivity or intolerance, is a non-IgE-mediated, delayed-type immune response that manifests with a variety of symptoms ranging from diarrhea to migraine.

Dr. Harumi Jyonouchi is a specialist in allergy and immunology at the University of Medicine and Dentistry of New Jersey in Newark. A major sub-specialty of her clinical and research practice is allergic disease in children with ASD, in which, arguably, she has an unparalleled experience. She has also published extensively on this subject in scientific and medical literature.[22] In 2010 she wrote: "It is our clinic's experience that ASD children tend to be **under-diagnosed and undertreated**[23] for common medical conditions such as allergic disorders."

She attributes this, at least in part, to these children's " . . . impaired expressive language, aberrant behaviors, and lower tolerance to diagnostic measures, compared with typically developing children . . . "

On the basis that IgE- and non-IgE-mediated food allergy are often confused by practicing general pediatricians and parents, she has provided an excellent "perspective" paper that reviews this topic and discusses food allergy in the context of ASD.[24] From the following narrative, it would seem that this confusion is shared by those who should know better.

Both types of food allergy, anaphylactic (or IgE-mediated) and delayed-type (non-IgE-mediated), have been recognized for many years and are well known to experts in the field. As described in Part 1, Chapter 3, the differential diagnosis of food allergy requires different approaches. The diagnosis of IgE-mediated food allergy is routinely made by measuring the inflammatory reaction following intradermal injection of extracts of a range of common foods. The diagnosis of non-IgE-mediated food allergy cannot be diagnosed by this method[25] and requires the approach described in Part 1, Chapter 3.

When they had been together as a family, the children had been on a strict diet that excluded gluten, casein, and other problematic foods. On this regimen, under the guidance of Dr. Schneider and others, the physical and mental health of the children is documented as having improved.

Such improvement is consistent with the expert opinion of Dr. Jyonouchi, who wrote, "We have found that treatment of common childhood illnesses, including allergic diseases, significantly improved behavioral symptoms and subsequent cognitive development."

With this background of the documented clinical facts and the claims of the parents' detractors, it is necessary to review the nature and findings of the food allergy testing that took place on the children in the hands of CPS. After they had been taken from their parents, special diets were stopped and only then were the children subjected to food allergy testing by Susan Symington, a physician's assistant at the Arizona Asthma & Allergy Institute.

As we have seen, her reports to Dr. Jacobsen on this testing included the categorical statement "FOOD ALLERGY: ruled out today."[26]

It was presumably on this basis that Dr. Stephens seemed to feel literally and figuratively emboldened to report on October 27, 2010, that *"None of the children have multiple environmental or food allergies."*[27]

It appears that Dr. Stephens was misled. While immediate-type, IgE-mediated allergic responses to forty common foods had been investigated and effectively excluded, the second major category of food allergy—non-IgE-mediated disease—had not been investigated at all. The job was half done, and food allergy had by no means been ruled out.

Somewhat disingenuously, Ms. Symington qualified her findings only later in her report when she wrote: " . . . the chance of a serious life-threatening reaction to the foods tested is highly unlikely."

Here, she was presumably referring only to immediate, anaphylactic reactions like peanut allergy, which *may* be life-threatening. Lower down, under the subheading "Testing Results," she confirmed this by providing an even narrower qualification of her findings, making her original statement all the more misleading: "Immediate hypersensitivity skin test negative."

At this stage and only at this stage did Ms. Symington make it clear that immediate-type food allergy testing alone was negative in the children who had been tested. But to the non-experts—and there were plenty of them—her message was clear: food allergy had been "ruled out," and this was the message that was carried forward, both to the court and to those who were responsible for managing the children's diets.

In fact, food allergies—either immediate or delayed-type—had not been studied for most of the children nor had the parents laid claim to food allergies in any but Child 3. The reintroduction of foods previously excluded on the basis of his positive allergy testing and his frank intestinal disease could have serious implications for this child's health.

In his ruling of January 6, 2011, Judge Brutinel threw in the unqualified observation that "the children have had a normal diet following removal without any negative effects."

In whose opinion? Certainly no one who had evaluated the children adequately for food allergy before and after their dietary intervention, including those doctors involved in the diagnosis and treatment of any GI and food allergic disease in these children. And it appears that not one single person who had made this determination had taken the trouble to read and assess the relevant medical literature on the merits of dietary intervention in autism.

In fact, it transpires that the children have not been asymptomatic having come off the diet following removal by CPS. Child 1 has had to go back to Dr. Jacobsen with recurrent abdominal pain; Child 5 said that pizza made him cough, a symptom of possible esophageal reflux or food allergy; and Child 2 said that, in relation to foods, she sometimes felt "sickened." When Dr. Sanders questioned Child 4 about the diet after it had been stopped, he said, "I do get stomach aches."[28]

When cross-examined on this point during her testimony, Dr. Sanders turned up the appropriate record. When granted permission to read the whole sentence, she continued, "Oh, I love this. 'I do get stomach aches, but not because of the foods. I just run into trees.' So cute."[29]

I am at a loss for words.

Could the prosecution's claim to an apparent lack of allergic symptoms on an unrestricted diet be accounted for by the children having grown out of their food allergies over time? Dr. Stephens was of the opinion that recovery from food allergy in response to dietary intervention did not occur.

Just for the record, with the exception of peanut allergy, children can and frequently do recover from food allergies[30] as Dr. Hellmers—the expert— confirmed in testimony.[31] Absence of previous symptoms following reintroduction of previously offending foods should not be taken as proof of an absence of food allergy in the first place.

It is my opinion that, for Child 3 in particular, the consequences of this medical malpractice are potentially serious. Because of the complex symptoms that may accompany non-IgE-mediated food allergy, the foster parents might well not recognize and report relevant problems as being food related. Serious symptoms such as ataxia, depression, behavioral deterioration, and seizures might not be recognized as reactions to food. In a litany of staggering professional incompetence this was just one more nail in this family's coffin.

Chapter 14

HELLMERS AND CARTER: PROFESSIONALS AT ODDS

For the Arizona 5, the diagnosis and treatment of an immune system problem—functional antibody deficiency—was to have provided Dr. Carter and CPS both a motive for the parents' behavior and a means for their entrapment.

At the core of Dr. Carter's allegations against the parents is that they were jointly engaged in abusing their children through sickness-seeking behavior and specifically that they had "falsely searched for a way to give their children this functional antibody deficiency diagnosis so that they can get IVIG therapy for their children AND get it paid for by Medicaid."[1]

Dr. Carter admitted to her professional colleagues that she was not "an autism specialist, immunologist, or psychiatrist."[2] However, it was her conviction that the parents were seeking experimental IVIG therapy for a nonexistent diagnosis of autism by contriving a disease—functional antibody deficiency—for which IVIG was a licensed treatment. She characterized her diagnosis of the parents further as "factitious disorder by proxy which is a perpetration of medical disorders by a caregiver in order to gain any variety of benefits including attention, sympathy, leniency, financial support, etc. parents with this disorder typically falsify the child's medical history and then enjoy the attention they get from having a sick child."[3]

Dr. Carter's description of FDBP was wrong, at least according to DSM criteria, since she had invoked financial gain as a possible motive. In a telephone call on April 23, 2010, Ms. Williams and Dr. Carter speculated further on the secondary gain for the parents from the purported abuse of their children, wondering "is it drugs, financial, or other problem[?]"[4]

While the parents' motives were uncertain, what was certain to Dr. Carter was their guilt. FDBP/MSBP is supposedly a very rare mental disorder and almost invariably affects only one of the parents, usually the mother. Moreover, it is unusual for the abusive behavior to be visited on more than one child at any one time. Here, in theory, was a situation where both parents were complicit—sharing, by necessity, the same psychopathology—abusing all five of their children simultaneously to satiate their perverse needs. Statistically, this scenario is extremely unlikely. Moreover, Dr. Carter's complex analysis required the telling of one lie to treat another, stealing from Medicaid as added gratification, and all this by both parents for all five of their children. Professor Roy Meadow, who first described MSBP, fell afoul of statistical fallacy, having concluded that the sudden deaths of two infant siblings must have been murder and backing up his conclusion with erroneous and disastrous mathematical reasoning (see Part 2).[5] Similarly, in the case of this family, where so many anomalies were required to operate in unison, any analysis demanded the utmost caution.

FUNCTIONAL ANTIBODY (IMMUNOGLOBULIN) DEFICIENCY

Functional antibody deficiency is usually defined by a significant inability to respond with IgG antibody production after antigenic (e.g., vaccine) challenge. Reduced levels of serum antibodies in patients with recurrent bacterial infections, coupled with a lack of response to protein or polysaccharide vaccine challenges (i.e., patients who cannot make IgG antibody against diphtheria and tetanus toxoids, pneumococcal polysaccharide vaccine, or both) is an indication for IgG replacement.[6] In this setting, IVIG therapy is appropriate for patients with difficult-to-manage recurrent otitis media with risk for permanent hearing loss, recurrent infections necessitating intravenous antibiotics, or multiple antibiotic hypersensitivities that interfere with treatment.

IVIG, the enriched antibody fraction of blood from multiple donors, is a complex therapy and can lead to adverse effects, which are not uncommon. Fortunately, most IVIG reactions are mild and non-anaphylactic. They are characterized typically by back or abdominal aching or pain, nausea, rhinitis, asthma, chills, low grade fever, myalgias, and/or headache. Slowing or stopping the infusion for fifteen to thirty minutes will reverse many reactions. Anti-inflammatory medication may also be helpful. More severe reactions can be treated with steroids. Rare serious reactions may also occur.[7] Expert monitoring of the patient receiving IVIG infusion is therefore necessary in anticipation of these potential complications. Prompt diagnosis and treatment of any adverse events is, therefore, required to ensure patient safety. There is also a theoretical risk of transmitted infection, although this has been greatly reduced after manufacturing processes were altered to screen and exclude hepatitis C virus after an earlier outbreak from a contaminated batch.

All IVIG infusions were administered under qualified supervision at PCH and none of the four children who received IVIG ever suffered even a slight adverse reaction to this treatment.

You will remember from Part 3, Chapter 3 that Dr. Carter's overriding medical concern was what she considered to be the inappropriate diagnosis and treatment of functional antibody deficiency in these children. In the case of Child 1, she had identified inconsistencies in his vaccination history that led her to question Dr. Hellmers's expert diagnosis. Having rejected the diagnosis of immunodeficiency for both Child 1 and Child 2, Dr. Carter subsequently refused to either prescribe or endorse IVIG as a treatment for their autism.

In order to understand the process by which the children came to receive a diagnosis of functional antibody deficiency and, therefore, receive treatment with IVIG, we must go back to the sentinel child, Child 3, who was the first to come to the attention of Dr. Hellmers.

Problems with Child 3's immune system first received comment from Dr. Katherine McCarthy, his pediatrician in New York, where he was hospitalized with pneumonia at the age of twenty-three months. According to the mother, her casual observation was that "this child has a crappy immune system."[8]

It was only after Dr. Ursea had made the diagnosis of eosinophilic gastroenteritis in Child 3 that she recommended he be assessed by an allergy specialist in order to determine the precise triggers for his food allergic disorder. Originally, Dr. Rose at the Arizona Asthma & Allergy Institute had been suggested, but the local autism community's list of preferred doctors recommended Dr. Hellmers.

Dr. Robert Hellmers graduated in medicine from the University of California, Irvine. After completing a pediatric residency at Children's Hospital Los Angeles, he undertook a fellowship in allergy and immunology at the University of Southern California Medical Center and obtained his diplomas from the American Board of Allergy and Immunology and the American Board of Pediatrics. He has been in group practice with Arizona Allergy Associates for approximately thirty-nine years.

The mother and Child 3 met with Dr. Hellmers on January 11, 2008. In an interview with her on February 6, 2011, the mother described how she had reported the key aspects of Child 3's medical history to Dr. Hellmers. This included a description of his recurrent infections and his immunization status. The mother had an immunization booklet to which Dr. Hellmers referred, noting specifically that he had received two doses of Prevnar, the *Streptococcus pneumoniae* vaccine. This is accurate according to his immunization administration record from Dr. McCarthy's New York office. The recommended schedule for this vaccine was for four doses at two, four, six, and twelve to fifteen months of age. Child 3 had stopped receiving vaccines in early 2003 after his autistic regression, having received only his first two doses of Prevnar. Child 3's blood tests, performed at this visit, confirmed that he had a non-protective antibody response to twelve of the fourteen (sero) types of *S. pneumoniae*. In addition, he had a deficient response to tetanus toxoid, despite having been vaccinated with it four times. Dr. Hellmers diagnosed him with a functional antibody deficiency and treated him with IVIG. He responded well; follow-up records from Dr. Hellmers on July 24, 2008, and January 27, 2010, documented a marked decrease in his infections. There is one further record, dated May 21, 2010, after his course of IVIG had stopped, in which Dr. Hellmers noted that his infections had returned and that he had developed obsessive behaviors.

Based upon information provided by the parents, there were several additional entries in his medical records that referenced Child 3's vaccination status, including the following: "Behind due to family wishes,"[9] "Exempt per mother and family wishes,"[10] "None per family wishes,"[11] "Absent due to family wishes,"[12] "Exempt,"[13] and "Exempt per family wishes."[14]

Notwithstanding the fact that the parents could not be held directly responsible for the precise form of words used by the doctors, all of these entries were consistent and accurate.

In light of Child 3's beneficial response to IVIG and similar histories of recurrent infections in Child 1 and Child 2, the latter children were seen by Dr. Hellmers on January 29, 2009, and April 8, 2009, respectively. In response to his questions about vaccination status, the mother remembers having reported that their immunizations were up to date until early 2003 but stopped following their younger brother's regression at eighteen months of age. Thereafter, none of their children were vaccinated.

In a letter to "whom it may concern" dated January 29, 2009, Dr. Hellmers described Child 1's history of recurrent infections and HSP. "Additionally, reviews of the youngster's laboratory work revealed that he has had all of his immunizations and boosters and **has virtually very little positive response to his strep pneumo titers, i.e., 12 of the 14 were abnormally low with no response to his vaccination**.[15] This generally suggests a functional antibody deficiency to polysaccharide-type bacteria. Additionally, his tetanus antibody titers were below normal as well, suggesting that he may have problems fighting bacteria that are protein encapsulated as well."

At follow-up on January 27, 2010, after a trial of IVIG, Dr. Hellmers reported that he had responded "very well" but, since stopping this treatment, the mother reported that Child 1 had been " . . . constantly sick with fevers of 104 lasting four to five days, sinus infections and bronchiolitis. He is also having difficulty with his Henoch-Schonlein purpura."

Dr. Hellmers recommended that IVIG be resumed. According to the mother, it was this treatment that enabled him to get off steroids for his refractory HSP, without relapse of disease, something that had invariably followed reduction of the steroid dose prior to the resumption of IVIG.

The problem was that Child 1 was too old to have received the Prevnar vaccine on schedule. Dr. Carter had noted in the emergency room on February 25, 2009, that Prevnar had not been part of the routine childhood immunization schedule until 2000. Since the four recommended doses were intended to be given by eighteen months of age, she concluded that Child 1, born in 1997, would have been unlikely to have received it. She was correct. Seeking clarification, she contacted Dr. Hellmers and subsequently wrote in the medical record, "Dr. Hellmers said that he made the diagnosis of immunodeficiency solely on Child 1's low *S. pneumoniae* titers."[16]

This is not correct; it is evident from the extract of Dr. Hellmers's letter of January 29, 2009, that, in fact, it was the combination of recurrent infections and low titers to both *S. pneumoniae* and tetanus toxoid that led his to this diagnosis in Child 1.

Nor is Dr. Carter's claim consistent with what she subsequently reported to her colleagues Heather Williams and Dr. Stephens. In an e-mail dated April 26, 2010, she wrote, "I called Dr. Hellmers back in February 2009 and asked how he made the diagnosis in [Child 1]. He told me that he had made it based on **low tetanus**[17] and strep pneumo antibody levels."[18]

Her story had materially changed; previously, she had accused Dr. Hellmers of making his diagnosis of functional antibody deficiency on the basis of low *S. pneumoniae* titers alone.[19] She made the case that Dr. Hellmers could not have made this diagnosis on titers for a vaccine—Prevnar—that the child didn't get. Now it appears that Dr. Hellmers made the diagnosis correctly on Child 1's low tetanus titers and recurrent infections and had told Dr. Carter as much.

Nonetheless, Dr. Carter had identified a material discrepancy that required explanation. Was this error over Prevnar the result of a genuine misunderstanding or was it something more sinister altogether?

Dr. Hellmers's initial handwritten records for Child 1 of January 28, 2009, made no mention of his vaccination status. In a letter written the following day, he had noted " . . . reviews of the youngster's laboratory work revealed that he has had all of his immunizations and boosters . . . ."[20]

It is not certain what laboratory work would have disclosed this information, and it is more likely to have been based on the mother's narrative; nonetheless, it was entirely correct. Child 1 had been fully vaccinated at age five to include his preschool boosters (see Table 5) and had stopped receiving further shots after his younger brother ran into trouble. This was consistent with the vaccine history for Child 1 that was documented by others at PCH during his various admissions to that hospital with HSP. For example, on February 24, 2009, medical resident Dr. Longhurst wrote, "Has most but stopped 2° [illegible] related to vaccination."[21]

Below this in the same ER record, there is a history taken by medical student Jason Samuel, who wrote in respect to Child 1's vaccines, "Had most but stopped."[22]

The parents never specifically claimed that their eldest son had received the pneumococcal vaccine. The parental reports of Child 1's vaccination status were consistent and accurate.

On February 25, 2009, Dr. Longhurst and Dr. Carter saw Child 1 again with his father. Despite her anxieties about his vaccination status, no further details were sought from the father by Dr. Carter at this time. Rather, she pursued the issue with Dr. Hellmers by telephone and subsequently wrote, "[Dr. Hellmers] was not sure of [Child 1's] vaccine record."[23]

The following day, February 26, 2009, Dr. Carter sought details from the father about the children's pediatrician in New York, Dr. McCarthy, who had vaccinated the three older children. The father also gave Dr. Carter permission to contact the local primary care physician, Dr. Sipes, for Child 1's vaccine record. This was sent to Dr. Carter and attached to Child 1's record. It confirmed that Child 1 had not received Prevnar. With respect to tetanus vaccine, the other vaccine exposure to which this child had inadequate immunity, Dr. Carter wrote, "Of note, [patient's] last tetanus vaccine was DTaP #4 given 12.28.98."[24]

While this would have supported her case, in fact, Dr. Carter was wrong; Child 1's last DTaP vaccine was given on March 22, 2002 (Table 5),[25] over three years later than she had claimed. This is not to suggest that Dr. Carter was dishonest; nonetheless, a pattern of inconsistency and contradiction has emerged not only from within her own reports but also between these reports and the facts as documented by others. It also makes the point that mistakes can be made quite easily. In this case there appears to have been no more than a simple misunderstanding: the mother had reported Child 1's vaccination status accurately to Dr. Hellmers. In turn, Dr. Hellmers had assumed that any child who'd had "all of his immunizations and boosters"[26] would have received Prevnar vaccine. In fact, Child 1 was too old by the time this vaccine was put on the routine childhood schedule in 2000 to have received it. It seems that Dr. Carter took this as evidence of dishonesty, by whom it is not certain, and it does not appear that she took any further steps to resolve the provenance of this discrepancy. In light of her own error in respect to tetanus vaccine, used as it was to reinforce her case against the parents, she may, in time, have cause to reflect.

To add further confusion, the details of Dr. Carter's call to Dr. Hellmers's office on February 26, 2009, were documented by a receptionist by the name of Emily who wrote with reference to Child 1, "Did receive copy of imm-record. **Did receive Prevnar vacc.**[27] Last tetanus 12/98."[28]

Whatever Child 1's actual exposure to Prevnar, based upon this record, Dr. Hellmers was entitled to believe that he had received it. Dr. Carter also made errors when documenting the family history in her review of Child 2 when she noted that "All sibs have . . . functional [antibody] deficiency."[29] The parents claim never to have reported this condition in Child 5, and this is consistent with the clinical records.

What had the parents reported to healthcare workers as far as Child 2's vaccination status was concerned? I could identify at least seven entries in the hospital records, representing encounters with different healthcare professionals on different occasions. Each of these entries correctly reported Child 2's vaccination status, including "Exempt,"[30] "Medically exempt,"[31] "Not up to date, needs,"[32] "None since age 4 per mom,"[33] and "None since 4 per mom."[34] All of these entries were accurate and not in the least bit contradictory.

For Child 2, and only for Child 2, did Dr. Hellmers have a copy of her immunization record from Dr. McCarthy's office in his medical chart. At the top, handwritten, it states "incomplete record." Once again, the mother reports having told Dr. Hellmers that her children received their scheduled vaccines up until Child 3's regression in early 2003, and beyond that, no vaccines had been given to any child. Once again, Dr. Hellmers was under the impression that Child 2 had received Prevnar. His record of April 8, 2009, included "PCV-7—felt to have been given and (Prevnar x4 per mother)."[35]

The reference to "incomplete record" on her immunization record was presumably due to the absence of any mention of Prevnar, since Child 2's vaccinations were up to date until age four. Post Prevnar's introduction in 2000, all four doses of this vaccine would have been given by age four.

Child 4's vaccinations stopped after he had suffered an adverse reaction to his two-month vaccines and his older brother had regressed following a vaccine reaction in early 2003. His vaccination record is shown in Table 5. There are only a few references in the medical records from PCH and Dr. Rice, the developmental pediatrician. These include "Exempt due to reactions to immunizations at 2 months"[36] and "Exempt due to reactions to immunizations at 2 months."[37] These are entirely consistent and accurate.

In light of his siblings' experiences, Child 5 received no vaccinations. The only entry in his PCH records was that of Dr. Ursea on January 26, 2010, where she stated, "Exempt per family wishes."[38]

This is also accurate. Child 5 did not have evidence of a functional antibody deficiency and, in light of his vaccine exemption, could not be tested for this in the standard way. He did not receive IVIG. The fact that he had received a diagnosis of ASD mitigated the notion that IVIG was either being given by Dr. Hellmers or requested by the parents for the treatment of autism.

In summary, the records reveal that this family started off fully compliant with the recommended childhood vaccine schedule. This changed following Child 3's adverse reaction with autistic regression at eighteen months and Child 4's behavioral changes following his two-month vaccines. Following these events, the children received no further vaccines. The narrative provided to successive healthcare professionals was consistent and accurate with respect to each child, with the exception of one instance for Child 1 and one for Child 2. These appear to have arisen as a result of a misunderstanding about when Prevnar was introduced into the routine schedule. There is no evidence, however, that the parents were the source of any deliberate misinformation.

The misrepresentation of the parents on the matter of immunization was to carry over into the courtroom. Dr. Stephens, when asked about her apparent discovery of the fact that the parents had given conflicting information to every healthcare provider, replied, "Yes, the records are filled with conflicting information."[39]

She appears to have inferred that this information was tailored by the parents, depending on what it was they wished to manipulate out of the doctor on any given day. She continued, "Every single note from the primary care physician documents 'immunizations refused again today by the parents.' And then when you go to see the note from Dr. Hellmers, the parents report that the children have had all of their immunizations."[40]

How these statements were allowed to go effectively unchallenged is a mystery. They are both utterly false. The primary care physician records for Children 1, 2, and 3 actually document the administration of their vaccines. As a further example, Dr. Hellmers documents the fact that Child 3 received only two of his Prevnar vaccines.

While a history of Prevnar exposure was material to their diagnosis of functional antibody deficiency, it was not exclusively so; added to it were these children's histories of recurrent infection and their laboratory evidence of a nonprotective level of tetanus toxoid antibody. Dr. Hellmers's clinical judgment was ratified by the documented beneficial clinical response that the children apparently experienced with IVIG.

But the story, according to the Sorority, was of the parents as wolves in sheeps' clothing. Its perception of events is captured in a string of e-mails that started with Heather Williams on April 23, 2010, who summarized Dr. Carter's encounter with the father during Child 1's presentation with HSP as "Dad came back with vague conditions such as joint pain. Dad was giving a history of pooping and vomiting blood and none of this was seen by the doctors at the hospital. Child 1 looked fine and no results were found."[41]

Despite blood in his stool and urine, swelling of his intestinal wall on abdominal ultrasound and CAT scanning, and ulceration of his stomach and duodenum, Ms. Williams' blatant misrepresentation stood in stark contrast with her dramatic picture of IVIG's potential hazards, both to the patient's health and the financial well-being of the State of Arizona. She wrote that IVIG " . . . runs the risk of infection, and a risk of horrible allergic life-threatening reactions. It always has to be given in hospital, it is extremely expensive."[42]

Dr. Hellmers was next in the firing line. Ms. Williams continued, "Problem one is that Dr. Hellmers is able to practice at PHX childrens [Phoenix Children's Hospital]. This Dr. she thinks is making money off this but they can't prove it."[43]

Ms. Williams' documentation is so poor and so inarticulate that it is quite impossible at times to know about what or whom she is referring. Here is an example: "She pulled him aside Her cousin is part of the autism coalition. She stated that if you want to do IVIG and if you want insurance to pay for it this Dr. Hellmers will get documentation to do this. He has been reported but there is not anything CPS can do about this."[44]

She continued, "Not only is [Child 1] getting this but all the children in the family are and **none of the children have been vaccinated**.[45] The family is using this diagnosis falsely."[46]

The second e-mail in the string consists of Dr. Carter's response to Ms. Williams, dated April 26, 2010. Dr. Carter confirmed her conviction of the abuse and dishonesty at the core of the parents' behavior: "I think the [family] have falsely searched for a way to give their children this functional antibody deficiency so that they can get IVIG therapy for their children AND get it paid for by Medicaid."[47]

It appears that the diagnosis of MSBP had, in the minds of Ms. Williams and her informant Dr. Carter, taken on an even more sinister aspect. The parents were using a dangerous therapy for a condition that their children did not have—one they had contrived as cover for treating a developmental disorder that they had also fabricated. Their crazy, attention-seeking behavior was apparently being facilitated by an apparently unscrupulous profiteer: Dr. Hellmers, a Phoenix Children's Hospital doctor, no less. The word in the parents' autism coalition was that this candy man could get their children an IV fix, regardless of the attendant hazards of death from infection and anaphylaxis, and was prepared to risk defrauding Medicaid in order to do so.

Later in court, the possibility was put to Dr. Hellmers that he had "been treating these children with IVIG under the guise of Functional Antibody Deficiency so the insurance would cover the treatment of autism."[48] He denied what would have amounted to insurance fraud.

Returning to Ms. Williams' e-mail, she held back the most bizarre scenario until last: "For arguments sake, if parents want to pay for IVIG treatment out of pocket or get it through insurance that is there business [sic]."

Was Ms. Williams suggesting that it was okay for people to either use their own dollar or defraud their private health insurance company in order to sponsor child abuse? Was the aim of this exercise actually to save the state money, a motive perhaps more obviously in keeping with a less humanitarian raison d'être of the Arizona Department of Economic Security?

For the first time, Ms. Williams also revealed Dr. Carter's true motive for having admitted Child 2 to the hospital on March 16, 2010, the occasion of her shoulder pain. The e-mail summary of her conversation with Dr. Carter read, "[Dr. Carter] said that they admitted the child to watch and see if they wanted the IVIG treatment and within 24 hours mom asked."[49]

This request was taken as clear vindication of Dr. Carter's suspicions of abuse. But there is far more to this than meets the eye. Dr. Carter's ER note of that same day recorded the fact that Child 2 had received IVIG up until November 2009, when it had been denied by the insurance provider, Capstone. Following Dr. Hellmer's intervention, IVIG had been reapproved by Capstone sometime in early 2010, whereupon, on February 10, 2010, Dr. Hellmers had written the next prescription and communicated this to the outpatient staff at PCH to schedule Child 2's treatment. The parents were to learn of this following their return from a trip to Mexico.

Dr. Carter noted in the ER on March 16, 2010, that IVIG had been reapproved and that there were plans to restart it for this child. So, the unstated fact in the e-mail string among Ms. Williams, Dr. Carter, and Dr. Stephens is that, at the time of her attendance at the ER, Child 2 was due for her routine IVIG according to Dr. Hellmers's resumed three-weekly treatment schedule. In fact, this treatment was somewhat overdue as a result of the family being out of town.

The stage had been set for the mother's entrapment; Dr. Carter had apparently arranged Child 2's admission to hospital—not for the treatment of her right shoulder pain, but as a sting, a snare for the unwitting mother to step into, by requesting—quite reasonably—that her daughter receive a prescribed and pending medication, one that was required to be given in the hospital, and, therefore, why not the same hospital in which it had always been given? Out of concern for her daughter and in compliance with Dr. Hellmers's orders, the mother had fallen into Dr. Carter's trap.

Ms. Williams closed her report on the conversation with Dr. Carter: "This case has got her [Dr. Carter] worked up and she has taken a risk and something is wrong. She said that this family is very scary and they threaten law suits but it is her duty to report concerns."[50]

It is not certain what risk Dr. Carter considered herself to have taken although, from the foregoing narrative, there are several possibilities. I questioned the parents about their threats of litigation. The father readily admitted that they had considered litigation after a series of prescribing errors involving their children at PCH. While this might have caused Dr. Carter some concern, it was not a criterion for MSBP according to any published definition.

Later in the same e-mail string, Dr. Stephens pitched in, casting the net of parental abuse across the larger autism community: "If the children really have autism, the concerns of Dr. Carter has about the IVIG are diluted by the fact that many families do all sorts of crazy, nonscientific, and potentially dangerous things to their children with autism. . . . None of these crazy 'autism therapies' including IVIG are alleged of child abuse."[51]

What was it that led Dr. Carter and others to believe that the diagnosis of functional antibody deficiency was the pathological contrivance of two disordered and dangerous personalities? For the parents' part, they claim never to have heard of this rare diagnosis before meeting Dr. Hellmers. In support of this, Dr. Hellmers confirms having first suggested and then diagnosed the condition in the children. CPS's position is largely invested in the alleged inconsistency with which vaccination histories were reported by the parents. Having extensively reviewed the children's vaccination histories above, it is instructive to take a closer look at the views of CPS and its agents, starting with the e-mail string wherein Dr. Stephens opened on May 27, 2010: "First of all, I totally agree with Dr. Carter's concerns and assessment of the family and the potentially harmful IVIG therapies these children are receiving! I reviewed the records from Dr. Hellmers (Peds Allergy and Immunology) and Dr. Carter is absolutely correct. **The children have not been immunized; however**, Mom reported to Dr. Hellmers in his initial evaluation of [Child 1] that he had had all of his immunizations including the pneumonia shot (PCV [streptococcus pneumonia]). This vaccine, however, was not released by the FDA until 2000, and [Child 1] would already have been over the age of 3 so he would NOT have received this vaccine as part of a routine immunization series."[52]

Dr. Stephens continued: "In addition, Dr. Sipes (the PCP) documents in every note on each child that the parents refuse immunizations. I pulled the children up in ASIIS[53] **and only one child has a single vaccine (Td)[54] recorded.**" Then, she added, "**The parents report conflicting information to every provider about immunizations.**"[55]

Dr. Stephens was to reiterate these allegations in her official report of July 10, 2010. In her later report of October 7, 2010, she also wrote, "Dr. Hellmers made the diagnosis of functional antibody deficiency on the basis of his lab work that in itself was **based on history from the parents** as:

a)   Frequent infections, especially chronic sinusitis and pneumonia. **This was not true, see above** (where she had set out the children's infection histories),

b)   Immunization history of children receiving immunizations when they were young. **This is not true**, see the following."

Bizarrely, Dr. Stephens then provides a printout, presumably from ASIIS, that documented not the vaccinations that children 1–4 had received, but those that were due or past due. For some reason Child 5, who was unvaccinated, was not included. It did not seem to cross Dr. Stephens' mind that ASIIS might record only vaccines administered in the state of Arizona.

What is conflicting and false, without doubt, was the reporting of the children's vaccination status by CPS and its agents. Dr. Stephens initially claimed that the children had not been immunized, and then in the next paragraph she identified that one child had in fact received one vaccine. The truth is that, among them, they had received at least sixty vaccines.

In her report, the prosecution's MSBP expert, Dr. Mary Sanders, limited her comments on vaccination to the notion of parental confabulation in the case of Child 3 by linking his "false" diagnosis of autism to false parental claims that it was caused by vaccines.[56] She then presented the parents' immunization choice for their children as evidence for irresponsible parenting if not outright abuse. "They are also partially immunized or not at all, leaving them vulnerable to serious illness or death."[57]

HISTORY OF INFECTIONS

In her idiosyncratic English, Ms. Williams' communiqué to the group[58] on April 23, 2010, described the parents as "reporting too many infections to count on each child which are not supported by the primary care physician."

In support of this position, Dr. Stephens provided summaries of the children's infections in her second report on October 7, 2010, as evidence that they were not prone to infections by virtue of defective immune systems.

Child 1: "He has had 5 episodes of sinusitis, 2 strep throats infections and has not had episodes of pneumonia over the past 4 years."[59]

In fact, a review of Child 1's medical records from April 3, 1997, to November 5, 2001, alone, shows thirty-four episodes of upper respiratory tract and ear infections. Rather than having been unsupported by the primary care physician, Dr. McCarthy, these episodes were diagnosed and documented by her.

Child 2: "She has had 1 episode of sinusitis and 1 strep throat. She has no documented pneumonia over the past 4 years. This number of infections is not considered excessive or abnormal."[60]

The GP records document at least ten infections between May 18, 2000, and June 7, 2004.

Child 3: "He has had 1 episode of sinusitis and 1 strep throat. He has no documented pneumonia over the past 4 years. This number of infections is not considered excessive or abnormal."

The GP records from December 17, 2001, to June 3, 2004, document twenty-four clinical infections, mainly of the ears, upper and lower respiratory tract, and intestine.

Child 4: "He has had 3 episodes of sinusitis and 1 strep throat. He has no documented pneumonia over the past 4 years. This number of infections is not considered excessive or abnormal."[61]

No GP records on Child 4 were available for review.

Child 5: "He has had only 2 episodes of strep throat and 1 episode of pneumonia over the past 4 years. This number of infections is not considered excessive or abnormal."[62]

The parents deny ever having reported a history of excessive infections for Child 5, and this is supported by the documents. His records document five respiratory tract infections from November 8, 2004, to January 3, 2006.

SUMMARY

In the context of immunodeficiency and IVIG, the cornerstone of Dr. Carter's concerns, Williams, Carter, and Stephens had to contrive a charge sheet that grossly underrepresented the vaccination status and infection history for each child, misrepresented the parents' reporting of the children's immunizations and infections, entrapped the mother in a sting operation, and implicated an expert in pediatric allergy and immunology in a criminal conspiracy to defraud. The source of this contrivance appears to have been, at most, confusion as to when Prevnar became part of the routine immunization schedule on the one hand, and a "worked-up" Dr. Carter on the other. In contrast, the parents' reporting of infections and vaccinations in their children was consistent with their medical records from one physician to the next. Their actions in respect of IVIG were to follow Dr. Hellmers's orders in compliance with what they considered to be their children's best interests.

"Fair is Foul and Foul is Fair."[63]
Nothing was quite what it seemed.

TABLE 5. The children's immunization status

Child 1[64]

Vaccine	Date	Age	Site	Manufacturer	Lot No.	Initials
DTaP 1	5.15.97	2 mo	L leg	Led[65]	444.256	KM
DTaP 2	7.25.97	4 mo	L leg	Led	444.256	KM
DTaP 3	10.1.97	6 mo	L leg	Led	445.539	KM
DTaP 4	12.28.98	18 mo	L arm	Led	454.759	KM
DTaP 5	3.22.02	5 yr	LA	?	516A2	AP
Hib 1	5.15.97	2 mo	R leg	Led	MO35PE	KM
Hib 2	7.25.97	4 mo	R leg	Led	MO35PE	KM
Hib 3	10.1.97	6 mo	R leg	Led	M265RF	KM
Hib 4	6.17.98	15 mo	L arm	Led	M240RK	KM
Hep B 1	4.3.97	2 wk	L leg	MSD[66]	1283D	KM
Hep B 2	5.15.97	2 mo	L arm	MSD	1554D	KM
Hep B 3	12.16.97	9 mo	L arm	MSD	0746F	KM
OPV 1	5.15.97	2 mo	po	Led	0754B	KM
OPV 2	7.25.97	4 mo	po	Led	0754B	KM
OPV 3	12.28.98	18 m	po	Led	0794C	KM
IPV 4	3.22.02	5 yr	LA	Aventis	40179	AP
MMR 1	6.17.98	15 mo	RA	M	0507H	KM
MMR 2	3.22.02	5 yr	RA	Merck	1207L	AP
VZV 1[67]	3.9.01	4 yr	LA	Mer 5–02	0760K	AP

Child 2[68]

Vaccine	Date	Age	Site	Manufacturer	Lot No.	Initials
DTaP 1	12.28.98	2 mo	L leg	Ced	454.759	KM
DTaP 2	4.15.99	4 mo	L leg	SKB[69]	a888A2	KM
DTaP 3	6.4.99	6 mo	L leg	SKB	a888A2	RR
DTaP 4	11.8.01	3 yr	LA	SKB	a998A2	AP
DTaP 5	-	-	-	-	-	-
Hib 1	12.28.98	2 mo	R leg	?	36–1453a	KM
Hib 2	4.15.99	4 mo	R leg	L	402253A	KM
Hib 3	6.4.99	6 mo	R leg	L	402250A	RR
Hib 4	11.8.01	3 yr	LA	Lederle	481–561	AP
Hep B 1	11.19.98	2 wk	L leg	SKB	2719A2	KM
Hep B 2	12.28.98	2 mo	L leg	SKB	2719A2	KM
Hep B 3	8.10.99	9 mo	LL	M 5–01	1393H	RR
IPV 1	12.28.98	P (?)	R arm	C[70]	N06991	KM
IPV 2	4.15.99	F (?)	L arm	C	N0726	KM
IPV 3	2.17.00	15 mo	LA	4–01 C	P05522	KM
IPV 4	-	-	-	-	-	-
MMR 1	2.17.00	15 mo	RA	M	19824	KM
MMR 2	-	-	-	-	-	-
VZV 1	11.8.01	3 yr	RA	Merck	1333K	AP
VZV 2	-	-	-	-	-	-
RVV[71] 1	4.15.99	?	po	WL[72]	4988046	KM
RVV 2	12.28.98	2 mo	po	WL	12–99	RR
RVV 3	6.4.99	6 mo	po	WL	12–99	RR

Child 3[73]

Vaccine	Date	Age	Site	Manufacturer	Lot No.	Initials
DTaP 1	9/01					OC*
DTaP 2	1/02					OC*
DTaP 3	3/02					OC*
DTaP 4	12.16.02		LLT	-	UC849DA	JP CAD
DTaP 5	-	-	-	-	-	-
Hib 1	9/01					
Hib 2	3/02					
Hib 3	7/02					
Hib 4	12.16.02		LLT	-	UA786AB	JP CAD
Hep B 1	7/01					OC*
Hep B 2	9/01					OC*
Hep B 3	1/02					OC*
OPV 1	9/01					OC*
OPV 2	1/02					OC*
IPV 3	1.28.03	-	LA	Aventis	W0013	BK
IPV 4		-	-	-	-	-
MMR 1	12.16.02		RUL	Merck	1485L	JP
MMR 2	-	-	-	-	-	-
VZV 1	7/02					OC
Prevnar 1	12.16.02		-	Led	485–045	JP
Prevnar 2	1.28.03		-	Led	485–991	BK

OC* given at outside center.

Child 4[74]

Vaccine	Date	Age	Site	Manufacturer	Lot No.	Initials
DTaP 1	1.28.03		LAT	?	V0846DA	BK
DTaP 2	-	-	-	-	-	-
DTaP 3	-	-	-	-	-	-
DTaP 4	-	-	-	-	-	-
DTaP 5	-	-	-	-	-	-
Hib 1	1.28.03			Aventis	UB3234A	BK
Hib 2	-	-	-	-	-	-
Hib 3	-	-	-	-	-	-
Hib 4	-	-	-	-	-	-
Hep B 1	12.16.02		LLT	?SKB	5346A2	?
Hep B 2	-	-	-	-	-	-
Hep B 3	-	-	-	-	-	-
IPV 1	1.28.03	-	RT	Aventis	W0013	BK
IPV 2	-	-	-	-	-	-
IPV 3	-	-	-	-	-	-
IPV 4	-	-	-	-	-	-
MMR 1	-	-	-	-	-	-
MMR 2	-	-	-	-	-	-
VZV 1	-	-	-	-	-	-
Prevnar 1	1.28.03		RAT		485–991	BK
Prevnar 2						

Chapter 15

DR. MARY J. SANDERS: EXPERT WITNESS FOR THE PROSECUTION

Iconfess from the outset that I have a problem with Dr. Sanders.[1] The following analysis may shed some light on the source of my dyspeptic chagrin. Dr. Sanders is a clinical associate professor and the program director of the Comprehensive Care Unit at Stanford. When not acting on behalf of CPS in the prosecution of alleged MSBP, she teaches and works with inpatients with eating disorders. She has, in her own words, "written extensively and presented nationally on the subject of the evaluation and treatment of eating disorders and also in the field of child abuse, specifically in the area of Münchausen by proxy."[2]

Dr. Sanders was an expert for CPS in the case of the Arizona 5. In 2002, she, in collaboration with her colleague Dr. Brenda Bursch from the University of California, Los Angeles, provided published guidance for the systematic forensic evaluation of possible MSBP cases for the purpose of providing expert testimony.[3] This guidance is referred to below in the context of her analysis and expert evidence in the case of the Arizona 5.

Incidentally, Dr. Bursch (Dr. Sanders's colleague) has also acted against parents on behalf of the prosecution in Arizona and currently faces an inquiry into her professional conduct in this respect.[4] She is subject to a complaint screening hearing in Arizona where she is alleged to have practiced without a license. The complaint involves a baby with a GI disorder and a mother who was accused of having MSBP. While this particular case does not involve autism, many of Dr. Bursch's Arizona cases apparently do. The common theme seems to be, as with the Arizona 5, biomedical treatment—including the use of special diets—being labeled as abusive.

It is worth noting with no small irony that even Professor Meadow, disgraced for abusing his brainchild MSBP, considered this to be a rare condition.[5] He emphasized that the diagnosis was itself vulnerable to abuse: ironically, the abuse of over-reporting. Sanders and Bursch seem to take the opposite view, speculating in their guidance that "many incidents of MSBP may go undetected and/or unreported."[6]

From the outset, this gave a flavor of the authors' bias; according to Sanders and Bursch, ascertainment of true MSBP is likely to be substantially incomplete, missing many cases. Alternatively, they acknowledge only that "some children are erroneously identified."[7] But, according to them, it is not like the many who may be missed. Sanders and Bursch recognized that false-positive diagnoses are made, but they seemed more concerned about those cases that slip under the radar. Their paper betrays little in the way of empathy for the victims of false allegations of MSBP.

In contrast, Professor Long reported the disquieting views of Dr. Loren Pankratz, an Oregon psychologist who is widely published on the subject of MSBP and whose concern was also for those falsely accused. On this topic, Dr. Pankratz wrote the following: "My clinical experience with MSBP has convinced me that the problems with this diagnosis are far more extensive than the concerns I raised in my earlier writings. The medical literature on MSBP often mentions false accusations, or the possibility of false accusations, but does not convey the prevalence of these misunderstandings or the devastating consequences of a wrong diagnosis."[8]

Set against MSBP/FDBP's short but turbulent history, including the fact that the diagnosis has now been withdrawn throughout the European Union,[9] when Dr. Sanders was asked in court if factitious disorder by proxy is a diagnosis surrounded by controversy, she answered, "I don't know about a lot. No. There's always some, yeah."[10]

Well, what is it, Dr. Sanders? In excess of 5,000 hits on Google for MSBP and controversy together would suggest that the "yeahs" have it. In fact, along with autism, MSBP is probably the most controversial diagnosis in medicine—the debate du jour. But in her report to the court on the Arizona 5 and their parents (as opposed to her oral testimony), there was no such equivocation. Dr. Sanders opened with a "Summary and Conclusions" section, where her indictment of the parents was delivered in the first line: "The present evaluation finds that both parents have falsified and exaggerated important, medically relevant information."

While a past history of wrongdoing is inadmissible in criminal proceedings, Dr. Sanders wasted no time in bringing to her readers' attention the fact that mother had, in the past, been "accused of sexually abusing her first daughter."[11]

The purpose of my analysis is to determine whether or not this family has been treated fairly and justly in the matter of alleged MSBP. For justice to be done and be seen to be done, both sides of any argument must be put before those who sit in judgment in order to avoid undue bias. In her forensic review, Dr. Sanders appears to have been keenly aware that matters of bias should be identified and dealt with. In her 2002 paper, when laying out the ground rules for forensic assessors, she wrote:

> The forensic evaluator must address only questions they are asked and qualified to answer and must do so in a scientific and **unbiased**[12] manner.
>
> Ideally, the evaluator is "court-appointed," which means that they are being asked directly by the court to provide information. As such, there is no appearance that the expert is **biased** for one side or another.
>
> Although an expert can legally be hired by one side, with or without the agreement of all parties, efforts to address the real and/or perceived presence of **bias** are important.[13]

In the case of the Arizona 5, Dr. Sanders was hired by CPS for the prosecution and was not appointed by the court; so, as far as being unbiased is concerned, she was not off to a good start.

Given Dr. Sanders' sensitivity to the issue of bias, real and perceived, and less than ideally in the pay of the State, it is perplexing as to why she allowed her reference to the accusation of sexual abuse by the mother to be left hanging, vulnerable, as it was, to prejudicial inference. This matter was mentioned briefly in Part 3, Chapter 1. In 1991 the mother, a single mom of twenty-seven years old, was imprisoned pending arraignment and her two-year-old daughter taken from her and put into foster care for one year after the mother called a community helpline in Syracuse, New York, to enquire as to whether, among other things, it was normal to feel sexually aroused by breastfeeding. Police immediately arrested the mother and criminal charges were filed. The case came to Criminal Court and was thrown out by the judge. CPS filed further charges in Family Court that were summarily dismissed by a second judge. CPS subsequently went judge shopping only to have the case rejected a third time. Finally the mother successfully sued CPS. Her accusers capitulated and CPS settled the case with an award of damages to the mother.

Nowhere in Dr. Sanders' report is there any mention of the mother's innocence on the one hand and the guilt of CPS on the other: findings in law that might have helped mitigate the perception of bias on the part of Dr. Sanders. In an interview, the mother had made Dr. Sanders fully aware of the facts of the case, but they appeared not to have suited the latter's case. Later, during cross-examination, it was put to Dr. Sanders that she was "aware that the Court found no evidence of sexual abuse by mother."[14]

Having acknowledged this, Dr. Sanders was asked why she had not included this information in her report. She claimed that she had. The fact is that, whereas she had given prominence to the issue of sexual abuse in the first paragraph of her twenty-page report, any facts about the outcome were buried enigmatically in a single sentence on page sixteen that explicitly did not say that two courts had found no evidence of sexual abuse by the mother. One may simply be left by Dr. Sanders with the impression of a recidivist child abuser looking for her next victim.

As her report progressed, Dr. Sanders continued to sow the seed of parental dysfunction. In her second paragraph, she wrote that "both [father and mother] have exaggerated their professional backgrounds. They have both stated they are nurses on numerous occasions."[15]

It is a matter of fact that the mother was a nurse. Confirmation that she was qualified as a licensed practical nurse (LPN, not "PVN" as written[16] or "LVN" as stated[17] by Dr. Sanders) was easily verified. Indeed, a copy of the mother's professional license had been provided to the prosecution, Dr. Sanders' employers in this matter, well in advance of the court proceedings. Nonetheless, Dr. Sanders' only disingenuous reference to the mother's nursing qualification is that "it has not been verified."

In light of the above, it must be concluded that Dr. Sanders made no effort to verify the mother's claim. It was easily done, and I have a copy of her license.[18] Instead, Dr. Sanders preferred to establish and maintain a climate of dishonesty and mistrust—one which she perpetuated in court where she stated, "I think that she was promoting herself as an RN [registered nurse] rather than LVN [sic] was my impression." Asked if there was any evidence for this, she responded, "I am not sure about that."[19]

The mother had never promoted herself as an RN. The prosecution's main expert was coming adrift. Despite this, in redirect examination by the prosecution lawyer it was put to Dr. Sanders that, as a matter of fact, the parents had actually admitted to her that they had falsified their nursing claims. In turn, Dr. Sanders acknowledged that this falsification was a good sign of factitious disorder by proxy.[20]

I can find no evidence at all in support of the claim that the father stated he was a nurse at any time, let alone "on numerous occasions." Dr. Sanders cites two examples of the father's alleged claims: i.e., that he once said (apparently at the time of Child 1's discharge from PCH) that he "could take over the nursing himself."[21]

When the time comes, I hope to be able to nurse my dying mother, but I make no claim to being a nurse. It is interesting that Dr. Mart provided a similar analogy of his own father, also not a nurse, nursing his dying wife during her final days, in rebutting Dr. Sanders' allegation. During cross-examination, Dr. Sanders reiterated the claim that the father had said he was a nurse multiple times.[22] As an example of this multiplicity, she cites only one further episode that, so far, I have not been able to identify in the medical records. She stated, "He indicated he was a nurse on February 27, 2009, he said—the father said that he should have pulled out the IV and left because he was a nurse."[23]

When questioned about this episode, the father explained that Child 1's discharge from hospital had been delayed by three hours because no one had come to remove his IV. What he had apparently said was, "I could take it out quicker than you guys."[24]

He denied ever having mentioned the word "nurse," let alone that he was one. So far, the gulf between what Dr. Sanders has alleged and what the documentary evidence does and does not show is very wide. At the heart of many of Dr. Sanders' problems with these parents is that, as vigorous advocates for their children, they had created friction. Where they had identified deficiencies in the system or in their children's care, they had taken issue. When, in 2005, they realized that their children's school had zero dollars for special education, they protested, and things improved. Where prescribed or recommended treatments were being withheld, as in the case of steroids for Child 1 and IVIG for Child 2,[25] they protested. As an example of their "troublemaking" (my word), Dr. Sanders cites a specific instance where "they fought with the school over situations they said could harm their children (i.e., protesting a mist medicine)."

Unfortunately, for those seeking to put this allegation into context, no further details were provided by Dr. Sanders. This incident actually involved the mass vaccination of pupils in Yavapai schools with the FluMist vaccine, delivered by nasal spray. This live-virus influenza vaccine is transmissible and, therefore, a potential danger to any person who is immunodeficient. This risk is documented by the vaccine's manufacturers and Dr. Schneider provided the parents with a letter to this effect for them to present to the school. In light of Child 3's physician-diagnosed immune system problems, the parents had asked to be notified by Child 3's school when the vaccinations were due to take place, but the school failed to do so. There was, however, no fight with the school; rather, the mother called an official of Yavapai County, requesting that the vaccination program be performed somewhere other than school since this would have been less disruptive. According to her, the response of county officials was to refer the parents to CPS for having taken Child 3 to school at the time of the immunization program (albeit unknowingly), thereby putting him in danger from FluMist exposure.

Any parent of a child with special needs, and autism in particular, will know the daily struggle of advocating for your child, running the seemingly infinite gauntlet of bureaucracy, and fighting a system that will sometimes only respond to the threat of litigation. Such parents should be commended, not vilified. Rather, Dr. Sanders appeared to interpret such advocacy as symptomatic of some malevolent psychopathology.

Dr. Sanders came next to the various diagnoses that the parents had apparently claimed for their children, diagnoses that "evaluations of the children since removal from the home indicate that none of the children have . . . "[26] Her claims related to autism, mitochondrial disorder, functional antibody disorder, and multiple environmental and food allergies. Errors and misrepresentations with respect to all of these issues have been discussed in previous chapters. My response may seem pedantic, but that is the nature of the law that presides over this issue. It is a matter of documented fact that they all *had* [tense: past imperfect] a diagnosis of an autistic spectrum disorder (ASD). Whether, at the time of their evaluation after removal from home, they continued to *have* an autistic disorder, the present tense used by Dr. Sanders, is a matter of interest but has no bearing on the parents' stated position. Can a patient with an ASD recover to the extent that they lose their diagnosis? Yes[27] is the answer, and if this were not the case, then the National Institutes of Health would not be studying children who have reportedly done so.[28]

In the matter of autism and Child 3, Dr. Sanders wrote that "[Child 3] was evaluated at 33 months in NY and was found not to have autism. However the parents went to Arizona and presented him as having autism."[29]

The unambiguous implication is that the parents had lied. In the light of this allegation, it is worth briefly reiterating Child 3's developmental history. Readers will remember that Child 3 *was* originally diagnosed in Syracuse, New York, on July 29, 2003, at twenty-four months old, with multiple developmental delays, motor delays, and a disorder of sensory regulation. The parents had sought out Dr. Schneider in Phoenix because of Child 3's possible lead poisoning and longstanding diarrhea. When the mother and son went to see Dr. Schneider, the latter's records, dated April 19, 2004, describe the stated reason for this clinical consultation as Child 3's "developmental delays and associated medical concerns."

This was an accurate representation of this child's prior assessment in New York, and the mother did not present him as having autism. Indeed, in view of his lack of aloofness (that is, his sociable nature), the mother had actually considered it unlikely that her son had an ASD. In light of his behavioral symptoms, including his later absence of joint attention, it was Dr. Schneider who diagnosed

Child 3 with ASD. There is absolutely no evidence of which I am aware to support Dr. Sanders' allegation that "the parents went to Arizona and presented him as having autism."[30]

Dr. Sanders made no mention of the fact that Dr. Schneider was the one who made the ASD diagnosis initially; in addition, she appears to have made no effort to interview Dr. Schneider on this crucial point—or at all. As presented, Dr. Sanders' report leads the reader to believe that the parents were confabulating to Dr. Schneider about the New York diagnosis. There is nothing in the records in my possession to suggest that the parents either questioned this initial diagnosis or took issue with it, and they deny ever having done so. Also inconsistent with Dr. Sanders' version of events is that, in her assessment on July 25, 2006, Dr. Rice makes no mention of the mother claiming that her child had autism. On this occasion and on the basis of her finding that Child 3 had deficits in the three core problem areas of autism—social skills, communication, and behavior—Dr. Rice also diagnosed this boy with an ASD.

Later in her report, pursuing the tack that the parents had preferred an autism diagnosis for their son and had rejected professional advice to the contrary, Dr. Sanders rendered the opinion that since "the evaluation at 33 months indicated that he was not autistic, they did not accept it and went to the Autism Center in Arizona."

This allegation has the effect of leading the reader to believe that, seeking reinforcement in their abusive mind-warp, Child 3's disgruntled parents took him to Arizona specifically in the hunt for an autism diagnosis. The records of Dr. Schneider and Dr. Rice make it clear that this was not the case at all. Moreover, Dr. Sanders' chronology is wrong: Child 3 had already received a diagnosis of an ASD from Dr. Schneider on April 19, 2004, before his second appointment with the developmental team in New York on April 29, 2004, when he was thirty-three months old. Dr. Sanders has completely misrepresented the basis for the family attending Dr. Schneider's autism center and has done so by omitting reference to Child 3's initial assessment in New York, thereby reversing events to put the visit to Dr. Schneider after the follow-up evaluation in New York.

Dr. Sanders continued with "I do not know the influence of the Autism Center on the parents' apparent dedication to the diagnosis of autism for [Child 3] and how this story may have spread to include all the children."[31]

The documentary evidence indicates that the parents accepted the initial diagnosis of developmental delay from New York. The evidence also supports the fact that they took issue with the second New York diagnosis only after Dr. Schneider had made a diagnosis of ASD in Child 3 and identified the inadequacy of the services being provided for him in New York. Dr. Sanders' interpretation of the facts is full of the most basic errors that color, at every turn, the reader's view of these parents. Her pejorative allusion on the one hand to the parents' "dedication to the diagnosis of autism,"[32] as though they were lashed to the helm of a ghost ship, and on the other, the possible spreading of this story to include all the children, like a septic contagion, has no basis in fact.

The matter is a simple one: did Child 3 have a developmental disorder? The answer is yes. Was this developmental disorder diagnosed as an ASD? The answer is yes, by two doctors, Dr. Schneider and Dr. Rice. Did the parents accurately report to doctors their understanding of the developmental diagnosis in Child 3? The answer, again, is yes.

Further on in her published guidelines on the forensic analysis of suspected MSBP, Dr. Sanders wrote that "the creation of a table is extremely helpful. The table should include the following information for each healthcare contact: name of patient, date, location, reason for contact, reported signs/symptoms as stated by caregiver, objective observations documented by healthcare provider, conclusions/diagnoses made, treatment provided, efficacy of treatment, and other comments or observations."

One of the most significant objective pathologic findings in Child 3 was his clinical, endoscopic, and microscopic diagnosis of eosinophilic gastroenteritis and gastroesophageal reflux disease, clearly consistent with food allergy. As discussed in some detail in Part 1, Chapter 3, food allergy may be integral to both GI and behavioral/developmental problems in some affected children. This subject had been described in considerable detail in the medical and scientific literature by 2010. Given the relevant contemporaneous literature and the significance of Child 3's GI pathology, these findings should have featured prominently in *any* forensic table compiled in the investigation of possible MSBP. They did not. Dr. Sanders made no reference to Child 3's positive food allergy testing under the care of Dr. Schneider and again under the care of Dr. Hellmers. She made no reference to the stool test undertaken by Dr. Bradstreet, the autism specialist, that was among the original pointers to food allergic intestinal disease. Dr. Sanders made no reference to Child 3's beneficial cognitive and GI responses to exclusion diet and acid blockers. In the matter of food allergy, she did, however, refer exclusively to the negative testing for IgE-mediated food allergy ordered by CPS.

Turning back to her published guidelines, Dr. Sanders' wrote that "the forensic evaluator must address only questions they are asked and qualified to answer and must do so in a scientific and unbiased manner."[33]

Dr. Sanders' opinion on food allergy, if only offered by proxy, was emphatic. Despite being a major plank of her allegations against the parents, it was also wrong. While it was quite clear that she was not qualified to address the issue of food allergy, it was unacceptable for her to have exceeded her duty as expert and cherry-picked the records in order to include the negative test results while omitting the overwhelmingly positive evidence of food allergic disease in Child 3. Therefore, her ability to accurately review such records more broadly must also be in doubt.

When questioned in court about the physical symptoms consistent with possible recrudescence of food allergies in Child 3, Child 4, and Child 5 following cessation of their exclusion diet in foster care, she offered as an alternative, "I am wondering if they have come to believe that these foods make them ill."[34]

She was pressed further: "Do you think those statements are indicative of allergies?"[35] She responded, "It wouldn't be my impression. My impression was that they thought that the foods made them ill."[36]

In the field of food allergy, Dr. Sanders is a know-nothing. Her willingness to opine on such symptoms shows lack of insight. It would have been a simple step, but vital in the assimilation of her evidence, to have spoken with Dr. Schneider and Dr. Ursea. Indeed, PCH's policy for the investigation of confirmed or suspected cases of MSBP required that they be "investigated and managed using a multidisciplinary team (MDT) comprised of involved professionals, including the assigned CPS specialist, the supervisor, **the treating medical doctor,**[37] a psychiatrist, Attorney General staff, and law enforcement."

Where was the treating doctor? Where in CPS' inquisition was there a physician who had been involved in the diagnostic process for the children's physical ailments—allegedly false ailments that for the inquisitors seemed to confound the diagnosis of autism? Where were Dr. Sanders' interviews with these key players? In fact, not one doctor who had seen and treated any of these children prior to their removal from home was called to give evidence by the prosecution, a fact that is itself astonishing.

Her apparent concern for thoroughness and objectivity is expressed in her guidance paper: "Also after completion of the record review, the evaluator may need to consult the medical team or other medical experts (in the specific area of symptom presentation) to address the unusual medical findings as to their differential diagnosis of the symptoms."[38]

Toward the end of her report, under the heading "Phone Consult with Physicians and Collaterals," Dr. Sanders listed the doctors in the specific area of symptom presentation that had been involved in the children's care and with whom she had spoken. Notable for their absence were Dr. Schneider, the treating physician, and Dr. Ursea, the gastroenterologist. These were two key figures in the children's medical management and, in particular, the diagnosis of their intestinal diseases and food allergies. Dr. Sanders sought to qualify her omissions by adding, "I called several others, but did not hear back in time. However, they have apparently given input to Dr. Stephens."[39]

Dr. Sanders did call Dr. Hellmers, apparently from her car when, according to Dr. Hellmers, he was busy with patients. She introduced herself as a doctor without mentioning that she was, in fact, a psychologist. This is uncannily reminiscent of passing oneself off as one thing, say a registered nurse (RN), while qualified as something materially different, say a licensed practical nurse (LPN). While, according to Dr. Hellmers, Dr. Sanders bombarded him with questions about the family, he correctly refused to answer on the basis that he would have been in violation of patient privacy under the Health Insurance Portability and Accountability Act (HIPAA). He reiterated his professional duties to the family later in court, when prosecution attorneys sought to present him as a less than cooperative witness.

Among those who apparently gave input to Dr. Stephens, Dr. Sanders listed Dr. Ursea but not Dr. Schneider. Unfortunately, there was nothing in the only two reports provided by Dr. Stephens, dated June 10, 2010, and October 7, 2010, respectively, or in the e-mail string referred to in Part 4, Chapter 1, that mentioned her having had any contact with Dr. Ursea at all. Between them, Dr. Sanders and Dr. Stephens had, in my opinion, ridden roughshod over the evidence and the Sanders-Brusch guidelines in their relentless pursuit of von Münchausen's mirage.

Given Dr. Sanders' lack of expertise in all medical matters—particularly gastroenterology and immunology—was there provision in her MSBP Forensics 101 for dealing with complex issues in which the evaluators were out of their depth? Fortunately, she and her colleague Dr. Bursch had provided for this eventuality: "It is important to note that a non-physician may compile, organize, and analyze the **behavior patterns**[40] revealed in medical records but may not make medical diagnoses unless they have a qualification that would allow them to do so. Therefore, it is useful to have a physician or other qualified medical care provider also review the records if needed."[41]

Given the complex medical matters in this case and the grave issues at stake, one would imagine that an independent expert review of the children's records would have been deemed essential before labeling them abused and irreparably damaging their family. This precautionary step would have allowed Dr. Sanders the opportunity to determine the extent to which objective, clinically documented medical disease in these children should have mitigated her enthusiasm for a diagnosis of MSBP. As Dr. Mart, a psychologist giving expert evidence of behalf of the parents, pointed out, if the medical evidence shows that these children are ill, then MSBP effectively becomes a moot point.

In support of this, a paper by authors Bass and Adshead reinforced the fact that the identification and confirmation of cases "relies heavily on pediatric assessment and investigation, and the exclusion of other causes for the child's 'symptoms.'"[42] While Bass and Adshead advocated for the reality of MSBP as an induced illness in the face of fierce criticism of the syndrome's validity following acquittal of mothers in the UK courts, they recognized and conceded that "detection requires detailed and painstaking enquiry involving the collection of data from many different sources." All and any such data have to be factored into whether an MSBP diagnosis is tenable.

The GI findings alone confirmed that the children were ill. These illnesses, which should have made the claim of MSBP moot, were not factored in by Dr. Sanders. Therefore, one has to ask why. Presumably it was because this would have disturbed her argument. Nothing in Dr. Sanders' report indicates that she had had any physician or suitably qualified healthcare professional, which she was not, review the records.

In contrast with her method of dealing with this case, her expert guidance continued with "the evaluator must be able to review all available medical records and any other records the evaluator deems important." Due, in her own words, "to the volume of records," it is not certain that Dr. Sanders reviewed the entirety of the medical records.[43] In the "Summary and Conclusions" to her report, she refers to a table (referred to as Appendix A) that incorporates "a partial review of the records that seem pertinent." Whether or not it is the case that the entire records were reviewed, given the earlier appearance of bias, the absence of an evaluation of what did not, to her, seem pertinent—such as Child 3's obvious intestinal disease—would be most unfortunate.

Dr. Sanders' guidelines continued with "common mistakes made when a medical record review is performed include failing to:

a)   identify or consider the source of information,
b)   examine primary data (test results, rather than simply the interpretation of test results),
c)   evaluate if healthcare provider diagnoses or conclusions match objective data,
d)   consider if objective findings could have been falsified or induced, and
e)   consider if the medical record makes sense."[44]

Given the myriad failings in Dr. Sanders' report to this point, it seems almost gratuitous to dwell upon the extent to which she had fallen afoul of her own points (a) to (e). Adding only confusion, her guidelines offered her readers a conundrum by way of warning: "It is strongly recommended that experts refrain from evaluating for possible illness falsification when this condition cannot be met."[45] It is difficult to understand how one is to determine whether or not the condition for a disorder can be met when this possibility has not been evaluated.

In my opinion, in court, her status as an expert also left a great deal to be desired. She rendered two key observations that inevitably would have had a profound effect on any judge ruling on dependency. First, she claimed that for MSBP, 3–20% of cases lead to the child's death. Secondly, she claimed that the likelihood of these parents reoffending was high.[46] When asked in cross-examination to cite her reference that supported these statements in the medical literature, she struggled, unable to remember the journal name. When pressed to quote the statistics that the study reported, she could not.[47] This is not what one expects of an expert.

DISEASE FALSIFICATION

Phoenix Children's Hospital and CPS, the Attorney General's Office and the Arizona Department of Economic Security, in collaboration with the Comprehensive Care Unit of Stanford School of Medicine's Child and Adolescent Psychiatry department, can lay claim to a new syndrome. It may be one that they would rather forgo and forget. The syndrome looks at first like a smiling braggart, the lying baron himself. But drawn from the cauldron of a quartet of well-meaning women, conjured from the confusion of smoke and steam, the specter is an illusion. It exists only on the basis of exaggeration, distortion, and fabrication. It has been allowed to ferment under a cloak of fear and secrecy, and the lives of seven innocent people have been denatured in its poisonous broth.

Chapter 16

RECHALLENGE: "THE MOST UNKINDEST CUT OF ALL."

Julius Caesar. Act 3, Scene 2.

US Court of Federal Claims: On March 14, 2005, Dillon Pearson received DTaP, MMR, and Hepatitis A vaccinations. Petitioners allege that Child Doe/87 suffered an acute allergic reaction immediately after receipt of the vaccinations and developed gastrointestinal and behavioral symptoms as a consequence of these vaccinations. The case was settled by the Secretary of the Department of Health and Social Services.[1]

Vaccines are a cause of ASD and autism-like symptoms. Why is the "and" necessary since autism is a diagnosis that is based exclusively upon the presenting behavioral and developmental symptoms? Because "autism-like symptoms"— language used in cases of compensated vaccine damage—may not have qualified for a diagnosis of full syndrome autism or even autism spectrum disorder. While helpful in some respects, the limitations of man-made criteria have been exposed by the increasing recognition that autism exists on a continuum of developmental disability and does not stand alone as an all-or-none disorder. The significance of this point is that the National Vaccine Injury Compensation Program, having conceded vaccine damage on a behavioral spectrum ranging from "behavioral symptoms"[2] through "autism-like symptoms" to full-blown autism, has also laid bare the potential that the repertoire of developmental damage caused by vaccines is a potentially vast continuum, ranging widely in the degrees of severity and disability.

The first probable vaccine-associated case of autism reported in the medical literature was that of Rutter et al. in 1994.[3] By 2010, the public domain boasted just a handful of cases of vaccine injury, conceded by the Department of Justice or won in vaccine court, where the damage—encephalitis (brain inflammation) or encephalopathy (non-specific brain damage)—resulted in an ASD.[4] Enthusiastically, but with, nonetheless, a tangible anxiety, officials dismissed these cases as rare and irrelevant to the autism-vaccine debate. But in 2011, in a landmark paper by Mary Holland and colleagues, who had gone behind the scenes of the US Vaccine Injury Compensation Program (VICP), it was revealed that the government had settled at least eighty-three cases of vaccine damage where the child was rendered autistic.[5] Vaccine damage had been masked by government officials, wittingly or unwittingly, as the precipitating acute vaccine reaction (e.g., encephalitis) and not the actual outcome—autism. The reason that many of these cases had been settled is because they represent injuries on the Vaccine Injury Table, that is, encephalitis, encephalopathy, or residual seizure disorder with onset in a short and specific time frame following vaccination.[6] The very restrictive criteria applied to such injuries are defined by the weight of the scientific evidence. It would be disingenuous, therefore, to argue that these cases are due to anything but true adverse vaccine reactions. Moreover, given the parsimonious conditions applied to the definition of table injuries and the absence of adequate safety data on combination vaccines in particular, the number of compensated children with autism and autism-like symptoms will be a substantial underestimate of the true state of affairs. Meanwhile, among the major networks, what should have been a news story of huge public interest with widespread coverage and analysis, Fox TV alone ran with it.

In my opinion, vaccines are very likely the proximate cause of the current autism epidemic. The evidence indicates a possible role for a number of vaccines and their components in ASD, possibly through a synergistic toxicity. Younger age of exposure to MMR is a risk factor for autism,[7] and an acute adverse reaction to MMR may predict a greater risk of autism.[8] Aluminum, the principal adjuvant in many vaccines, kills brain cells.[9] The likelihood that the ethylmercury based preservative/adjuvant Thimerosal is a contributing cause to autism is high. A recent scientific review showed that 74% of the published studies supported such a link, while the official doctrine/public relations fantasia is that the link has been ruled out by the science.[10] Most importantly, perhaps, aluminum, Thimerosal, and MMR drive the immune system into a state of potentially synergistic imbalance favoring allergy and autoimmunity; however, shamefully, their interaction remains unstudied.

The senior architects of the US vaccine program, the US government, ex-regulators, the Institute of Medicine, and a growing cadre of scientists have conceded that vaccines are not simply unavoidably unsafe,[11] as the CDC has claimed, but that the safety studies have simply not been done[12]—studies that could have helped to avoid many injuries in the first place. But manufacturers are not liable for damage from recommended vaccines. And if you face no liability, why be unnecessarily vigilant in matters of safety? In fact, there has been a conscious, deliberate, and cynical neglect of the necessary science in dereliction of a moral, ethical, and professional duty on the part of those responsible. Many doctors have forsaken their primary duty to their patients in what has become a relentless march of dollars.

Adverse rulings in vaccine court against autism test cases in the Omnibus Autism Proceeding hearings[13] have been compounded more recently by a Supreme Court ruling that protects manufacturers from vaccine design defects. Recourse to civil litigation by plaintiff parents of vaccine-injured children is no longer possible.[14] These events have, barring an act of Congress, removed any safety net for parents who wish to file a claim for damages on the basis that their children's autism was caused by vaccines.

Arizona, in common with many other states, still has philosophical, medical, and religious exemptions to vaccination that allow parents to make vaccination choices on behalf of their children. As we have seen from an analysis of their medical records, at least some of the children in the case of the Arizona 5 have what appears to be a vaccine injury. From the perspective of someone who has been involved with thousands of similar cases and who has observed recovery, to a greater or lesser extent, from a gut-immune-brain injury, the records show that, in this case, the parents' diligence and perseverance paid off. Years of effort, education, advocacy, determination, and hard cash had improved their children's well-being and developmental status. Child 3, the most obviously vaccine injured, lost his diagnosis of autism by the age of approximately nine years, very likely through biomedical intervention.

In light of these factors—the established vaccine-autism link, inherent vaccine defects, the recognized deficiencies in vaccine safety science, the lack of a legal safety net, Arizona laws that allow parental vaccine choice, and the children's painstaking recovery—state-enforced vaccination of these children would seem like an act of barbarism.

But even before the parents had got to court, the State, having seized their children, was straining at the leash to have them caught up on their vaccines. In fact, depriving their children of protection from vaccines against disease and death has been cited by agents of the state as evidence of parental abuse.[15] The State's case was something of a logical fallacy, however: usually in MSBP it would be the norm that craving excess medical resources and interventions was part and parcel of the parents' abusive malady. On this very point, the father had been accused of urging, indeed forcing doctors to stick needles into his children.[16] And yet when it came to needles on the ends of syringes that contained vaccines, they had resisted their craving? Was the parents' presumed motive in forgoing this gratification and not vaccinating in order to deliberately have the children fall seriously ill upon contact with contagious disease? And yet, if this were the case, then why had the parents expressly asked to be informed about the mass FluMist immunization program in the children's school in order that they might avoid exposing their most vulnerable child, Child 3? And if they had wanted to harm their children, if only subconsciously, then, in the knowledge that mercury is a powerful poison, would they not have embraced the administration of Thimerosal? What unnatural precedent in medical and legal history were these parents hoping to set?

For the clear-thinking Dr. Jacobsen, head of Ambulatory Pediatrics at PCH, the parents' rights were irrelevant, presumably redundant in his eyes for their having curdled the milk of human kindness.[17] For him, vaccination was not a matter of "if" but of "when." On July 15, 2010, he wrote, "Once we have a court-ordered approval from CPS we will begin immunizations. General Pediatrics @ Phoenix Children's Hospital follows the AAP and CDC recommendations for immunizations."[18]

He attached the relevant schedule. Ironically, in 2011 it required many new vaccines; because the older children, in particular, had been exempt they now faced getting more vaccines as part of a catch-up than they would have done if their parents had complied with state mandates in the first place. The parents were understandably terrified for the well-being of their children. On July 20, 2010, Jennifer Kupiszewski, the father's lawyer, filed an objection to the State's motion to vaccinate the children. The objections were based upon the parents' personal experience with Child 3, in particular, and on the fact that vaccines can harm as evidenced by compensation awarded to nearly two and a half thousand children in the VICP to the tune of almost two billion dollars.[19] They argued that parenting was a fundamental right and that, according to legal precedent,[20] parents retain residual rights and responsibilities over vaccine choice even when their children are in state custody.[21] They presented medical exemptions for their children from Dr. Schneider and cited a clearly documented medical rationale for such exemptions. Ms. Kupiszewski concluded that "The parents have a fundamental right to control the upbringing of their children and that right did not evaporate when the State took legal custody. Arizona law affirms and honors the parents' rights regarding the decision to vaccinate their children."[22]

She ended by pointing out the willingness of the State and its medical appointees to ride roughshod over the Constitution and its citizens' rights: "The request to vaccinate the children, an irreversible procedure, indicates that ADES and the children's treating physician do not respect the parents' constitutional rights, their beliefs, or their relationship with their children."[23]

On August 3, 2010, ADES responded by putting out their case for why it was in their interest to " . . . invade the rights of the parent."[24] They cited ADES' requirements to provide comprehensive medical care for each child placed in a foster home and consent to a minimum of mumps, rubella, smallpox, and polio vaccination. They argued that, in the case of dependent children, legal precedent for exemption was confined to objections on religious grounds. The compelling state interest, however, was a utilitarian one: protection not only for the children but for those who come into contact with the children from potentially dangerous contagious disease.

They dismissed the children's medical exemptions on the basis that these had relied on parental fabrication, e.g., misdiagnosis based on falsified immunization histories, citing as an example Dr. Stephens' letter of June 10, 2010. Inevitably, ADES rejected the parents concerns over Child 3's adverse vaccine reaction, the parent's principal reason for having abandoned further vaccination and obtaining exemptions. ADES claimed that the parents " . . . do not provide any medical documentation of the described reaction."[25]

Consistent with ADES' version of events is Dr. Sanders' expert report of September 27, 2010, when she documented, under "Phone Consult with Physicians and Collaterals," her conversation with Dr. Katherine McCarthy, the children's pediatrician from New York. It was in this medical practice, and often by the hand of Dr. McCarthy herself, that vaccines had been administered to Children 1, 2, and 3. With reference to this conversation, Dr. Sanders wrote, "When asked about immunizations . . . it is her memory that they had immunizations with no problems reported."[26]

This is simply not true, as Dr. McCarthy's own records on Child 3 confirmed. She had documented his progressively severe behavioral and physical problems, ascribed contemporaneously to his eighteen-month immunizations [see Part 3, Chapter 4]. According to Dr. Sanders, Dr. McCarthy also stated that "she is certain that she would not have allowed the parents to refuse immunizations. If the parents refuse to immunize, she does not treat them in her practice."[27]

This is also complete fabrication as the medical records confirmed that on September 11, 2003, Dr. McCarthy documented that "Parents want to hold vaccines."[28]

And from that point on, they ceased vaccinating any of their children. Rather than refusing to treat them in her practice, Dr. McCarthy did not document any objections to this choice and continued to see Child 3 until at least April 7, 2004, without requiring him to have any further immunizations. It may be that without the relevant medical records to hand, Dr. McCarthy just "misspoke" to Dr. Sanders. This exchange was, nonetheless, used as evidence against the parents by Dr. Sanders when a simple but mandatory perusal of Child 3's records would have identified Dr. McCarthy's error. The failings here are both Dr. McCarthy's for providing evidence without the documentary record to hand and Dr. Sanders' who failed in her duty as an expert and in defiance of her own guidelines for reviewing and reporting on the relevant medical records.

Despite Ms. Kupiszewski's pleadings on behalf of the family, the planets were not aligned for justice: when delivering his ruling of January 6, 2011, on the children's dependency, Judge Brutinel ordered that "ADES is authorized to consent to evaluation and treatment for medical and dental procedures."[29]

The parents' rights had been stripped away, and the State was handed the power to vaccinate their children. If this cannot be stopped at appeal, then "present fears are less than horrible imaginings."[30] "Imaginings" is, perhaps, too abstract, since there is science that supports my concern that with revaccination, these children stand tiptoe at the edge of an abyss.

There are two specific issues that I would like to raise with respect to vaccination/revaccination in this family. The first addresses the issue of rechallenge: what are the likely consequences of re-exposing a child to a vaccine(s) that probably triggered his or her injury in the first place? The second is the unfortunate but predictable—and now officially acknowledged—problem of transmission of live vaccine viruses from one person to other susceptible (nonimmune) individuals, a process termed horizontal transmission.

THE POTENTIAL HAZARDS OF VACCINE RECHALLENGE

Rechallenge refers to a situation where re-exposure of an individual to an agent such as a drug or vaccine elicits a similar adverse reaction to that which was seen following the initial exposure. The secondary reaction, associated with rechallenge, may either reproduce the features associated with the primary challenge, or it may lead to worsening of the condition that was provoked or induced by the initial exposure. Alternatively, the risk of an adverse outcome may increase with repeated exposure, possibly because the immune system has been put on alert by previous exposure(s). During the course of our clinical investigations in the UK between 1995 and 2000, we observed that some children who received a second dose of MMR or boosting with the combined measles, rubella[31] (MR) vaccine experienced onset of further deterioration in their physical and/or behavioral symptoms following re-exposure.

The importance placed upon rechallenge in determining causation is evidenced by the proceedings of the US Institute of Medicine's (IOM) Immunization Safety Review Committee, where judgment favoring acceptance of a causal relationship has been based solely on one or more convincing case reports. For example, Coulter and Fisher[32] reported one case of hemolytic anemia in a two-year-old boy that occurred six days after a fourth dose of DPT vaccine. The boy returned to health until six days after his fifth DPT vaccine when he was rehospitalized with the identical symptoms that accompanied his initial reaction plus loss of consciousness. Fortunately, the boy recovered.

In April 2001, that same Immunization Safety Review Committee stated that, in the context of MMR vaccine as a possible cause of autism, "challenge re-challenge would constitute strong evidence of an association."[33] Subsequently, a study was conducted to test the hypothesis that for children with likely MMR-induced regressive autism and GI pathology, those who got an MMR booster may exhibit a different pattern and degree of severity of GI disease than those children who received only one dose.

Comparison with a similar, once-exposed group was necessary to exclude the possibility that secondary regression was something that just happened in these children without the need for a further trigger. With respect to the bowel disease, the comparison group helped to rule out the possibility that disease severity varied from child to child in a random way, regardless of what vaccines they had received.

Twenty-three children with normal early development and autistic regression who had received more than one dose of an MMR/MR vaccine, the re-exposed group, were compared with twenty-three children with normal early development and autistic regression who had received only one MMR/MR, the once-exposed group. Each re-exposed child was matched for sex, age, and time elapsed from first exposure to endoscopy with a once-exposed child. Exposure groups were compared on their histories of development and behavior, GI and related physical symptoms, and scores of endoscopic and microscopic disease, judged without knowledge of the children's vaccination status. The GI findings have been reported previously.[34] The findings are set out on the following page.

TABLE 6. A summary of the demographic details and developmental and physical history in each re-exposed and once-exposed child. Key to vaccines is outlined below.

Abbreviation	Description
MCV	Polyvalent measles containing vaccine (1 and 2 refer to first and second dose respectively)
MVM	Monovalent measles vaccine
MMR	Measles mumps rubella vaccine (1 and 2 refer to first and second dose respectively)
MR	Measles rubella vaccine

Re-exposed Children

Case no.	Sex	Vaccine & age given in months	Clinical Summary
1v	M	MMR 12 MMR 48	Pre-MMR1: cow's milk intolerance & asthma; required multiple antibiotic courses. Normal development to 12m. Following MMR developed repetitive behaviors & preservation, repeating the same word up to 100 times, with partial complex seizures. Became socially unresponsive & isolated. Parents could no longer "reach him." Refused all foods except wheat & dairy. Suffered progressive behavioral deterioration until introduction of GFCF diet. No secondary regression after MMR2.

Once-exposed Children

Sex	Vaccine & age given	Clinical Summary
M	MMR 13	Normal development to 18m. One week after MMR became very floppy "like a rag doll." By 18m he had lost all speech, social interaction, eye contact & developed obsessive behaviors. From 18m he developed chronic constipation with soiling.

2	M	MMR 14 MMR 52	Normal development to 14m with a vocabulary of 50–60 words. Two days after MMR, went limp & was "never well following this." Immediately suffered two episodes of mouth ulceration & intermittent bouts of constipation & diarrhea. By 18m, hardly slept, had lost speech, & developed asthma. Loss of words started with shortening of words (e.g., helicopter to copter) progressing to loss of entire word. Became antisocial & suffered violent outbursts. Booster MMR led to recurrence of mouth ulcers, return of alternating constipation/diarrhea, & loss of all bowel control that persisted.	M	MMR 13	Pre-MMR1: cow's milk intolerance from 3m. Normal development to 12m. Was using a few words appropriately from 4–5m, was walking at 11m, & by 12m was inquisitive & pointing. Regression from around 13m. By 15–18m all speech had gone. Developed uncontrollable hyperactivity, sleep disturbances & smearing of feces.
3	M	MMR 12 MR 52	Normal development to 12 months, using words & phrases. Between 12 & 16 months suffered increasing social withdrawal & lack of responsiveness. Following diphtheria/pertussis/polio booster at 43m, suffered further deterioration with regression in speech & language, & lost bowel & bladder control, but was still managing in mainstream school. In 5th year, following booster he suffered further deterioration ("his worst year ever") and required	M	MMR 15	Pre-MMR1: eczema. Normal development to 15 months with 60 words and singing nursery rhymes. From 15m insidiously lost eye contact, stopped pointing, singing and social interaction. Vocabulary reduced to a few words and became echolalic. Became clumsy, falling and walking into things. Developed excessive thirst and disturbed sleep

(Continued)

TABLE 6. (*Continued*)

	Re-exposed Children			Once-exposed Children		
Case no.	Sex	Vaccine & age given in months	Clinical Summary	Sex	Vaccine & age given	Clinical Summary
3	M	MMR 12 MR 52	institution of one-on-one care. Described as having disintegrative disorder.	M	MMR 15	pattern. GI symptoms started at 17m with diarrhea. Suffered cow milk intolerance & eczema from 18m, with recurrent ear infections and tonsillitis requiring antibiotics from 2 years of age.
4	M	MMR 16 MMR 30	Normal development to 16m. Vaccinated with MMR when unwell with a cold. Developed diarrhea & tremendous thirst within 2 weeks of MMR. By 20m demonstrated evidence of clear regression with a glazed look & loss of speech. Following booster MMR rapidly lost remaining speech & became increasingly hyperactive, & lost bladder & bowel control, associated with fecal smearing.	M	MMR 16	Normal development to 16m. By 18m had lost speech, language & communication skills. Stopped eating with a knife & fork, pointing to parts of his body & pretend play. From being able to walk normally he started toe walking, & lost the ability to throw & catch a ball. Suffered constant ear infections for next 13m. From 19m developed stomach pains associated with screaming attacks & diarrhea.

#	Sex	Age		Sex	Age	
5	M	MMR 14 MR 58	Normal development to 15m. At 15m he became unresponsive. Hearing was investigated & found to be normal. At 18 months mother realized that he no longer understood things. Diarrhea & pain developed progressively. No obvious change in GI or behavioral symptoms following MR booster.	M	MMR 14	Pre-MMR1: cow's milk intolerance. Multiple ear infections & antibiotic courses in first year. Normal development to 14m. Two weeks after MMR went from being a happy baby to being "continuously sad." Stopped using words & language, stopped sleeping, pointing, & wanting to be cuddled. Became clumsy and has a continuing gait abnormality. Also developed eczema. GI symptoms appeared by 20m with constipation & overflow diarrhea.
6	F	MMR 14 MR 35	Pre-MMR1: cow's milk intolerance, asthma & ear infections requiring multiple antibiotic courses. Normal development to 14m. Following MMR suffered developmental regression with loss of speech & understanding, & deterioration in motor skills. Suffered loss of eye contact & socialization, & aggression with self-injurious behavior. Improved on GFCF diet with return of some verbalization, pointing & social skills.	F	MMR 13	Pre-MMR1: delivered electively at 36 weeks due to maternal proteinuria. Apgars 7 at 1min and 10 at 5min. Suffered necrotizing enterocolitis that resolved on conservative management. Normal development to 13m and was a very happy sociable child. Immediately following MMR she developed a continuous

(Continued)

TABLE 6. (*Continued*)

	Re-exposed Children			Once-exposed Children		
Case no.	Sex	Vaccine & age given in months	Clinical Summary	Sex	Vaccine & age given	Clinical Summary
6	F	MMR 14 MR 35	By one month after MR booster her school reported deterioration in behaviour, with no social interaction and a marked increase in aggression. GI symptoms, with abdominal pain & fecal soiling, started after MR booster.	F	MMR 13	high-pitched scream. Underwent a complete personality change. She stopped speaking, socializing, and feeding herself with a spoon. Lost all facial expression and looked blank and distant. Grand mal seizures started 2.5m after MMR. Alternating constipation & "extreme" diarrhea & abdominal pain started at 13m.
7	M	MMR 12 MMR 54	Pre-MMR1: cow's milk intolerance & eczema. Normal development to 12m. Cruising around furniture & playpen at 11 months and had 6 words at one year. Following MMR speech regressed; health visitor (nurse) noted that within 3 months of MMR he had stopped speaking & returned to babbling. Reverted to sitting only with no further attempt to mobilize in any way. Had become very constipated by 24m. After booster, behavior & sleep pattern deteriorated; stopped all socialization & exhibited tantrums	M	MMR 14	Normal development to 14m. Developmental regression started from 1 week after MMR with onset of head banging, hand flapping, & eating wallpaper & carpet. Sentences of 4–5 words were all gone by 2. Suffered onset of severe constipation that developed progressively over 6 months following MMR that was associated with occasional rectal bleeding.

No.	Sex	MMR	Clinical history
8	M	MMR 13, MMR 49	Pre-MMR1: multiple antibiotic courses for recurrent ear infections; antibiotics associated with episodic diarrhea. Normal development to 14m. Developmental regression started from 15m, associated with obsessive & repetitive behaviors, loss of words and imaginative play, & only fleeting eye contact. He became clumsy and his grip weakened so that he could no longer hold things. After MMR he developed bilateral glue ear requiring grommets. Following booster MMR his behavior deteriorated with development of further autistic behaviors so that referral to a clinical psychologist was required in order to help the family cope. Following booster he also developed alternating constipation & diarrhea, progressing to severe chronic diarrhea.
	M	MMR 14	Normal development to 16m. Walking 11 months and at 14m he had at least 6 words used appropriately. Pointed to parts of body. Started "growling" speech by 16m & by 18 months exhibited definite regression. Stopped obeying simple instructions and was no longer able to identify body parts. By 23 months he had lost eye contact & all social interaction. Abdominal pain started at 24m, progressing to chronic diarrhea.
9	M	MMR 12, MMR 48	Pre-MMR1: cow's milk intolerance. Normal development to 18m. Had speech & socialization that stagnated at 18m & from being a happy sociable infant he became increasingly isolated. Also after 12m suffered multiple ear infections, eczema and impetigo
	M	MMR 16	Normal; development to 16m. First word at 11m. Feeding himself at 11m. Very sociable with excellent social skills & eye contact.

(Continued)

TABLE 6. (*Continued*)

	Re-exposed Children			Once-exposed Children		
Case no.	Sex	Vaccine & age given in months	Clinical Summary	Sex	Vaccine & age given	Clinical Summary
9	M	MMR 12 MMR 48	(one dose of antibiotics given before 12m and 7 per annum for 2 years afterwards). Speech improved with therapy but he remained socially isolated. Following MMR at 48m he experienced further regression, with loss of the speech he had gained, & development of aggression, insomnia & constipation.	M	MMR 16	Within 2 months of MMR, sleep disturbances started. He developed obsessive behaviors such as lining up sweets. Stopped responding to his name. A fear of women developed. Speech stopped. Eye contact went. Restricted diet developed & he became increasingly constipated from this time.
10	M	MMR 14 MR 46	Maternal chickenpox during pregnancy. Normal development to 15m. Following MMR he suffered 2 weeks of ill health & fever. Within 6 weeks of MMR he had lost speech & stopped responding to parents, with hand flapping & loss of imaginative play. Following booster MR he showed marked deterioration in GI symptoms with bowels open up to 12 times per day. Since first MCV,	M	MMR 25m	Pre-MMR[1]: ear infections from 15m requiring multiple courses of antibiotics, therefore MMR deferred. Required grommets for glue ear with impaired hearing at 22m. Otherwise, normal development to 25m. Vaccinated when unwell with an ear infection. Within 2m of MMR he stopped walking & reverted to

#	Sex	MMR	Clinical history
			crawling, stopped understanding simple instructions, lost urinary continence & developed diarrhea and abdominal pain. Suffered major secondary regression following severe chickenpox at 30m. Lost almost all residual skills.
			behaviour & development has regressed in a "progressive rather than step-wise fashion."
	M	MMR 12	Normal development to 12 months when he had 10 words, was sleeping through the night, & was very sociable with good eye contact. Vaccinated with MMR soon after course of amoxicillin that produced diarrhea. Suffered developmental regression within 3 weeks of MMR when he started ignoring things & stopped talking. Also developed screaming & temper tantrums & his sleep pattern became very disrupted. Exhibited hyperactivity with craving for milk & bread &
11	M	MMR 13, MMR 76	Normal development to 13m. Became increasingly withdrawn socially at 15–16 months, associated with loss of language skills. He started to suffer temper tantrums, antisocial behaviour, screaming & repetitive behaviour, obsessively watching the washing machine going around. After booster MMR, suffered severe abdominal pain & exhibited no weight gain, no increase in height and no increase in shoe size for 18m. He only started to grow again upon the introduction of GFCF diet. Developed asthma from 60m.

(Continued)

TABLE 6. (Continued)

	Re-exposed Children			Once-exposed Children		
Case no.	Sex	Vaccine & age given in months	Clinical Summary	Sex	Vaccine & age given	Clinical Summary
11	M	MMR 13 MMR 76		M	MMR 12	obsessive traits developed. Developed severe alternating constipation & diarrhea with continual soiling. Some speech has returned and behavioral improvements have occurred on GFCF diet.
12	M	MMR 18 MR 53	Pre-MMR1: cow's milk intolerance. Normal development to 16m with large vocabulary. By 20m became obsessive, started lining things up, refused to wear clothes with buttons, & eating a restricted diet. He passed developmental tests at 3 years, & school tests at 52m. Frank autistic features developed after MR booster. Straight after booster stopped sleeping, started soiling at night, stopped learning & developed self-injurious behavior and oral ulceration. His IQ, measured serially after booster, went from 143 to 103.	M	MMR 13	Normal development to 13m. Onset of developmental regression within 2–4 weeks of MMR with loss of language. Went from sleeping through the night to a very disturbed sleep pattern. Developed many ear & chest infections post-MMR. Became clumsy, particularly on walking. Suffered onset of GI symptoms at the same time with progressively severe abdominal pain and slow weight gain.

			Also developed severe constipation & immediately after booster developed leg pains that were diagnosed as juvenile arthritis with positive anti-nuclear antibodies.			
13	M	MMR 13 MMR 71	Normal development to 13m. Thereafter, developed learning difficulties with particular problems in drawing, writing & language, the latter requiring speech therapy. Stopped walking at 16m until 24m of age. Marked deterioration at 71m with development of obvious autistic behaviors. He became mute for 6m following booster, with marked loss of eye contact, attention, and communication. He suffered sleep disturbances, developed strange hand and foot movements, & suffered episodes of urinary incontinence. Constipation with abdominal pain developed from this time. Diagnosed with disintegrative disorder.	M	MMR 13	Normal development to 12m. Three weeks after MMR started to suffer panic attacks & agoraphobia. Strange behaviors developed including head banging. No further skills developed beyond this time.
14	M	MMR 14 MMR 74	Pre-MMR1: cow's milk intolerance. Normal development to 16m. Cruising furniture & had a few words at 1 year. From 14m became withdrawn & frustrated. Stopped	M	MMR 14	Pre-MMR1: cow's milk intolerance with esophageal reflux. Normal development to 15m. After MMR lost speech &

(Continued)

TABLE 6. (*Continued*)

	Re-exposed Children			Once-exposed Children		
Case no.	Sex	Vaccine & age given in months	Clinical Summary	Sex	Vaccine & age given	Clinical Summary
14	M	MMR 14 MMR 74	talking & started rocking, toe walking, & ceased interest in mobilization. Developed an "ataxic gait." Improved behaviorally on GFCF diet. Asthma started at 15m. Within "days" of booster MMR became very distressed, with high-pitched screeching & hyperactivity. Behaviour deteriorated markedly. Developed severe chronic diarrhea after booster.	M	MMR 14	acquired no new words. High-pitched screaming started. Lost the ability to identify flash cards & became withdrawn with loss of eye contact. Echolalia & other repetitive behaviors developed. GI symptoms, including alternating constipation & severe diarrhea started at around 18m. After one year of no developmental progress, started very slow improvement, gaining a few words.
15	M	MMR 4 MMR 15	Vaccinated with MMR at 4m when unwell with cold. Normal development to 16m. Diarrhea started within one week of booster MMR at 15m & became chronic. Developmental regression started within 4 weeks of booster MMR. Developed clumsi-	M	MMR 14	Pre-MMR1: suffered ear infections & required multiple antibiotic courses. Normal development to 14m. Had 50 words. Suffered onset of regression & diarrhea by 2 weeks after MMR.

#		MMR/MR		
	M	MMR 14 MR 59	Normal developmental to 14m. Could count to 10 & had 50 words at 12m of age. By 16m had lost all speech and was grunting only. Recovered slowly with speech therapy and regained speech and language to the point where he was talking in sentences. First GI symptoms started at 19m with abdominal pain & alternating constipation & diarrhea. Following MR booster his speech deteriorated & he reverted to grunting sounds. He became clumsy, with loss of balance & falling. Also developed excessive thirst. Within a few days of booster he developed Henoch-Schönlein purpura, and was later diagnosed with erythema nodosum.	ness, thirst & head banging. Particularly food sensitive & suffered episodes of behavioral deterioration associated with gluten exposure while on diet, with recovery following reinstitution of diet.
16	M	MMR 19	Pre-MMR1: as one of triplets he was followed closely to 12m. Had eczema as infant. Developed normally to 18m with speech & language. Following MMR developed recurrent ear infections, lost language & stopped playing & communicating. From the same time he developed severe chronic diarrhea with intermittent rectal bleeding and abdominal bloating. Improved on GFCF diet.	Did not speak again until five years of age when he became echolalic. Also suffered recurrent pyrexia of unknown origin.

(Continued)

TABLE 6. (*Continued*)

	Re-exposed Children			Once-exposed Children		
Case no.	Sex	Vaccine & age given in months	Clinical Summary	Sex	Vaccine & age given	Clinical Summary
17	F	MMR 18 MR 70	Normal development to 19m. Following MMR, developed rash, fever, mouth ulcers and abdominal pain. Regressed with decreased socialization & loss of words. Speech development stopped completely until 2.5–3 years of age. Ten days after booster MR, became febrile & started hallucinating with photophobia. Underwent major physical deterioration thereafter. Constantly unwell with rashes, fevers & abdominal pain mouth ulcers & blood & mucus in stool. Developed anger & frustration at loss of ability to learn.	F	MMR 13	Normal development to 18m. By one year knew colors & alphabet. Used potty & was well on the way to potty training. Clear regression from 18–22m. Suffered loss of speech & onset of abnormal hand movements. GI symptoms started by 20m with chronic alternating constipation & diarrhea. Clumsiness started following MMR associated with a gait abnormality that has since required corrective surgery. Suffers asthma, eczema, & hay fever.
18	M	MMR 15 MMR 49	Normal development to 15m. Following MMR stopped walking round furniture & regressed to crawling. Appeared to stop learning & by 20 months, stopped talking	M	MMR 12	Pre-MMR1: multiple courses of antibiotics for ear & upper respiratory tract infections. Received MMR 10 days after an antibiotic

No.	Sex	MMR	Clinical history
			...altogether. General ill health developed with ear, chest, & throat infections. Suffered loose motions & abdominal pain. Following 2nd MMR "disappeared" within 2 weeks & "lost all skills & communication." Started head banging & repetitive behaviors & could no longer hold a cup.
			...course. Normal development to 12m. Started speaking at 10m & was sociable and loved music. Soon after MMR, stopped talking and became isolated, unresponsive & attention became poor. Became terrified by music and sounds that he had previously enjoyed. Chronic diarrhea and abdominal pain started at 36m. Developed chronic otitis media & candida skin infections.
19	M	MMR 18, MMR 88	Normal development to 18m. At 18m suffered developmental arrest & lost speech, which became incomprehensible, deteriorating into a yell. Bowel symptoms started after 1st dose with constipation & blood in stool. After booster MMR he suffered marked deterioration in behavior, concentration became very poor and had uncontrollable temper tantrums & episodes of "blanking out." Diagnosed ADHD with autistic features and complex learning disorder.
	M	MMR 15	Pre-MMR1: very colicky baby with cow's milk intolerance. Normal development to 16m. Pointed & named parts of body. Following MMR, became unresponsive & lost words. Stopped pointing. "Huge" improvements on GFCF diet.

(Continued)

TABLE 6. (*Continued*)

| Case no. | Re-exposed Children | | | Once-exposed Children | | |
	Sex	Vaccine & age given in months	Clinical Summary	Sex	Vaccine & age given	Clinical Summary
20	M	MVM 12 MMR 15 MR 72	Normal development to 18m. At 18m lost words & developed hyperactivity & sleep disturbances. ASD at this stage was reported to be relatively mild. Progressed well at infant school with considerable improvement in behaviour & development. Following MR booster he deteriorated within 2 weeks with upper respiratory infections & discharging ears, requiring multiple courses of antibiotics. Suffered developmental regression with return of behaviors that had resolved, such as lining things up & reverted to crawling. Started new aberrant behaviors including self-injury (head banging & pinching until badly bruised). Required removal from special school due to behavior following 2nd developmental regression.	M	MMR 14	Normal development to 14m. Two weeks after MMR, developed clumsiness with unsteadiness on his feet & walking into things. Suffered speech & language regression, developed poor eye contact with social isolation & solitary play, with head banging & tic. No GI symptoms were evident until 8 years.*

No.	Sex	Vaccines	History	Sex	Vaccines	History
21	M	MMR 13 MR 73	Normal development to 18m. Developed increasing distress & behavior problems and hyperactivity over the next year leading to exclusion from crèche. Lost all interest in communicating or socializing. Underwent speech therapy & was placed on special needs. Subsequently withdrawn from Special Needs Register due to behavioral and developmental improvement. Urinary and fecal continence was achieved both day & night. After MR booster suffered "stepwise regression" & severe constipation. ASD became obvious & violent behavior developed. Started fecal soiling. Special needs status required reinstating within 2.5m of booster.	M	MMR 13	Described as being developmentally advanced at 8 months. Normal development to 12m. Chickenpox just prior to MMR. Suffered regression starting 3 weeks after MMR with loss of speech & pointing. Explosive diarrhea started from 17–18m. Symptoms stabilized and improved from 5 years after steroids were given following a diagnosis of Landau-Kleffner syndrome (LKS). GFCF was introduced at 7 years of age, leading to further improvements.
22	M	MVM 12 MMR 51 MR 108	Received measles vaccine at 12m with no reaction. Developed normally to 51m. MMR at 51 months following which he regressed to "ASD." Suffered episodes of fecal soiling and smearing. Booster MR at 9 years was followed rapidly by loss of residual speech & language, & loss of bowel & bladder control. Following booster MR, suffered 12.7 kg weight loss with anorexia & abdominal pain. Failed to gain weight for 5 years.	M	MMR 15	Normal development to 15m. From 15m, became disinterested in surroundings, suffered a general loss of skills, bad-tempered, & withdrawn. Developed obsessive traits with preoccupation with electrical appliances, toilets, & water in general. Suffered chronic constipation from 8 weeks of age, with no obvious change following MMR.

(Continued)

TABLE 6. (*Continued*)

	Re-exposed Children				Once-exposed Children		
Case no.	Sex	Vaccine & age given in months	Clinical Summary		Sex	Vaccine & age given	Clinical Summary
23	M	MVM 12 MR 168	Normal early development to 12m. During 2nd year after measles vaccine developed hyperactive response to food colorings, obsessive behaviors, sleep disturbances & general ill health. Improved over the intervening years to become completely well and a successful student & musician. Following MR, suffered acute photophobia. Dramatic behavioral change within 2 weeks of booster MR vaccine, with anxiety attacks, marked obsessive-compulsive symptoms, hallucinations, & violent behavior. Also physical health deteriorated from this time with onset of asthma. GI symptoms developed, starting with chronic diarrhea, abdominal pain, and vomiting, progressing to episodic bloody diarrhea.		M	MVM 16	Normal development to 16–18m. Gradual deterioration with obvious regression by end of 2nd year. Mother (Health Visitor) contemporaneously linked onset of regression to measles vaccination. By 3 years had developed severe constipation with abdominal pain & bloating.

The first thing to appreciate from the brief narratives in Table 6 is the consistency of symptoms that are also shared with the Arizona 5. There is even one case of HSP. What is also clear is that a high proportion of children who developed problems after their first exposure fared very badly after the second.

PHYSICAL SYMPTOMS FOLLOWING RECHALLENGE

The following figures illustrate changes in physical status of children comparing the events following re-exposure with the once-exposed children. Secondary incontinence refers to loss of continence in a child who has previously achieved this developmental milestone. Re-exposed children scored significantly higher than once-exposed for secondary physical (GI) symptoms,[35] including incontinence.[36] Secondary incontinence is an important feature of developmental regression and a hallmark of childhood disintegrative disorder,[37] a condition that is otherwise indistinguishable from ASD.

BOWEL DISEASE FOLLOWING RECHALLENGE

In support of a rechallenge effect, the severity of bowel inflammation in the children re-exposed to a measles vaccine was significantly greater in a number of important respects: (1) re-exposed children scored significantly higher than once-exposed children for the following: presence of severe ileal lymphoid hyperplasia,[38] (2) number of children with eosinophilic inflammation,[39] (3) number of biopsies with epithelial damage,[40] and (4) number of children with acute inflammation. Significant markers of acute inflammation included number of children affected,[41] proportion of biopsies affected,[42] and greater severity.[43] The data identify a rechallenge effect on symptoms and a biological gradient effect on intestinal pathology and support a causal association between regressive autism and GI disease.[44]

This study provided evidence of a range of systematic, negative effects associated with re-exposure to measles vaccines in this population. Several aspects of this study strengthen the conclusion that there is a causal association between these vaccines and the syndrome described, the first of which is an effect of rechallenge on behavioral and physical symptoms. The second is a biological gradient seen, for example, in the severity of mucosal inflammation, where more severe inflammation was significantly more common in those who received more than one measles-containing vaccine.

Reports of clumsiness (ataxia) and associated gait disturbance, recurring issues in the narratives of the Arizona 5, were evident in a high proportion of the

UK study children; from parental reports, these symptoms were most prominent during the early phase of regression, consistent with an evolving brain injury.[45] These symptoms may be relevant to the observation of gait disturbance and ataxia following MMR by Plesner et al. in Denmark.[46] In Denmark, this association had not been associated with any other vaccine administered to children of the same age prior to the introduction of MMR in 1987, indicating that a novel adverse reaction might be associated specifically with this vaccine. In a recent review of the mandatory passive reporting[47] system for vaccine adverse events operated in Denmark, Plesner not only confirmed the previously observed association between MMR and ataxia but, crucially, also documented that the more severe ataxias following MMR may be associated with residual cognitive deficits in some children.[48] These were not short-term injuries. The precise nature of these residual deficits is not known.

If the Arizona 5 are forcibly revaccinated the prospects for their physical and developmental well-being are not good. Child 3 and Child 4, who are likely to have already suffered major adverse vaccine reactions, are particularly at risk in my opinion. An MMR booster in Child 3 would, based upon the evidence presented above, be sufficient to produce major deterioration in his condition and should be resisted at all costs. It is likely, however, that he will not be given MMR in isolation, but in combination with all the other vaccines that the CDC in its wisdom considers necessary for a nine-year-old boy to have had. The toxic load in aluminum and mercury exposures alone would be sufficient to cause mass neuronal suicide.[49]

MMR AND HORIZONTAL TRANSMISSION[50]

There is another issue that merits consideration, one that may have an important bearing on revaccination of the Arizona 5 and the younger two siblings in particular. At first sight, the children are a mixed bunch in terms of the pattern of onset of their developmental problems. Child 1 regressed at three and a half years, Child 2 regressed at two and a half years, and Child 3 at eighteen months. Child 4 and Child 5, on the other hand, had developmental problems in their first year of life.

Regression in Child 3 was clearly vaccine related, and his adverse reactions were documented contemporaneously by his primary care physician. In her expert report, Dr. Sanders brought attention to the distinct histories of the various children in an effort to discredit any parental claims of a link between vaccination and autism. She wrote that "they then reported that the autism [in Child 3] was due to immunizations. As a result, [Child 4] had only one vaccine (according to parents) and developed autism, so they did not get vaccines for [Child 5]. However they later presented [Child 5] as having autism."[51]

I was unable to identify where the parents had reported that Child 4 was the recipient of one vaccine only. In fact, he had received seven vaccines, with six of these given on one day (Part 4, Chapter 3, Table 5). Nonetheless, her point was that, in view of the parents' claim to Child 5's "autism" and the fact that he had received no vaccines, this meant that vaccines could not be the cause of *any* developmental problems that the parents had claimed for their children. One is led to infer that either they didn't have ASD or that if they did, vaccines had nothing to do with it.

Alternatively, is it possible that autism is, on occasions, contagious? Crohn's disease may be contagious,[52] so why not the bowel disease in autism? While this may sound preposterous, over a five-year period we have identified up to twenty families in one clinical practice who may have been affected in this way. The older children with ASD and GI disease, with onset following MMR vaccine, had younger siblings also with ASD and confirmed GI disease. But the younger siblings were different; for reasons of parental concern due to the experience with their older child, the younger ones had not received MMR or any other measles-containing vaccine, nor did they have any documented exposure to natural measles. What also distinguished them from their older siblings is the fact that their developmental trajectory was quite different. They had either regressed early, within the first year of life, or not at all; their development had simply plateaued. Within this group of unvaccinated, affected siblings some had antibodies against measles, often at high titer and on repeated measurement. Given the wide geographic distribution of these cases and lack of any other obvious mode of exposure to measles, it is possible that these children were infected by their vaccinated autistic siblings.

Live polio virus vaccine can and does cause paralysis and death.[53] It can do so when excreted in the feces of recently vaccinated infants and spread to susceptible contacts such as a nonimmune mother changing a dirty diaper. If measles vaccine virus can be shed from an inflamed intestine, it might similarly infect susceptible siblings, children who are likely to be younger (unvaccinated), who come into close contact with the source. If this is the case, then we would expect certain conditions to influence the sibling factor. Taking the child who regressed and developed GI disease after MMR as the index case and the unvaccinated ASD child as the secondary case, one would predict the secondary case to be younger. This is not only because younger sibs are less likely than older sibs to have been vaccinated because of their age but also because any vaccine link in the index case will put parents off vaccinating the younger sibling. The closer in age the secondary case is to the index case, the greater the risk. Why? Because siblings closer in age share a closer environment; e.g., bathing together and being together with mother when she changes the other's diaper.

Can this happen? Yes. Millson first reported a probable case of brother-to-sister transmission of measles after measles-mumps-rubella (MMR) immunization in 1989.[54] A four-year-old boy had onset of clinical measles with Koplick spots, little white measles ulcers in the mouth, ten days after MMR vaccination. His eight-month-old sister developed an almost identical clinical picture two days later. Both children followed the same clinical course with complete recovery. No laboratory tests were undertaken to confirm measles infection. Campbell responded on behalf of the Joint Committee on Vaccination and Immunization (JCVI), stating that "extensive testing and experience with measles vaccine and MMR vaccine had not shown evidence of vaccine virus transmission to susceptible contacts."[55]

This evidence was neither provided nor cited; the truth is, there was none. Despite this, he concluded that "there is no risk of virus transmission following measles, mumps, or rubella vaccine."

Like so many public health pronouncements on vaccines, both before and since, Campbell's was foolish and the case is simply made. Following maternal rubella vaccination, vaccine virus transmission from mother to infant in infected breast milk is not only established but is declared as a warning on the MMR product insert. Horizontal transmission of mumps vaccine virus from a vaccinated to a susceptible sibling has been reported.[56] The likely vertical transmission of measles vaccine through breastfeeding is described by Yazbak and Diodati,[57] and a critical review of the data indicates the possibility of horizontal transmission even in the limited early trials of measles vaccine.[58]

The position on measles vaccine virus transmission has undergone an about face from Campbell's wishful fallacy. Since the availability of sensitive techniques for virus detection, it has become apparent that following vaccination measles vaccine virus can be shed in urine and the upper respiratory tract[59] for in excess of three weeks post-exposure.[60] The reality of sporadic outbreaks of clinical measles originating from a vaccine source have now been confirmed worldwide and have been supported by the findings of independent laboratories.[61]

In such cases, the molecular characterization of the vaccine virus and its distinction from wild (natural) strains of measles virus led Christensen and colleagues to conclude that "a small number of clinical manifestations of measles virus worldwide from which strains similar to the vaccine strain were identified, were vaccine related rather than being caused by members of a persistently circulating ancient genome type."[62]

Transmission of measles vaccine virus is a real, if apparently uncommon, occurrence, at least if the frequency of this event is judged by the presentation of typical clinical measles infection in susceptible contacts. Any estimate of the frequency of these atypical cases will also be limited by the completeness of their recognition, reporting, and investigation. If the cases don't present like measles they won't be reported as such.

It would be a game-changer if, for example, MMR vaccine caused a novel disease—one not recognized as typical measles—such as an intestinal disease with fecal shedding of the virus, as with poliovirus. Neopathogenesis, the emergence of a new clinical disease or syndrome, arising as a consequence of vaccination and horizontal transmission would be likely to escape detection for some time. It is important to bear these things in mind when reading of the Yanomami's experience described below. Moreover, little consideration has been given to the potential for delayed transmission from prolonged virus shedding by immunodeficient individuals in whom the virus is able to replicate, a factor of potential concern for four of the Arizona 5 children.

HORIZONTAL TRANSMISSION: EVIDENCE FROM NONHUMAN PRIMATES

Measles infects nonhuman primates, reproducing key aspects of the human disease, including fever, rash, infection of the body's immune cells, and immunodeficiency, followed by induction of specific protective immune responses. Chen and colleagues described sporadic measles-associated colitis in captive Tamarins (*Saguinus mystax*) following a measles outbreak in their colony.[63] Similarly, measles vaccination of captive rhesus macaques at the University of California facility at Davis was associated with a sporadic diarrheal disease with failure to thrive and apparent behavioral disturbances (unpublished observations). Surgical pathology of ileal and colonic tissues revealed an enterocolitis consistent with moderate-to-severe human inflammatory bowel disease. Molecular analysis of gut tissues for measles virus gene sequences was positive in these animals (unpublished observations).

A similar problem occurred at the Brookfield Zoo in Illinois with their colony of new world primate *Callimico goeldii*, some of whom had received measles vaccine prophylaxis. Previously thriving, the population of *C. goeldii* in American zoos has been in decline since the 1990s, with mortality rates exceeding those of live births. Some animals were developing chronic diarrhea, failure to thrive, and apparent (if somewhat poorly characterized) behavioral disturbances. This is of interest, given reports of the propensity of new world primates to intestinal complications following measles, with depression, loss of appetite, and high mortality.[64] Tissues from sick Brookfield animals were submitted to microscopic and virological examination. This identified Moraten measles vaccine-strain-specific gene sequences in the monkey tissues. What was unexpected is that nonvaccinated cagemates of vaccinated, diseased *Callimico* monkeys had the same intestinal pathology and the same virological findings as their sick, vaccinated cagemates. Irrespective of any role for measles virus in the intestinal pathology, the data provide direct evidence of horizontal transmission. The implications are self-evident for spread of a vaccine-derived measles virus at close quarters.

HORIZONTAL TRANSMISSION: EVIDENCE FROM THE FIELD

Patrick Tierney's compelling account of the violation of the indigenous peoples of Venezuela in *Darkness in El Dorado* raised the question of whether measles vaccine has become transmissible among so-called virgin-soil populations.[65] Vaccination experiments were conducted by the geneticist James Neel among the Yanomami Indians in 1968. Despite an apparent prohibition by the Venezuelan government, Neel employed the most reactive of the early measles vaccines, the Edmonston B, on the Yanomami. The results were unexpected. He recorded the highest temperatures for any measles vaccine among any population. Then a measles epidemic, of unknown origin, spread in Neel's words "as a wave away from the original point"—the point from which, in fact, the vaccinations had started. And within two months of the first case, measles had spread to fifteen villages.

Steinvorth-Goetz, a physician and anthropologist, described measles morbidity and mortality among the Yanomami during this epidemic: "Many Indians fled deep into the forests, but for most of the people living near the Orinoco it was already too late. They carried the disease germs with them, infecting others and dying by the score. They had absolutely no resistance. Only a very few even developed the characteristic rash, which is a sign of the skin's fight to throw off the disease. Mucous membranes became horribly inflamed, with extreme toxic vomiting and diarrhea. Many had hemorrhaging of the inner walls of the larynx. Many developed pneumonia and died from it. All too often even relatively mild cases failed to respond to penicillin."[66]

An independent investigation by the Venezuelan Congress found that Yanomami survivors blamed the vaccine for the epidemic.[67] Is it unlikely, indeed untenable, that villagers who had lived without epidemic measles exposure but with regular outside contact should first experience a natural measles epidemic at precisely the same time and apparently, in precisely the same place as they were first exposed to a highly reactive measles vaccine, one capable of being shed. And as Neel confirms, it had the same pattern of spread as the vaccination procedures.

PERSISTENT INFECTION AND WANING IMMUNITY

The possibility that measles outbreaks may occur from a point source such as a persistently infected individual whose immune system has failed to control and kill the virus, for whatever reason, is a real concern.[68] The associated immune dysregulation in some individuals with autism and GI disease, in particular with immunoglobulin deficiency, lymphopenia, and impaired NK cell cytotoxicity,[69] may provide a reservoir of persistent viral infection.

CONCLUSIONS

For ethical, constitutional, and, above all, medical reasons, the Arizona 5 should not be revaccinated. They are at high risk for developing further neurological and GI damage, and while the issue remains controversial and the subject of wide-ranging debate, these children must be given the benefit of the doubt.

It may be that the younger children have been exposed to the components of the MMR vaccine through horizontal transmission from their vaccinated siblings. If the State of Arizona continues on its current tack and is determined to violate the ethical, constitutional, and medical imperatives for not vaccinating these children, then at a minimum, certain demands must be made.

All five children should be formally assessed behaviorally, developmentally, and physically, before and at three and six months after vaccination. Antibody levels for all vaccine antigens should also be measured before and after vaccine administration at these same assessments.

This process would allow the determination of the following:

i.   The children's current level of health and function and whether these are adversely impacted by revaccination.
ii. Whether the children, particularly those who omitted certain vaccines, have antibody immunity to the respective infections.

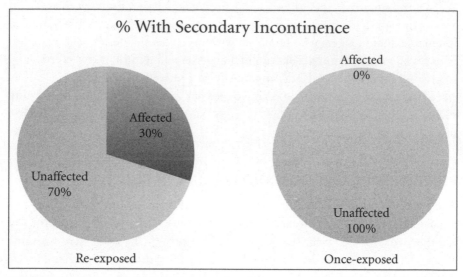

FIGURE 1. The percentage of re-exposed and once-exposed children with secondary fecal and/or urinary incontinence (having previously been continent). The risk is significantly greater in re-exposed children p = 0.009.[70] The relative risk (infinite) cannot be calculated with zero in the once-exposed group.

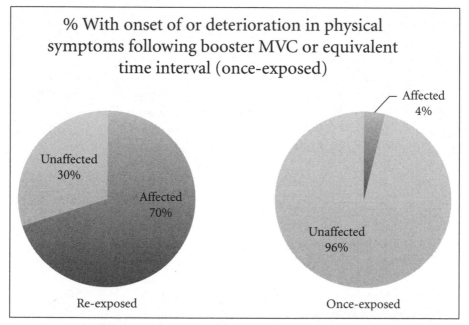

FIGURE 2. The percentage of re-exposed and once-exposed children with onset of or deterioration in physical symptoms following re-exposure. The risk is significantly greater in re-exposed children (p < 0.0001); only one once-exposed child suffered secondary physical deterioration, following a severe chickenpox infection.

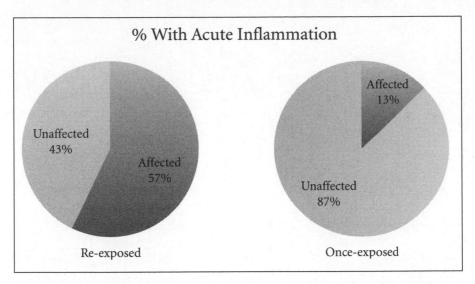

FIGURE 3. The percentage of re-exposed and once-exposed children with acute ileo-colonic inflammation. The risk is significantly greater in re-exposed children. *RR 4.67 (1.55–14.09); $p < 0.05$.

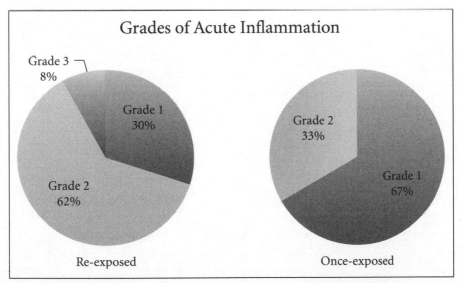

FIGURE 4. The percentage of re-exposed and once-exposed children with one of three graded levels of acute ileo-colonic inflammation. Re-exposed children presented significantly lower levels of mild inflammation compared with once-exposed children. RR 0.48 (0.24–0.94); $p < 0.05$.

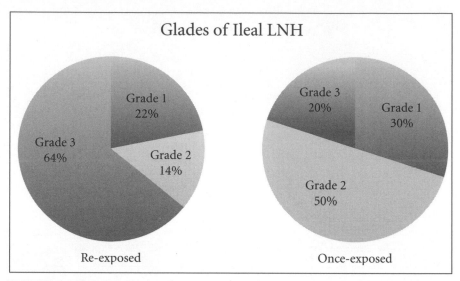

FIGURE 5. The percentage of re-exposed and once-exposed children with one of three graded levels of ileal LNH. The risk of severe ileal LNH is significantly greater in re-exposed children. RR 2.44 (1.30–4.58); p < 0.005.

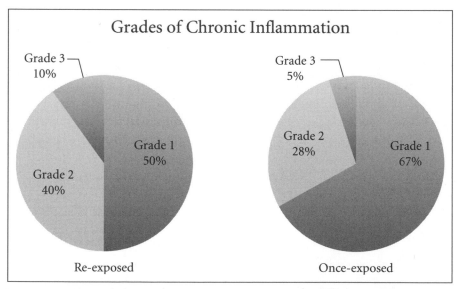

FIGURE 6. The percentage of re-exposed and once-exposed children with one of three graded levels of chronic inflammation. Fifty percent of re-exposed children presented moderate to severe levels of chronic inflammation compared with thirty-three percent of once-exposed children. These differences are not statistically significant.[71]

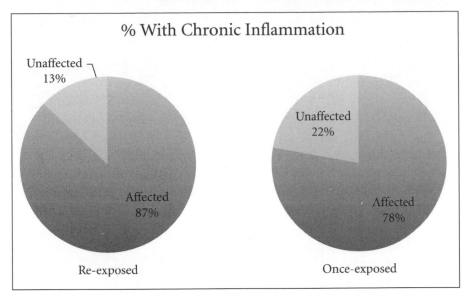

FIGURE 7. The percentage of re-exposed and once-exposed children with chronic inflammation. Eighty-seven percent of re-exposed children presented chronic inflammation compared with 78 percent of once-exposed children. These differences are not statistically significant.

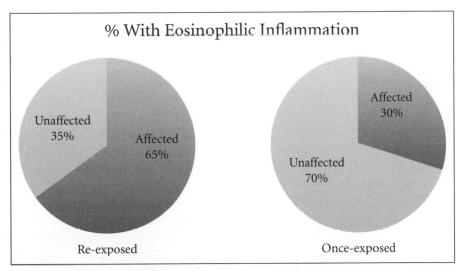

FIGURE 8. The percentage of re-exposed and once-exposed children with eosinophilic inflammation. The risk of eosinophilic inflammation is significantly greater in re-exposed children. RR 2.05 (1.09–3.86); $p < 0.02$.

PART V

Chapter 17

THE ANALYSIS

"Come, you spirits . . . . Come to my woman's breasts,
And take my milk for gall . . ."

MacBeth Act 1, Scene 3

Applied behavior analysis (ABA) is a behavior modification technique for treating children with autism. It was conceptualized in its original form by Dr. Burrhus Frederic Skinner[1] and adapted clinically by Dr. Ivar Lovaas to reinforce good behaviors and extinguish bad. The case of the Arizona 5 is the antithesis of this methodological approach and the outcomes it seeks to achieve. The good behavior—parental advocacy on behalf of sick children—has been all but extinguished in this case. Bad—sometimes very bad—behavior has been endorsed and indeed rewarded. The latter behavior is likely, therefore, to be repeated and become progressively more embedded unless it is immediately extinguished.

April 2011. Since justice has not been served, the decision of Judge Brutinel is to be appealed. The outcome may even find its way into a postscript in this book, although at the time of writing this analysis, no date for the appeal has been set, and the book—with the parents' blessing—cannot wait. Whatever the outcome of the appeal this battle will not stop here. The only acceptable conclusion to this matter will be the return of *Perpetual Sunshine*—Child 1—and his siblings to their parents and the prevention this kind of violation in the future.

First, as a general comment, it must be said that the case for the existence of MSBP as a rigorously defined and reproducible entity has never been made or even come close. No standardized methodology has ever been used to validate this quasi-syndrome. Even in the present case, the prosecution's medical witnesses could not agree on whether it was the children who suffered from MSBP, in line with Meadow and Rosenberg, or the parents who were afflicted, according to the official manual, DSM-IV.[2] The syndrome is a confusing experimental construct that is open to abuse and misuse in the wrong hands. Its footings turned to quicksand for its originator, Professor Meadow. It is my opinion that the Sorority of Williams, Carter, Stephens, and Sanders has built its case for the Arizona 5 on those same perilous sands in pursuit of the mirage of children suffering at the hands of their parents.

In drawing the case to its logical conclusion, let us start with the most serious allegation, one that characterized the mindset of Dr. Stephens in particular. It was her contention that " . . . on many occasions the parents may have . . . induced illness in the child."[3]

Could the parents have deliberately induced the disorders suffered by their children? The merit of rehearsing this argument, for which no evidence was presented, is that it provides a yardstick for the mentality, a swelling chant in the village square of "kill the beast" that fueled the assault on this family. Despite Dr. Stephen's efforts to lead this chant, the Arizona situation had none of the hallmarks of Professor Meadow's original cases, where the children's problems were caused by deliberate falsification of tests and fatal poisoning. Forensic analysis of the records and witness testimony provided no supportive evidence for the induction of illness. Judge Brutinel was forced to conclude that the parents were not guilty on this count.

The finding of guilt on lesser charges and the removal of these children from their parents will, I imagine, have assuaged the conscience of Dr. Stephens for having made such a disgraceful claim.

Implicit in the remaining arguments of Dr. Stephens and others was that even if the illnesses had not been directly induced by their parents, the latter's "fabrication" and "exaggeration" of symptoms had put the children at risk of harm from "unnecessary . . . invasive procedures."[4]

Here, on the issue of invasive procedures, I must disclose a potential conflict: Those who have read *Callous Disregard*[5] or followed my case in the UK will know that I was found guilty by the UK's General Medical Council (GMC) on a similar charge, of causing children to undergo invasive procedures, in this case for the purpose of experimentation (rather than clinical care). My "crime" was indifference to the children's suffering—children identical in so many ways to the Arizona 5—as opposed to these parents, who, it is alleged, sought to bring attention, by proxy, to their own deranged personas. Our circumstances were otherwise similar: others—clinicians—had ordered diagnostic tests in order to elucidate the origins of the children's symptoms. The respective physicians had explicitly, and for good reasons, also conducted and interpreted those diagnostic tests and treated according to their findings. We identified an apparently new disease syndrome, the discovery of which has improved the lives of thousands of children. Dr. Ursea and her colleagues reaffirmed this syndrome in the Arizona 5. In both instances, the well-being of the children had improved as a consequence. But that did not suit the respective inquisitors, the UK's GMC and Arizona's Attorney General's office, which held there to be one truth and one truth only. I empathize with the parents and, therefore, I disclose this conflict on the basis that objectivity is elusive.

On the objective evidence, however, did the parents cause or contrive, for example, the GI pathology in order to have their children undergo endoscopy, the most invasive of the diagnostic procedures? Or rather, did they interpret the children's symptoms correctly and seek appropriate care that led to a treatable diagnosis? Let me take Child 1 as case in point: did he hemorrhage from his intestine, and was this represented accurately by the father? The progressive fall in his blood level of hemoglobin, his repeatedly positive stool tests for blood, his swollen intestine on repeated abdominal scanning, and his residual gastric and duodenal erosions and mucosal inflammation despite heavy anti-inflammatory treatment, all in the setting of severe HSP, are entirely in keeping with the father's story of black, tarry stools and a description of his vomitus that was interpreted as having contained blood. It is, in my opinion, an embarrassment for any healthcare professional to have pitted the suggestion of confabulation of this blood loss against such objective evidence. A similar case has been made in the foregoing narrative for each of the children.

Despite the objective evidence, this argument—putting the children at risk from fabrication and exaggeration—did find traction with Judge Brutinel in his decision to remove the children from their parents. Surprisingly, in finding against the parents, other than to reiterate the allegations of ADES, no analysis on the part of the court was provided.

To a non-lawyer, what is most perplexing about the ruling is its lack of analysis, the absence of any reasoning such as that provided here, that should, surely, have formed the cornerstone of ADES's case and Brutinel's decision. Instead, there were just multiple, false allegations that came like spitballs, fast from every direction, in the hope that some would stick. Clearly, some did. The invidious position of the judiciary, when faced with a controversial diagnosis and a prosecution expert prophesying the likelihood of further abuse and possible death, harmonized, in this case, with the frenzied accompaniment of Dr. Stephens and others, strongly suggests to me that those who judge these cases require dual qualification in medicine and law and that they should be valued accordingly.

Better, therefore, to step back from the absence of judicial analysis, angry cries of the mob, the medical malpractice and possible misconduct, and view this case from ten thousand feet. It is a parent's biological and instinctive imperative to sense and act upon symptoms of distress and sickness in their children. If this were not the case then we, as a species, would not exist. These parents did just that: starting with their sentinel child, Child 3, they reported their concerns about his progressive adverse vaccine reactions that led them to a diagnosis of a developmental disorder, whatever the name or diagnostic nuances might have been. The State of New York, in its genuine wisdom, has a policy of screening children routinely for lead poisoning, and Child 3 was found to be lead-toxic. With time and the right doctors, the multisystem disease complex from which Child 3 was suffering started to emerge. As the light fell onto the uncut crystal of his disorder, it was refracted, split into many colors that when viewed by ADES and its cohorts appeared distinct, rare, and incredible to the extent that his disorders must have been illusory. However, from what was known at the time of the trial—of heavy metal poisoning, vaccine reactions, encephalopathy, mitochondrial dysfunction, oxidative stress, MTHFR deficiency, food allergy, immunodeficiency, and enterocolitis as a likely integrated, multisystem disorder—a very different interpretation was possible. The refracted spectrum, its many colors followed back into the crystal, may have entered as a single incident shaft of white.

Between the more easily discernable colors were shades that further beguiled the unwary and uninformed. Alteration in pain perception in children with developmental disorders on the autism spectrum is but one example. The emerging science of gut-immune-brain interactions in food allergic disorders such as celiac disease is another. The related benefits of exclusion diets in ameliorating aberrant behaviors in children is yet a third.

And then among the shadows there is possible medical misconduct. This matter demands further scrutiny because, on its face, in their joint and several desire to secure a conviction, some opposed to the parents may have variously falsified evidence, defamed colleagues, forsaken their duty of care, and sought to re-engineer diagnoses, thereby abandoning their training, their integrity, and the family in the process.

It is interesting to review who among the cast came closer to fulfilling the DSM-IV criteria for MSBP: those criteria that Dr. Sanders referred to in making her case against the parents.

- Intentional production or feigning of physical or psychological signs or symptoms in another person who is in the individual's care.

I have found no evidence that the parents met this criterion. Heather Williams of CPS, with her mumbo-jumbo English, came closer by a thousand times, while Dr. Stephens' facility for feigning by exaggeration was unparalleled. In turn,

Dr. Sanders, the expert, played loose with the facts, moved events around in time, insinuated, cherry-picked the evidence by omitting crucial information, let accusations hang, broke her own rules of engagement, and ignored key witnesses. The net effect was a feigned psychopathology in the parents who were thereby condemned.

- The motivation of the perpetrator's behavior is to assume the sick role by proxy.

Since psychological motive is so difficult to discern in the absence of a frank confession, this criterion sets an almost impossibly high bar for making the diagnosis of MSBP. ADES, on the advice of their expert Dr. Sanders,[6] has sought to extract this confession from the parents retroactively. Apparently, ADES has, in effect, threatened them with permanent loss of their children should they refuse to admit their guilt by "taking responsibility for their abusive actions."[7] On the basis of "simply no research,"[8] in the opinion of Dr. Mart, the MSBP expert for the defense, Dr. Sanders, claimed that parental admission of wrongdoing should be a precondition to redemption and return of the children. Presumably, in going into the appeal proceedings, ADES also requires this admission since the prosecution actually has no other evidence of MSBP. Obtained, as it would be, under extreme duress—nothing less than mental torture—I imagine that it would breach Article 5 of the United Nations Universal Declaration of Human Rights,[9] and should, in my opinion, be a criminal offence. So far the parents have withstood their torment and refused to sign a document that would forever condemn them. In short, there is no evidence that the parents fulfilled this criterion.

Based upon the progressive clinical course in the rare historical cases of MSBP, the evidence does not support the idea that the parents were seeking attention by proxy. Implicit in this criterion is that the sicker the child appears, the closer the abusive parent comes to fulfilling his or her motive. In contrast, these children, the Arizona 5, improved over time and with intervention. For every action that the parents took on their children's behalf, the reaction was intended to be and often was improvement in the children's health. They improved, whether it was from HSP, an ASD, recurrent infection, or food allergy, rather than spiraling ever downward into intractable—if factitious—illness that would have given the parents the attention that they were alleged to have craved.

It is ironic that the sicker the children really were, the more complex their genuine disorders, and the greater the multitude of their valid diagnoses, the closer the Sorority came to fulfillment. If, in addition, the parents' accusers could cast doubt upon these diagnoses by ascribing further diagnoses to children where none had in fact been claimed—immunodeficiency in Child 5, asthma in Child 1 and Child 4, food allergies in all but Child 3—then the Spirit of Abuse might come to life. If they could present the parents' concerns as deliberately overstated—Child 1's "self-limiting" disorder for which the passage of blood in stool and vomit was claimed but never witnessed, "an arm thing that was nothing" in Child 2, and "too many infections to count" for all the children—then the specters drawn from their rank cauldron had spoken true. If they could insinuate into the collective consciousness of the court the image of dysfunctional parents, charges of sexual abuse, false claims to be nurses, shopping the breadth of the country for an imaginary diagnosis, refusing generously offered services, regaling every doctor with a different story, and antagonizing every state employee with whom they came in contact, the court would do the rest; it did. And when, upon this, the most abstract of the four criteria, the battle had been won, the Sorority doubtless drew strength for a new fight with the bar set lower than ever before.

• External incentives for the behavior (such as economic gain) are absent.

On the face of it, the parents do not fulfill this criterion. They received state assistance for their children's special educational needs, on the one hand, needs determined by medical and other healthcare professionals. The Sorority seemed also of the opinion that this criterion was not fulfilled. When Ms. Williams and Dr. Carter speculated on the "secondary motivation" for the parents, among the possibilities they considered were "drugs, financial or other problems. Dr. Carter feels that it is money to some degree, attention, it allows them not to have to work, they get free babysitting."[10]

There were, on the other hand, considerable material disadvantages to their healthcare-seeking behaviors on behalf of their children. The gasoline bill alone for the well-traveled road to Phoenix must have placed considerable strain on their limited resources.

Neither does the Sorority fit this criterion easily. Dr. Stephens acts for and is funded by a state Department of Economic Security—how strange a role is child protection for this department? (How did the incongruous phenomena of MSBP and fiscal rigor find themselves under the same blanket?) Nonetheless, one need not look further than the monthly paycheck to cede economic gain for Dr. Stephens. But there may also be genuine altruism in her actions. By her own admission, she had a "great deal of expertise" in the field of autism and seemed dismayed by desperate parents indulging in "crazy" therapies. Here was an opportunity for her to put a stop to what she considered to be clear evidence of abusive behavior.

Dr. Sanders is the expert. As a consequence, she writes and travels, speaking and testifying on the subject of MSBP. When ADES put its reputation on the line in this case, she delivered for them. Likely as not, she has already been invited back to assist in one or more of the many cases of MSBP that are pending litigation in Arizona. Although she is not licensed to practice in Arizona, she is doubtless well paid for her troubleshooting, hit-and-run role and does not fulfill this criterion either. The more cases that are exposed, the more her expertise and profile swell, and the closer the diagnosis of MSBP, despite its quicksand footing, edges toward inclusion in the full diagnostic bible of psychiatric maladies.[11] There is glory here.

Dr. Carter is something of a mystery. Like Dr. Stephens, I can discern altruistic motive here too; she was a concerned and critical pediatrician. "What person," she asked, "could put their children through these problems?"[12]

But was her judgment in error? Did she miscalculate or underplay the seriousness of Child 1's HSP while over-focusing on his allegedly factitious antibody deficiency and risky IVIG treatment? Was she so offended at having been fired by the father that she was motivated, even subconsciously, by revenge? She suspected malpractice and financial motivation in Dr. Hellmers but seemed to lack insight into her own shortcomings. And potentially, most serious of all, in a hospital corridor on the evening of March 16, 2010, did she forgo an essential examination of Child 2, only to fabricate it later that same night? Is this the risk that she had taken, referred to in the later e-mail exchange of April 23, 2010, in her determination to entrap the mother by putting her in a situation where she would request IVIG, a treatment prescribed for her child by a medical expert?

•   The behavior is not better accounted for by another **mental**[13] disorder.

Assessment of the parents by Dr. Mart, a psychologist retained by the defense— and someone whose opinion was, on the whole, sound—referred to the parents as having a "borderline personality disorder."[14]

Given the extraordinary circumstances in which they had been placed when Dr. Mart made this observation—the stress, the trauma of separation, the sleepless nights aching for the children's return while fearing for their safety and their perseveration on the possibility of permanent loss—a little upheaval in the psyche is to be expected.[15] And the extreme allegations, the isolation, and the

assumption of guilt might fuel a creeping paranoia that would be entirely justified. Grief, trauma, fear, insomnia, and paranoia—these are powerfully destabil-
izing; these can unbalance the stoutest mind.

Anger too—righteous anger—violated and threatened: this family is under
attack. It is their view and mine that they have been put in this position, at least
in part, by unsafe vaccination practices. They have every reason to be angry.
Despite this, they have, by all accounts, defended themselves with dignity and
a stoic reserve. I have found them to be charming and sincere. Any "borderline
personality disorder," a diagnosis that was milked for all it was worth in the
prosecution's final analysis, is better accounted for, in my opinion, by blunt
trauma: repeated blows to the head. This is not simply a metaphorical trauma;
it took the mother's therapist, psychologist Sarah Edmonds to point out to
the court that according to the DSM, a personality disorder should not be
diagnosed as it was in the mother by Dr. Sanders and Dr. Mart in the presence of "rule outs"—pre-existing conditions that preclude the diagnosis of a
personality disorder—like her previous head trauma and post-traumatic stress
disorder.[16]

It would be wrong to ascribe any formal diagnosis of mental disorder to the
Sorority. As far as I am aware, there is nothing in the DSM that fits their behavior. While DSM describes the manifestations of disease in affected individuals,
here the behavior is more of a collective hysteria—a drumbeat with a contagious
rhythm. Starting with Dr. Carter's being worked up, the volume rose to a level
that drowned out doubt, dissent, and reason.

So who best fit the uniform of Baron von Münchausen? Not the parents, for sure. And for the future, one overriding question should determine
the outcome of any enquiry of this nature: is the behavior of parent and/or
child better accounted for by the presence of organic disease(s) in the child?
According to this criterion the parents of the Arizona 5 are innocent. Indeed,
as Ms. Kupiszweski, the father's attorney, observed in her opening address, they
should be celebrated.

As I considered the closing of this book I sat, on the afternoon of March
11, 2011, in a meeting of the British Society of Ecological Medicine in London's
Hallam Street. The venue for the conference was the historical home of the
UK's medical regulator and my *bête noir*,[17] the GMC. The remit of the GMC has
always been to protect patients by the appropriate governance of doctors and
their practice. They have failed, certainly on behalf of the autism community.
Never was there a more bogus, compromised, and self-aggrandizing group of
committee men and women than those with whom I came in contact. But that's
only my opinion, and I'm biased, having been erased from the Medical Register

in May of 2010 in the process of acting to help children whose plight was very similar in many respects to the Arizona 5, children who have been all but forsaken by British medicine.

In the main council chamber, surrounded by the ghosts of doctors who, since 1885, had handed down or received judgment, a brave mother stood and told her halting, painful story of being falsely accused of MSBP. The elements of her son's narrative were virtually identical to those of the Arizona 5: developmental disorder, ataxia, GI disease with confirmed gastritis and colitis, a beneficial response of all of the above to a gluten- and casein-free diet, and of course, the allegation of abuse. And I realized then just how pervasive, how endemic this problem is in an era that marks the decline and fall of classical medicine—medicine that puts the patient first. The New Age, the age of public health and its delusion of utopia, the age of mandatory mass vaccination driven by Pharma's broken pipeline of drug discovery, for which vaccines are the only succor, a low-to-no-risk $35 billion annual succor by 2014.[18] This age will be mercifully short in the great scheme of human evolution, although brevity on an evolutionary scale is of little comfort to those affected.

The Arizona 5 should never have been taken from their parents. The strength of the family, their love for each other, and the devotion and quality of the parenting was confirmed in spades by witness Betty Jordan, a veteran of caring for handicapped children since the 1950s and a foster parent to no fewer than 326 children.[19] Judging by the enduring impact of separation at the hands of CPS on their older sister, Cherilyn, an event that still haunts her twenty years on, the effects upon these children will be long-lasting. If they are re-vaccinated, the effects may put them beyond repair.

On the issue of the impact of separation, Dr. Carter almost gets the last say: "The children would be so mentally damaged if they were removed [from their parents] that she is unsure what is best."

Dr. Carter may have cause to reflect that there was a time when that damage might have been prevented. But it began and should end with the children. In his closing argument, Mr. Horton, the children's attorney, pleaded with Judge Brutinel, "What I know is that these children want to go home . . . I ask that the Court listen to these children. The two older children [Child 1 and Child 2] and even [Child 3] to the extent that he is able have consistently told me that they want to go home. They feel safe at home, they are fine at home. They love their parents."[20]

It goes without saying that they should be immediately returned to their parents before further harm is done.

Today, in Jamaica, from the beautiful home of Al and Claire Dwoshkin, I left these pages and the palms to bend in the early morning breeze, the sun to rise over Montego Bay, and went to yoga. On the road—a gauntlet of bougainvillea and hibiscus—I walked past an heiress of a major pharmaceutical empire and vaccine manufacturer.

Time slips away—like light into a dark star—for one Arizona family.

I wanted to say something, but where do you start?

EPILOGUE

For over 20 years, the federal government has publicly denied a vaccine-autism link, while at the same time its Vaccine Injury Compensation Program (VICP) has been awarding damages for vaccine injury to children with brain damage, seizures and autism. Coming out just after the prevalence study of autism in South Korea [1 in every 38 children], this investigation, based on public, verifiable government data, breaks new ground in the controversial vaccine-autism debate.

Holland M et al.[1]

* * *

My friend, a researcher from Cuba who is also working on toxicity of vaccine adjuvants had one of his papers rejected from a journal with this explanation: *The article was not accepted under the **criteria**[2] [sic] that it open[s] doubts regarding the safety of vaccines and it is inadmissible.*

Dr. Lucija Tomljenovic
July 5, 2011

* * *

Today, May 31, 2011, I tried a little harder to understand where things had gone so badly wrong. I left the annex building of the United Nations Educational, Scientific, and Cultural Organization (UNESCO) on Rue Miollis, Paris, and hailed a cab. Despite the proximity of the Pasteur Institute and the mausoleum of the great Louis Pasteur, it was not my intention to seek answers there—at least on this occasion. On a perfect spring day I traveled west, staying south of the Seine, to the womb of Renaissance neuropsychiatry—the Hôpital de la Salpêtrière in Paris' 13th arrondissement.

First commissioned and designed in 1656 by Louis XIV, it was here that, in the latter half of the nineteenth century, Professeur Jean-Martin Charcot led the avant-garde of clinical neurology with medical assistants such as Georges Gilles de la Tourette, Pierre Marie, and Joseph Babinski. But among his many contributions to our recognition of such diseases as multiple sclerosis, amyotrophic lateral sclerosis (Lou Gehrig's disease), and neurosyphilis, he also opened a grimy window on the mysterious and evanescent malady of *hysteria*. Among those of his students attracted to this disorder, including Charcot's use of hypnosis on his comely and compliant patient "Blanche"[3] in an effort to get closer to hysteria's organic origins, was Sigmund Freud. For a human affliction of any significance, hysterics had their hour upon this Parisian stage, went on tour to Vienna with Freud's "Theatre of the Absurd," and are heard no more, except, perhaps, by proxy in the deceptive guise of psychoanalysis. Was there ever a condition that got more play from less substance? Olmsted and Blaxill have offered an attractive proposition and an ironic etiological counterpoint for mercury's toxic role in this enigmatic condition. In turn, however, the derivative field of psychoanalysis, with its requisite box of hidden desires and repressed hostilities, put another infinitely more important disorder—autism—in the hands of the wrong people. There, from Bedlam[4] to Baltimore,[5] not only has it languished, but blame for this disorder has been borne by parents for their genes and their glacial souls. And when these parents set about solving the mystery of autism's organic ins and outs, when they started to heal their damaged children, leaving most doctors speechless and emasculated in their wake, some in the Arizona medical system retrenched in MSBP—a bogus remedy for Medicine's own maladies. Why, Professor Charcot, why did it go wrong? Why did you hand over to these people the art of meticulous clinical observation—the mysteries revealed in the patient's history and examination?

My reason for having been at UNESCO was to present an overview of fifteen years of autism research at the invitation of Professeur Luc Montagnier and the scientists and doctors in his CHRONIMED group; autism has become one of their areas of research interest. Modest in height, Montagnier is a colossus in medical science, having received the Nobel Prize in 2008 for the discovery of human immunodeficiency virus. Despite the fact that we—le Professeur and I—exist at opposite poles of scientific respectability, I left his office with a collaboration agreed upon, a radically new view of molecular biology performing cartwheels in my neocortex, and a copy of his book *Les Combats de la Vie*—Life's Battles.[6] Inside he had written, "To Andy, with my great respect for his remarkable and courageous work." Forgive me such immodesty, but in a year when

I was described by the world's richest man as a "child killer,"[7] I was deeply moved by Professeur Montagnier's comment and wished to share it.

"One in 38 children in South Korea now has autism;"[8] 43–54% of US children have a chronic health condition;[9] time to get over myself.

On my third day in Paris, I walked through the Cimetière de Montmartre to pay my respects at the last resting place of Charcot, the Napoleon of the Salpêtrière, and to seek some spiritual guidance. The cemetery itself is like an elaborate gothic village for small people with agoraphobia. It is a wonderful testament to a France that has clung to its innate sense of social hierarchy, despite a revolution or two, intended to extinguish such recidivism. And the ability for name-dropping—even in death—must be irresistible: "My great-grandmother decays next to Emile Zola," or "I have a little plot between Vaslav Nijinsky and Hector Berlioz." Here, star of the Moulin Rouge Louise Weber—"*La Goulue*," inventor of the cancan—undoubtedly sleeps with a few old lovers. Over there, Edgar Degas,[10] perhaps the greatest artist of them all, is at peace. It is an extraordinary place; how the other half die. Now, however, because they are a health hazard, the *nouveau mort* must rest forever outside the limits of their beloved city.

I sat on some ancient stone steps and reflected upon a story recently told to me by my great friend and partner in the Autism Media Channel,[11] Polly Tommey. The French would love her—Polly—Eugene Delacroix's *Liberté* scaling the barricade to repel an enemy assault, her bare bosom striking, well . . . confusion into their hearts. Her passion is irrepressible and I have come across no combatant with more stomach for the fight.

Polly told me of a meeting of autism healthcare professionals and parents that she had addressed two months earlier in Cheshire in the North of England. There she had related her experience of having appeared with her husband, Jon, on a BBC news program with anchor Trevor MacDonald not long after their son Billy had been diagnosed with autism. The Tommeys had described their son's immediate seizure and regression into autism following his MMR vaccine. His medical records subsequently went missing from his GP's office. Familiar with the shortcomings of the National Health Service and not unduly concerned, the Tommeys contacted Paul Shattock at the Autism Research Unit in Sunderland where a duplicate set of records were held. Unfortunately Paul had to report to Polly that there had been a break-in; Billy's records, from among the many hundreds that they held, were the only things to have been stolen.

At the end of Polly's talk, a GP, who shall be known only as "Dr. Deb," raised her hand and addressed the meeting. She told of how, before her own child became autistic, she had been paid by a pharmaceutical company to destroy the medical records of children with autism in her practice. Apparently, *they* had approached her and *she* had accepted the bribe. Clearly, abuse comes in many guises. Dr. Deb's come-to-Jesus moment in Polly's audience— presumably her need to confess before this congregation following her own child's diagnosis—needs to be resolved; if not, such disgraceful actions including those of the drug company to whom, in effect, she sold these children's futures, will continue. It is a criminal offence to destroy evidence and an act of serious professional misconduct for "Dr. Deb" to have betrayed any patient in this way, let alone one whose damage and lifelong disability might otherwise have been due compensation for possible vaccine damage. Such records might even have been necessary for a defense against a charge of MSBP leveled at the child's parents. But for the pharmaceutical company involved, it was probably just all in a day's work.

The local autism community has rallied to Dr. Deb's support on the basis that she now provides for their children, reconciled as it appears to be in the fact that "we all make mistakes." Although some might not care to see it, there is a very clear line in the sand. The pharmaceutical company and the continuing violation of children with autism are on one side of this line and war is inevitable; it is time to decide where you stand.

On the Rue des Martyrs, walking south from Montmartre to the Rue des Moulins, I called my friend Dan Olmsted, editor of the daily autism newsblog *Age of Autism*. He and another friend—his fellow editor Mark Blaxill— had spent considerable time and effort doing what Brian Deer and the *British Medical Journal* (*BMJ*) had distained to do in their recent assault on me. Olmsted and Blaxill had conducted a thorough review of the *Lancet* paper, including face-to-face interviews with parents of the *Lancet* children on both sides of the Atlantic, analysis of the original documents from the parents, their doctors, the children's clinical records, the GMC transcripts, and the reports of the pathologists involved in the original description of bowel disease in these children. These had been compared with the claims of Deer and Dr. Fiona Godlee, the *BMJ*'s editor-in-chief. The factual findings of the Olmsted-Blaxill analysis and the colorful fantasy of the Deer-Godlee collaboration bear no relation. Independently, others reached the same conclusions as the Olmsted-Blaxill analysis, including Martin Hewitt and Clifford Miller in the UK and Dr. David Lewis, an ex-US Environmental Protection Agency (EPA) senior scientist who was himself subjected to false claims of scientific misconduct in an agency-industry act of gross indecency. Dr. Lewis, a fellow traveler, was innocent and has been completely exonerated; the EPA and their industry conspirators were not.[12]

On June 19, 2011, in a twist of 360 excruciating degrees, Dan Olmsted presented Dr. Godlee and her editorial team with the evidence of Deer's fraud and their own egregious editorial failings. Seven years earlier, in February 2004, Deer had presented his own "findings" to Dr. Richard Horton at the offices of the *Lancet*—and so it was the carousel with its garish, grinning characters, like Jack Nicholson's Joker and the dwarf from *Death in Venice*, were set upon their macabre bobbing pole dance—their ride, in my opinion, paid for by a pharma-government mutual fund.

And talking of small people with attitude, I have learned from the BBC that based upon the Deer-Godlee fantasia, Professor Mark Pepys—once, but briefly, my professor of medicine at the Royal Free Hospital School of Medicine—is to conduct a full review of my research. Below is a copy of a letter that I sent in response to this information to the vice-provost of University College, London, Sir John Tooke.

Dear Sir John,

I understand from his statements on BBC Radio 4, that Professor Mark Pepys is to conduct an investigation of my research while at the Royal Free Hospital School of Medicine. May I suggest that he is not a good choice for this task, for the following reasons:

1. He has a real conflict of interest—having initially declined his appointment at the Royal Free until I had been removed. The following are extracts from Professor Pepys' attendance note with Kate Emmerson of Field Fisher Waterhouse, the GMC's lawyers, on 12th April 2005.

    "He [Pepys] accepted the job on the condition that Wakefield was removed (this didn't happen)."

    "MP would have dismissed W but others at the Royal Free were unwilling to do so. MP was really the only person at the Free who was putting forward anti-W views."

2. Having taken up this appointment (his above condition having been rejected [Pepys' bluff had been called]), in the company of the Dean and the School Secretary, he confirmed to me that, despite having strong negative opinions about my research, he had never actually read any of it.

3. A book is due to be published later this year covering Professor Pepys' activities in relation to my work. It will allege, supported by documentary evidence, conspiracy to execute a bribe with a senior academic from

another institution in order to destroy peer-reviewed grant-awarded research looking at vaccine safety. This book will unfortunately be a source of major embarrassment for UCL and The Royal Free. May I suggest that you ask Professor Pepys to provide you with his email traffic from the relevant period October 1999 to 2002? This traffic has already been examined by third parties.

4. Professor Pepys' extreme bias against me has been evident throughout my dealings with him. He expressed this in public in his Harverian oration, as well as on the BBC.

5. He is deeply conflicted due to his relationship with vaccine manufacturers GlaxoSmithKline.[13] He is totally unsuited to leading any investigation of my research.

Finally, I will forward a copy of my book covering events at the Royal Free in the late 1990s and beyond—events that, sadly, will haunt that institution for many years to come. I do hope that you can find time to read it.

Yours sincerely,

Now it is almost time to return to the New World where the battle will be won. Like the lingering memory of good wine on the tongue, however, the narrative's Gallic roots cling tightly, reluctant to let the story go.

Latitude: 40°68' North, longitude: 74°04' West is a crime scene. The victim, a handsome woman of uncertain age, was actually conceived in France (after a reputedly excellent dinner hosted by Monsieur Edouard-Rene Lefebvre de Laboulaye at his mansion near the Palace of Versailles). As a newborn she moved to the New World, and it is here that she was violated. The crime itself—of neither passion nor insanity—was extreme, repeated, and took place in full daylight. Like many crimes, albeit usually of a lesser degree, there were witnesses, in this case thousands—hundreds of thousands. In the face of her violation, a gang-rape of the coldest and most callous measure, she stood—yes, stood—proud, apparently unmoved, appealing not even to God for an end to her suffering. Had you stared into her unblinking eyes for one hundred years you would have discerned nothing of her distress. She maintains, to this day, the illusion of her native *sang-froid:* she is stoic as she is vulnerable, vital but badly wounded—and we need her to survive. As for the witnesses, they paid to watch—can you believe it? They stood in line, jostling, laughing, and taking pictures to show to all their friends. And some were even paid to bring order to the ecstatic mob.

Surrounded by the bright waters of the Western Atlantic blending with the East River's final eddies they were dazzled, seeing only what they chose to. How could they have missed her tears? She weeps still, while staring with a sightless longing, back from whence she came. Her violation must end but those who have had her, those who have gorged upon her virtue, who violate her still, have become insatiable. She is in desperate need of the best medical care that money cannot buy.

Bearing northwest and leaving the Statue of Liberty off the port bow, one passes between Manhattan Island's Battery Park to the west and to the east, Brooklyn Heights, sitting on the western reach of Long Island. Whether you or your predecessors came to this great country by sea or air, for many the waters of Long Island Sound and the land masses of Manhattan and Long Island were the first encounter and a reason for excitement—heady hope. It is time to reclaim that hope.

Rue Yonne Letac, Montmartre, Paris. June 5, 2011

POSTSCRIPT

Following an analysis of the family's prospects for reunification by the Foster Care Review Board, part of the Judicial Branch of the Arizona Supreme Court, on May 23, 2011, the findings and recommendations were prepared for submission to the new judge—Judge Brutinel's successor—Judge Ethan Wolfinger. The Board's clear view was that the children's biological parents should forfeit all rights and that the children should be placed in permanent foster care. With echoes of the treatment of Soviet dissidents, they urged the Court to order psychiatric evaluation of the parents in light of their alleged anti-social behavior with paranoid and histrionic features. Moreover, the biological parents had not shown meaningful progress, which included a signed confession of their guilt— guilt of medical, emotional, and psychological abuse of their children.[1]

But before these recommendations had found their way into court, Judge Wolfinger, showing a wisdom that has been otherwise lacking in this story, ordered that the children be returned home to their parents. Amid considerable protest from the prosecution, he gave CPS a deadline to comply with his order.

On Tuesday June 7, 2011, after 359 days in care—extraordinarily, the exact number of days that Cherilyn had been removed from her mother by CPS over twenty years ago—the children came home. The mother likened the scene to the winning players' Superbowl celebration seconds after the final whistle. Unlike at the Superbowl, however, the children also asked for and were granted permission to bounce on their beds. At this stage the beds were just mattresses and box springs on the floor. To have erected the children's beds before this day would have been tempting fate.

Chisos Mountains, Big Bend National Park, Texas. June 30, 2011

* * *

This was written June 16, 2010. The day after my five siblings were taken away from their parents by Child Protective Services.

Cherilyn

We all have our childhood fears.
The monsters under the bed and the troll that lived in the basement.
Our parents tell us that we don't need to be afraid. That it will be Ok.
What do you do when you find out that your deepest fear has come true?
Mine just has.
The shakes start and I find that I just can't breathe.
I gasp for air praying that it isn't true.
My heart breaks with 4 simple words.
They took the kids.
The nightmare starts all over again.
However when I open my eyes it doesn't go away. It is real.
My deepest childhood fear has come to life and it feels like it is going to eat me alive.
The same nightmare that haunted me for 14 years has come true.
The monsters that chased my family in my dreams have caught them.
They tore them away and put them into a small car.
As in my dreams I am helpless to save them. All I can do is watch.
My deepest pain that became my deepest fear has been realized.
What do I do now? There is no one to tell me that I am going to be OK.
No one can tell me that it is just a dream.
My nightmare has turned into my brothers' and sisters' nightmare.
I sob wanting to be able to take their pain and situation on myself.
They were never supposed to see what happened in my nightmare.

I want to charge into battle and save the day.
I want to be the knight in shining armor that sweeps in and makes it all Ok.
I pick up the sword only to find that it is too big . . .
I can't pick it up. I can't wield it against my enemy . . .
Tears roll down my face as I realize that this is a battle that I can't fight.
I turn around and see God standing there with His arm outstretched.
He asks me to give Him back His sword.
His sword? But this is my battle!? It is my family!
He kneels down with tears in His eyes.
"Little one, do you think that I love them any less than you?

They were mine long before they were yours.
Let me fight this battle that only I can win.
This sword it too heavy for you because it was never meant for you to bear."
He wraps His arms around me as I cling to the sword sobbing.
I know what He says is true but I still feel like I have to do something.
He whispers in my ear, "Just trust me."
I look up into His eyes and know that I have to trust Him.
I slowly release my grip on the sword and place it in His large calloused hands.
He takes the sword and turns to walk away.
Then he looks back and says something that I will never forget.
"You had to give me the sword before I could fight this battle.
When you held onto it I was helpless. Your release has guaranteed victory, for when I fight on your behalf I can not lose."

God you have to take control of this. You have to be the knight in shining armor,
I can't save them, I can't protect them. Only you.
You saved me from the dragon and now I need you to save them.
They are the hardest thing that I have ever given you.
I want to be able to save them, but I can't.
This darkness that is trying to take them is bigger than me.
But it isn't bigger than you.
You are light, and where light is darkness can not be.
Please God; bring your light into this situation.
You are the only one that can make this nightmare end.
You can take it and turn it into a "Happily ever after."
Please God, let your mercy reign over them and your justice fall on their accusers.
Bring truth to the situation and peace over their hearts.

~Cherilyn Derusha

ACKNOWLEDGMENTS

I would like to express my gratitude to my publisher, Tony Lyons of Skyhorse Publishing, for allowing this important story to be told; my wonderful editor, Teri Arranga, who always took the helm in times of crisis; my valiant and inspirational wife, Carmel; and our wonderful children, James, Sam, Imogen, and Corin—I am very proud of you. My gratitude is also extended to the Autism Media Channel and Polly Tommey for the opportunity to share the plight of the Arizona 5 and my interpid cameraman, Erik Nanstiel, for helping me to do so. The brave doctors Robert Hellmers, MD, and Cindy Schneider, MD, for sharing their observations; Cynthia Macluskie, mother of a recovered child, for sounding the alarm; and, most of all, to the Derusha family, for providing a beacon of courage and love in the midst of great adversity. Beyond this is that army of supporters and fellow travelers to whom we are all related by blood, sweat, and tears; once again, my sincere thanks are extended to you also.

NOTES

PROLOGUE

1   It is uncertain quite how one subjects another person to developmental delays.

2   *Age of Autism.* (March 7, 2010). "Danish scientist absconds with $2 million, Poul Thorsen 'proved' vaccines don't cause autism." Retrieved from: www .ageofautism.com/2010/03/danish-scientist-absconds-with-2-million-poul-thorsen-proved-vaccines-dont-cause-autism-.html.

3   Handley JB. (April 18, 2011). "*OC Register* corrects Autism Science Foundation founder Dr. Paul Offit's lies (finally)." Retrieved from: http://www.ageofautism .com/2011/04/oc-register-corrects-autism-science-foundation-founder-dr-paul-offits-lies-finally.html.

4   Kirby D. (May 5, 2011). "Government and many scientists agree: vaccine-autism research should continue." Retrieved from: http://www.huffingtonpost .com/david-kirby/government-and-science-ag_b_853910.html.

5   *Age of Autism.* (May 9, 2011). "Investigators and families of vaccine-injured children to unveil report detailing clear vaccine-autism link based on government's own data." Retrieved from: http://www.ageofautism .com/2011/05/investigators-and-families-of-vaccine-injured-children-to-unveil-report-detailing-clear-vaccine-auti.html.

INTRODUCTION

1   *Arizona Department of Economic Security et al. v. Anon.* October 29, 2010. Page 24.

2   Allen Frances. *The Autism Generation*: "The most likely cause of the autism epidemic is that autism has become fashionable—a popular fad diagnosis." Available at: www.project-syndicate.org/commentary/frances1/English. Last accessed: January 27, 2012.

Chapter 1

1   For the purpose of this report, includes autism, Asperger's syndrome, pervasive developmental disorder—not otherwise specified (PDD-NOS), and childhood disintegrative disorder.

2   Kanner L. "Autistic disturbances of affective contact." *Nervous Child*. 1943; 2:217–50.

Wakefield AJ, Puleston JM, Montgomery SM, et al. Review article: "The concept of entero-colonic encephalopathy, autism, and opioid receptor ligands." *Alimentary Pharmacology and Therapeuticsapeutics*. 2002; 16:663–74.

Gastrointestinal symptoms are common in children with developmental disorders, a fact that was recognized by some of the earliest commentators on pathobiological mechanisms in autism; in 1986, Dohan was reported to have written: "K. Soddy (University College Hospital, London) wrote me that he noted that recurrent gastrointestinal upsets were a constant feature of autistic children and that, among other symptoms, the deteriorating autistic child often has acute diarrhoea." These observations feature prominently in parental accounts, but have been largely ignored in the autism literature.

Goodwin MS, Cowen MA, Goodwin TC. "Malabsorption and cerebral dysfunction: a multivariate and comparative study of autistic children." *Journal of Autism and Child Schizophrenia* 1971; 1:48–62. Walker-Smith J, Andrews J. Alpha-1-antitrypsin, autism, and coeliac disease. *Lancet*. 1972; 2:883–4.

Two studies published almost four decades ago identified GI problems in some children with autism. In 1971, a report of fifteen randomly selected autistic cases described six children who had bulky, odorous, or loose stools, or intermittent diarrhea; one patient had coeliac disease. The other study described low serum concentrations of a-1 antitrypsin in some patients with autism, an indication of pathological loss of protein from the intestine.

3   Sandler RH, Finegold SM, Bolte ER, et al. "Short-term benefit from oral vancomycin treatment of regressive-onset autism." *Journal of Child Neurology*. 2000; 15:429–35.

4   Balzola F, et al. "Beneficial behavioural effects of IBD therapy and gluten-/casein-free diet in an Italian cohort of patients with autistic enterocolitis followed over one year." *Gastroenterology*. 2008; 4:S1364.

Whitely P, Haracopos D, Knivsberg AM, et al. "The ScanBrit randomised, controlled, single-blind study of a gluten- and casein-free dietary intervention for children with autism spectrum disorders." *Nutritional Neuroscience* 2010; 13:87–100. Knivsberg AM, Reichelt KL, Høien T, Nødland M. "A randomised, controlled study of dietary intervention in autistic syndromes." *Nutritional Neuroscience*. 2002; 5:251–61.

5   Long WR. (2008, July 12). "Münchausen syndrome by proxy/factitious disorder by proxy: A critical assessment for judges and lawyers." Retrieved from: www.autism.com/pdf/families/MBSP_unabridged.pdf.

6   Blaxill M. What's going on. "The question of time trends in autism." *Public Health Reports.* 2004; 119:536–551.

Hertz-Picciotto I, Delwiche L. "The rise in autism and the role of age at diagnosis." *Epidemiology.* 2009; 20:84–90.

DeSoto MC, Hitlan RT. "Sorting out the spinning of autism: heavy metals and the question of incidence." *Acta Neurobiologiae Experimentalis (Wars).* 2010; 70:165–76.

7   Deykin EY, MacMahon B. "Viral exposure and autism." *American Journal of Epidemiology.* 1979; 109:628–638.

Ring A, Barak Y, Ticher A, et al. "Evidence for an infectious etiology in autism." *Pathophysiology.* 1997; 4:91–6.

Johnstone JA, Ross CAC, Dunn M. "Meningitis and encephalitis associated with mumps infection: A 10-year survey." *Archives of Disease in Childhood.* 1972; 47:647–51.

Chess S. "Autism in children with congenital rubella." *Journal of Autism Child schizophrenia.* 1971; 1:33–47.

8   Hertz-Picciotto I. "It's time to start looking for the environmental culprits responsible for the remarkable increase in the rate of autism in California." Quoted in: Kirby D. (January 8, 2009). UC Davis study authors: "Autism is environmental (Can we move on now?)." Retrieved from: http://www.huffingtonpost.com/david-kirby/uc-davis-study-autism-is_b_156153.html

Hallmayer J, Cleveland S, Torres A, et al. "Genetic heritability and shared environmental factors among twin pairs with autism." *Archives of General Psychiatry.* 2011; 68:1095–102.

9   Palmer RF. Blanchard S, Wood R. "Proximity to point sources of environmental mercury release as a predictor of autism prevalence." *Health Place.* 2009; 15:18–24.

Oberts EM, English PB, Grether JK, et al. "Maternal residence near agricultural pesticide applications and autism spectrum disorders among children in the California Central Valley." *Environmental Health Perspectives.* 2007; 115:1482–9.

Volk HE, Hertz-Picciotto I, Delwiche L, et al. "Residential proximity to freeways and autism in the CHARGE study." *Environmental Health Perspectives.* 2011; 119:873–7.

10   Reviewed in *Callous Disregard: Autism and Vaccines—The Truth Behind a Tragedy.* New York: Skyhorse Publishing, 2010. Chapter ten, pp. 143–68.

11 Ibid.

12 Fombonne E, Chakrabarti S. "No evidence for a new variant of measles-mumps-rubella-induced autism." *Pediatrics*. 2001; 108:E58.

13 Ashwood P, Wills S, Van de Water J. "The immune response in autism: A new frontier for autism research." *Journal of Leukocyte Biology*. 2006; 80:1–15.

14 Rutter M, Bailey A, Bolton P, et al. "Autism and known medical conditions: myth and substance." *The Journal of Child Psychology and Psychiatry*. 1994; 35:311–22.

15 DeSoto MC, Hitlan RT. "Sorting out the spinning of autism: Heavy metals and the question of incidence." *Acta Neurobiologiae Experimentalis (Wars)*. 2010; 70:165–76.

    Holland M, Conte L, Krakow R, et al. "Unanswered questions from the Vaccine Injury Compensation Program: A review of compensated cases of vaccine-induced brain injury." *Pace Environmental Law Review*. 2011; 28:480. Available at: http://digitalcommons.pace.edu/pelr/vol28/iss2/6.

16 Buie T, Campbell DB, Fuchs GJ III, et al. "Evaluation, diagnosis, and treatment of gastrointestinal disorders in individuals with ASDs: A consensus report." *Pediatrics*. 2010; 125:S1–S18.

17 Taylor B, Miller E, Lingam R, et al. "Measles, mumps, rubella, vaccination and bowel problems or developmental regression in children with autism: Population study." *British Medical Journal*. 2002; 324:393–6.

    Ming X, Brimacombe M, Chabaan J, et al. "Autism spectrum disorders: Concurrent clinical disorders." *Journal of Child Neurology*. 2008; 23:6–13.

    Fombonne E, Chakrabarti S. "No evidence for a new variant of measles-mumps-rubella-induced autism." *Pediatrics*. 2001; 108:E58.

18 Horvath K, Perman JA. "Autistic disorder and gastrointestinal disease." *Current Opinion in Pediatrics*. 2002; 14:583–587.

    Melmed R et al. "Metabolic markers and gastrointestinal symptoms in children with autism and related disorders." *Journal of Pediatric Gastroenterology and Nutrition*. 2000; 31:S174.

    Reviewed by Buie T, Campbell DB, Fuchs GJ, et al. "Evaluation, diagnosis, and treatment of gastrointestinal disorders in individuals with ASDs: A consensus report." *Pediatrics*. 2010; 125:S1–18.

19 Valicenti-McDermott M, McVicar K, Rapin I, et al. "Frequency of gastrointestinal symptoms in children with autistic spectrum disorders and association with family history of autoimmune disease." *Journal of Developmental and Behavioral Pediatrics*. 2006; 27:S128–S136.

20   Wakefield AJ, Puleston JM, Montgomery SM, et al. Review article: "The concept of entero-colonic encephalopathy, autism, and opioid receptor ligands." *Alimentary Pharmacology and Therapeutics*. 2002; 16:663–74.

"Long-standing intestinal symptoms, including pain, oesophageal reflux, diarrhoea, chronic constipation with overflow, and provocation of both gastro-intestinal and behavioural symptoms by certain foods, are typical of this group of children and have been described by others. Frequently, careful attention needs to be paid to the history in order to adduce these symptoms; an autistic child in pain who is unable to communicate normally may be distressed, aggressive and self-injurious; our early findings that bowel clearance often abrogates these behavioural symptoms is a clue to their likely intestinal origin."

21   Horvath K, Perman JA. "Autistic disorder and gastrointestinal disease." *Current Opinion in Pediatrics*. 2002; 14:583–7.

22   Krigsman A, Boris M, Goldblatt A, et al. "Clinical presentation and histologic findings at ileocolonoscopy in children with autistic spectrum disorder and chronic gastrointestinal symptoms." *Autism Insights*. 2010; 2:1–11.

23   Buie T, Campbell DB, Fuchs GJ III, et al. "Evaluation, diagnosis, and treatment of gastrointestinal disorders in Individuals with ASDs: A consensus report." *Pediatrics*. 2010; 125:S1–S18.

24   American Psychiatric Association. *Diagnostic and Statistical Manual of Mental Disorders*, Fourth Edition, Text Revision (DSM IV-TR). Washington, DC: American Psychiatric Association, 2000.

25   Axelrod FB, Chelimsky GG, Weese-Mayer DE. "Pediatric autonomic disorders." *Pediatrics*. 2006; 118:309–21.

There is sufficient evidence of autonomic dysfunction in autism that Axelrod and colleagues classify it as a *pediatric autonomic disorder*.

26   Reviewed by Wakefield AJ and Stott CM. "Autism—an epicenter in the brainstem." *The Autism File Global*. 2010; 37:120–9.

27   Brusch B, Ingman K, Vitti L, et al. "Chronic pain in individuals with previously undiagnosed autistic spectrum disorders." *Journal of Pain*. 2004; 5:290–5.

28   Kellow JE, Ekersley GM, Jones MP. "Enhanced perception of physiological intestinal motility in irritable bowel syndrome." *Gastroenterology*. 1991; 101:1621–7.

Van Ginkel R, Voskuul WP, Benninga MA, et al. "Alterations in rectal sensitivity and motility in childhood irritable bowel syndrome." *Gastroenterology*. 2001; 120:31–8.

Hyman PE, Bursch B, Sood M, et al. "Visceral pain-associated disability syndrome: A descriptive analysis." *Journal of Pediatric Gastroenterology and Nutrition*. 2002; 35:663–8.

29 Peristalsis is a radially symmetrical contraction and relaxation of muscles which propagates in a wave down the muscular tube. In humans, peristalsis is found in the contraction of smooth muscles to propel contents through the digestive tract. http://en.wikipedia.org/wiki/Peristalsis.

30 Hansen MB. "Small intestinal manometry." *Physiological Research*. 2002; 51:541–56.

Recordings of intraluminal intestinal pressures are performed using a multi-lumen polyvinyl catheter, which detects pressures resulting from phasic contraction of the circular muscle layer. The probe is introduced via the mouth and positioned under fluoroscopic (X-ray) control in such a way that the different sensors are located in the antrum of the stomach and in different regions of the small intestine. The catheter is continuously perfused with water by means of an infusion pump at a low rate and connected to external pressure transducers and recorded at a sampling frequency not less than 4 Hz, for later analysis of motor patterns.

31 Anuras J, Anuras S. "Pseudo-obstruction syndromes." In *Motility Disorders of the Gastrointestinal Tract*. S. Anuras (Ed). New York: Raven Press, 1992, pp. 327–44.

32 Emphasis added.

33 Cucciara S, Borrelli O, Salvia G, et al. "A normal gastrointestinal motility excludes chronic intestinal pseudoobstruction in children." *Digestive Diseases and Sciences*. 2000; 45:258–64.

34 Rosenberg DA. "Web of deceit: A literature review of Münchausen syndrome by proxy." *Child Abuse and Neglect*. 1987; 11:547–63.

35 Carter KE, Izsak E, Marlow J. "Münchausen syndrome by proxy caused by ipecac poisoning." *Pediatric Emergency Care*. 2006; 22:655–6.

36 Hyman PE, Bursch B, Beck D, et al. "Discriminating pediatric condition falsification from chronic intestinal pseudo-obstruction in toddlers." *Child Maltreatment*. 2002; 7:132–7.

37 Gardener H, Spiegelman D, Buka SL. "Prenatal risk factors for autism: Comprehensive meta-analysis." *The British Journal of Psychiatry*. 2009; 195:7–14.

38 Of unknown cause.

39 Altaf M, Werlin S, Sato T, et al. "Colonic volvulus in children with intestinal motility disorders." *Journal of Pediatric Gastroenterology and Nutrition*. 2009; 49:59–62.

40 Hyman PE, Bursch B, Sood M, et al. "Visceral pain-associated disability syndrome: A descriptive analysis." *Journal of Pediatric Gastroenterology and Nutrition*. 2002; 35:663–8.

41   CIP (7), idiopathic or post-viral gastroparesis (paralysis) (5), Crohn's dis-
      ease (3), GERD (5), biliary dyskinesia (impaired bile flow) (2), and superior
      mesenteric artery syndrome (GI symptoms due to intermittent occlusion
      of the blood supply to the small intestine) (2).

42   Sabra A, Bellanti JA, Colón AR. "Ileal-lymphoid-nodular hyperplasia, non-
      specific colitis, and pervasive developmental disorder in children." *Lancet.*
      1998; 352:234–5.

            Sabra A, Hartman D, Zeligs BJ. "Linkage of ileal lymphoid nodular
      hyperplasia (ILNH), food allergy, and CNS development: Evidence for a
      non-IgE association." *Annals of Allergy, Asthma and Immunology.* 1999; 82:8.

43   Buie T, Campbell DB, Fuchs GJ III, et al. "Evaluation, diagnosis, and treat-
      ment of gastrointestinal disorders in individuals with ASDs: A consensus
      report." *Pediatrics.* 2010; 125:S1–S18.

44   Thompson WG. "Factitious gastrointestinal symptoms and Münchausen
      syndrome." *American Journal of Medicine.* 2003; 31:115–8.

Chapter 2

1   Chong S, Blackshaw AJ, Boyle S, et al. "Histological diagnosis of inflam-
      matory bowel disease in childhood." *Gut.* 1985; 26:55–9.

2   Gonzalez L, López K, Martínez M, et al. "Endoscopic and histological
      characteristics of the digestive mucosa in autistic children with gastro-
      intestinal symptoms." *Archivos venezolanos de puericultura y pediatria.* 2005;
      69:19–25.

            Balzola F, Barbon V, Repici A, et al. "Panenteric IBD-like disease in a
      patient with regressive autism shown for the first time by wireless capsule
      enteroscopy: Another piece in the jig-saw of the gut-brain syndrome?" *The
      American Journal of Gastroenterology.* 2005; 100:979–81.

            Galiatsatos P, Gologan A, Lamoureux E. "Autistic enterocolitis: Fact or
      fiction." *Canadian Journal of Gastroenterology.* 2009; 23:95–8.

            Krigsman A, Boris M, Goldblatt A, et al. "Clinical presentation and
      histologic findings at ileocolonoscopy in children with autistic spectrum
      disorder and chronic gastrointestinal symptoms." *Autism Insights.* 2009;
      1:1–11.

            Chen B, Girgis S, El-Matary W. "Childhood autism and eosinophilic
      colitis." *Digestion.* 2010; 81:127–9.

3   Crohn's disease and ulcerative colitis.

            Balzola F, et al. "Beneficial behavioural effects of IBD therapy and gluten-/
      casein-free diet in an Italian cohort of patients with autistic enterocolitis
      followed over one year." *Gastroenterology.* 2008; 4:S1364.

4   Wakefield AJ, Anthony A, Murch SH, et al. "Enterocolitis in children with developmental disorders." *The American Journal of Gastroenterology*. 2000; 95:2285–95.

5   Horvath K, Papadimitriou JC, Rabsztyn A, et al. "Gastrointestinal abnormalities in children with autistic disorder." *Journal of Pediatrics*. 1999; 135:559–63.

6   Krigsman A, Boris M, Goldblatt A, et al. "Clinical presentation and histologic findings at ileocolonoscopy in children with autistic spectrum disorder and chronic gastrointestinal symptoms." *Autism Insights*. 2010; 2:1–11.

7   Balzola F, Daniela C, Repici A, et al. "Autistic enterocolitis: confirmation of a new inflammatory bowel disease in an Italian cohort of patients [abstract]." *Gastroenterology*. 2005; 128:Suppl 2;A–303.

8   González L, López K, Martínez M, et al. "Endoscopic and histological characteristics of the digestive mucosa in autistic children with gastrointestinal symptoms." *Archivos venezolanos de puericultura y pediatria*. 2005; 69:19–25.

9   Torrente F, Anthony A, Herushkel RB, et al. "Focal-enhanced gastritis in regressive autism with features distinct from Crohn's and helicobacter pylori gastritis." *The American Journal of Gastroenterology*. 2004; 4:598–605.

10   Torrente F, Ashwood P, Day R, et al. "Small intestinal enteropathy with epithelial IgG and complement deposition in children with regressive autism." *Molecular Psychiatry*. 2002; 7:375–82.

11   Kushak RI, Lauwers GY, Winter HS, et al. "Intestinal disaccharidase activity in patients with autism: Effect of age, gender, and intestinal inflammation." *Autism*. 2011; 15:285–94.

12   Audit of Royal Free cases and abstract presented by Dr. Anthony to the British Society of Gastroenterology.

13   Farmer M, Petras RE, Hunt LE, et al. "The importance of diagnostic accuracy in colonic inflammatory bowel disease." *The American Journal of Gastroenterology*. 2000; 95:3184–8.

    Theodossi A, Spigelhalter DJ, Jass J, et al. "Observer variation and discriminatory value in biopsy features in inflammatory bowel disease." *Gut*. 1994; 35:961–8.

14   Wakefield AJ, Murch SH, Anthony A, et al. "Ileal lymphoid nodular hyperplasia, non-specific colitis and pervasive developmental disorder in children." *Lancet*. 1998; 351:637–41.

15   Wakefield AJ, Anthony A, Murch SH, et al. "Enterocolitis in children with developmental disorders." *The American Journal of Gastroenterology*. 2000; 95:2285–95.

GMC v. Wakefield, Walker-Smith, and Murch. Evidence of Dr. Susan Davies. Day 32.

Report of Dr. Noam Harpaz, Mount Sinai Hospital NY, in the UK MMR litigation.

16 Letter from AW to John O'Leary. September 28, 1998.

17 Wakefield AJ, Anthony A, Murch SH, et al. "Enterocolitis in children with developmental disorders." *The American Journal of Gastroenterology.* 2000; 95:2285–95.

18 Horvath K, Papadimitriou JC, Rabsztyn A, et al. "Gastrointestinal abnormalities in children with autistic disorder." *Journal of Pediatrics.* 1999; 135:559–63.

Furlano RI, Anthony A, Day R, et al. "Colonic CD8 and α T-cell infiltration with epithelial damage in children with autism." *Journal of Pediatrics.* 2001; 138:366–72.

Torrente F, Ashwood P, Day R, et al. "Small intestinal enteropathy with epithelial IgG and complement deposition in children with regressive autism." *Molecular Psychiatry.* 2002; 7:375–82.

Torrente F, Anthony A, Herushkel RB, et al. "Focal-enhanced gastritis in regressive autism with features distinct from Crohn's and helicobacter pylori gastritis." *The American Journal of Gastroenterology.* 2004; 4:598–605.

19 Ashwood P, Murch SH, Anthony A, et al. "Intestinal lymphocyte populations in children with regressive autism: evidence for extensive mucosal immunopathology." *Journal of Clinical Immunology.* 2003; 23:504–17.

20 $p < 0.01$.

21 Personal communication.

22 *The Gary Null Show.* Available at: http://www.progressiveradionetwork.com/the-gary-null-show-wnye/.

23 Ibid.

24 Ibid.

25 *GMC v. Wakefield, Walker-Smith, and Murch.* Testimony of Professor Walker-Smith. Transcript. Wednesday July 16, 2008.

26 "In my new discipline, paediatric gastroenterology, there was virtually no literature when I started; this is what it was about, actually making detailed observations on individual children, often—I could take the example of coeliac disease—vague reports of partial villus atrophy by routine labs and then when we looked at it and did detailed observations, we found there were a number of features in which you could either prove or disprove the diagnosis of coeliac disease, just by careful observation." *GMC v. Wakefield,*

Walker-Smith, and Murch. Testimony of Professor Walker-Smith. Transcript. Wednesday July 16, 2008.

27   Ibid.

28   Emphasis added.

29   *GMC v. Wakefield, Walker-Smith, and Murch.* Testimony of Professor Walker-Smith. Transcript. Wednesday, July 16, 2008.

30   Ibid.

31   Ibid.

32   Ibid.

33   Ibid.

34   Notes of Professor Walker-Smith prepared for a presentation at the Wellcome Trust in December 1996.

35   *GMC v. Wakefield, Walker-Smith, and Murch.* Statement of Dr. A. P. Dhillon. July 28, 2006. Reproduced in *Callous Disregard: Autism and Vaccines— The Truth Behind a Tragedy*, Skyhorse Publishing, 2010, pp. 214–215; and Wakefield's complaint about Brian Deer to the UK's Press Complaints Commission at www.cryshame.org.

36   Davies S. "Caution in assessing histopathological opinions." *British Medical Journal Rapid Responses.* April 30, 2010. Available at: http://www.British Medical Journal.com/content/340/British Medical Journal.c1127/reply#235073 [last accessed June 2010].

37   *GMC v. Wakefield, Walker-Smith, and Murch.* Examination of Dr. Davies by Mr. Hopkins, counsel for Dr. Murch. GMC transcripts, Day 32, pp. 36–7.

38   Wakefield AJ, Murch SH, Anthony A, et al. "Ileal lymphoid nodular hyperplasia, non-specific colitis and pervasive developmental disorder in children." *Lancet.* 1998; 351:637–41.

39   *GMC v. Wakefield, Walker-Smith, and Murch.* Testimony of Professor Walker-Smith. Transcript. Wednesday, July 16, 2008.

40   Ibid.

41   Wakefield AJ, Murch SH, Anthony A, et al. "Ileal lymphoid nodular hyperplasia, non-specific colitis and pervasive developmental disorder in children." *Lancet.* 1998; 351:637–41.

42   Wakefield AJ, Anthony A, Murch SH, et al. "Enterocolitis in children with developmental disorders." *The American Journal of Gastroenterology.* 2000; 95:2285–95.

43   Wakefield AJ. "Autistic enterocolitis: Is it a histopathological entity?" *Histopathology.* 2007; 50:380–4.

44   Deer B. Wakefield. 'Autistic enterocolitis' under the microscope." *British Medical Journal.* 2010; 340:838–41.

45 Ibid.

46 Davies S. "Caution in assessing histopathological opinions." *British Medical Journal Rapid Responses.* April 30, 2010. http://www.British Medical Journal .com/content/340/British Medical Journal.c1127/reply#235073.

47 Ibid.

48 *Callous Disregard: Autism and Vaccines—The Truth Behind a Tragedy,* Skyhorse Publishing, 2010; and Wakefield's complaint about Brian Deer to the UK's Press Complaints Commission at www.cryshame.org.

49 "Left Brain/Right Brain." (February 10, 2009). *Autism News Science and Opinion.* http://leftbrainrightbrain.co.uk/?p=1849andcpage=3#comment-56579.

50 Ibid.

51 Wakefield AJ, Anthony A, Murch SH, et al. "Enterocolitis in children with developmental disorders." *The American Journal of Gastroenterology.* 2000; 95:2285–95.

    Jarocka-Cyrta E, Wasilewska J, Kaczmarski MG. "Eosinophilic esophagitis as a cause of feeding problems in autistic boy. The first reported case." *Journal of Autism and Developmental Disorders.* 2011; 41:372–4.

    Balzola F, Barbon V, Repici A, et al. "Panenteric IBD-like disease in a patient with regressive autism shown for the first time by the wireless capsule enteroscopy: Another piece in the jigsaw of this gut-brain syndrome?" *The American Journal of Gastroenterology.* 2005; 100:979–81.

52 Sbeih F, Abdullah A, Sullivan S, et al. "Antral nodularity, gastric lymphoid hyperplasia and Helicobacter pylori in adults." *Journal of Clinical Gastroenterology.* 1996; 22:227–30.

53 Zanardi LR, Haber P, Mootrey GT, et al. "Intussusception among recipients of rotavirus vaccine: Reports to the vaccine adverse event reporting system." *Pediatrics.* 2001; 107:E97.

54 Konno T, Suzuki H, Kutsuzawa T, et al. "Human rotavirus infection in infants and young children with intussusception." *Journal of Medical Virology.* 1978; 2:265–9.

55 Sbeih F, Abdullah A, Sullivan S, et al. "Antral nodularity, gastric lymphoid hyperplasia and Helicobacter pylori in adults." *Journal of Clinical Gastroenterology.* 1996; 22:227–30.

56 Konno T, Suzuki H, Kutsuzawa T, et al. "Human rotavirus infection in infants and young children with intussusception." *Journal of Medical Virology.* 1978; 2:265–9.

57 Montgomery EA, Edwina J. "Intussusception, adenovirus, and children: A brief reaffirmation." *Human Pathology.* 1994; 25:169–74.

58   Hermans PE, Huizenga KA, Hoffmann HN, et al. "Dysgammaglobulinaemia asscociated with nodular lymphoid hyperplasia of the small intestine." *American Journal of Medicine.* 1966; 40:78–89.

Webster ADB, Kenwright S, Ballard J, et al. "Nodular lymphoid hyperplasia of the bowel in primary hypogammaglobulinaemia: Study of in vitro lymphocyte function." *Gut.* 1977; 18:364–72.

Levendoglu H, Rosen Y. "Nodular lymphoid hyperplasia of gut in HIV infection." *The American Journal of Gastroenterology.* 1992; 87:1200–2.

59   Zanardi LR, Haber P, Mootrey GT, et al. "Intussusception among recipients of rotavirus vaccine: Reports to the vaccine adverse event reporting system." *Pediatrics.* 2001; 107:E97.

60   Kokkonen J, Karttunen TJ, Niinima KA. "Lymphoidnodular hyperplasia as a sign of food allergy in children." *Journal of Pediatric Gastroenterology and Nutrition.* 1999; 29:57–62.

Kokkonen J, Karttunen TJ. "Lymphoidnodular hyperplasia on the mucosa of the lower gastrointestinal tract in children: An indication of enhanced immune response?" *Journal of Pediatric Gastroenterology and Nutrition.* 2002; 34:42–6.

61   The institution where Dr. Burrill Bernard Crohn first described his eponymous disease with colleagues Dr. Ginsberg and Dr. Oppenheimer in 1932. Crohn BB, Ginsburg L, Oppenheimer GD. "Regional ileitis: A pathologic and clinical entity." *Journal of the American Medical Association.* 1932; 99:1323–9.

62   Krigsman A, Boris M, Goldblatt A, et al. "Clinical presentation and histologic findings at ileocolonoscopy in children with autistic spectrum disorder and chronic gastrointestinal symptoms." *Autism Insights.* 2009; 1:1–11.

63   Wakefield AJ, Ashwood P, Limb K, et al. "The significance of ileo-colonic lymphoid nodular hyperplasia in children with autistic spectrum disorder." *European Journal of Gastroenterology and Hepatology.* 2006; 17:827–36.

64   Ashwood P, Anthony A, Torrente F, et al. "Spontaneous mucosal lymphocyte cytokine profiles in children with autism and gastrointestinal symptoms: Mucosal immune activation and reduced counter regulatory interleukin-10." *Journal of Clinical Immunology.* 2004; 24:664–73.

65   Ashwood P, Wakefield AJ. "Immune activation of peripheral blood and mucosal CD3+ lymphocyte cytokine profiles in children with autism and gastrointestinal symptoms." *Journal of Neuroimmunology.* 2006; 173:126–34.

66   Jyonouchi H, Sun S, Le H. "Proinflammatory and regulatory cytokine production associated with innate and adaptive immune responses in children with autism spectrum disorders and developmental regression." *Journal of Neuroimmunology.* 2001; 120:170–9.

67 Horvath K, Papadimitriou JC, Rabsztyn A, et al. "Gastrointestinal abnormalities in children with autistic disorder." *Journal of Pediatrics*. 1999; 135:559–63.

68 Kushak RI, Lauwers GY, Winter HS, et al. "Intestinal disaccharidase activity in patients with autism: Effect of age, gender, and intestinal inflammation." *Autism*. 2011; 15:285–94.

69 $p < 0.05$.

70 Kushak RI, Winter HS, Farber NS, et al. "Gastrointestinal symptoms and intestinal disaccharidase activities in children with autism." Abstract of presentation to the North American Society of Pediatric Gastroenterology, Hepatology, and Nutrition Annual Meeting, October 20-22, 2005, Salt Lake City, Utah. *Journal of Pediatric Gastroenterology and Nutrition*. 2005; 41:508.

71 D'Eufemia P, Celli M, Finnochiaro R, et al. "Abnormal intestinal permeability in children with autism." *Acta Paediatrica*. 1996; 85:1076–9.

72 De Magistris L, Familiari V, Pascotto A, et al. "Alterations of the intestinal barrier in patients with autism spectrum disorders and in their first-degree relatives." *Journal of Pediatric Gastroenterology and Nutrition*. 2010; 51:418–24.

73 Horvath K, Zielke H, Collins J, et al. "Secretin improves intestinal permeability in autistic children." *Journal of Pediatric Gastroenterology and Nutrition*. 2000; 31:S30–S31.

74 Collins S, Bercik P, Denou E, et al. "The influence of commensal bacteria on the gut-brain axis: Implications for understanding and treating functional GI disorders." *Bioscience and Microflora*. 2010; 29:179–83.

75 Ibid.

76 Bolte ER. "Autism and Clostridium tetani." *Medical Hypotheses*. 1998; 51:133–44.

77 Finegold SM, Molitoris D, Song Y, et al. "Gastrointestinal microflora studies in late-onset autism." *Clinical Infectious Diseases*. 2002; 35(Suppl 1):S6–S16.

78 Ibid.

79 Wall JL. "The characterization of gut microflora and gastrointestinal symptomatology in children ages 3–9 years with autism spectrum disorders." Master of Science Thesis. Ohio State University, 2010. http://etd.ohiolink.edu/view.cgi/Wall%20Jody.pdf?osu1275488429.

80 $p = 0.006$.

81 $p = 0.008$.

82 $p = 0.008$.

83 $p = 0.007$.

84   $p = 0.034$.

85   $p = 0.002$.

86   $p = 0.00002$ (a factor that may be explained, in part, by probiotic use).

87   Adams JB, Johansen LJ, Powell LD, et al. "Gastrointestinal flora and gastrointestinal status in children with autism–comparisons to typical children and correlation with autism severity." *BMC Gastroenterology.* 2011; 11:22.

88   Li W, Dowd SE, Scurlock B, et al. "Memory and learning behavior in mice is temporally associated with diet-induced alterations in gut bacteria." *Physiology and Behavior.* 2009; 96:557–67.

89   $P = 0.0008$.

90   $p = 0.0008$.

91   $p < 0.0001$.

92   $P = 0.0004$.

93   Li W, Dowd SE, Scurlock B, et al. "Memory and learning behavior in mice is temporally associated with diet-induced alterations in gut bacteria." *Physiology and Behavior.* 2009; 96:557–67.

94   Heijtz RD, Wang S, Anuar F, et al. "Normal gut microbiota modulates brain development and behavior." *Proceedings of the National Academy of Sciences of the United States of America.* 2011; 108:3047–52.

95   Thomas RH, Foley KA, Mepham JR, et al. "Altered brain phospholipid and acylcarnitine profiles in propionic acid infused rodents: Further development of a potential model of autism spectrum disorders." *Journal of Neurochemistry.* 2010; 113:515–29.

96   MacFabe DF, Rodríguez-Capote K, Hoffman JE, et al. "A novel rodent model of autism: Intraventricular infusions of propionic acid increase locomotor activity and induce neuroinflammation and oxidative stress in discrete regions of adult rat brain." *American Journal of Biochemistry and Biotechnology.* 2008; 4:146–66.

97   Shultz SR, MacFabe DF, Ossenkopp. KP, et al. "Intracerebroventricular injection of propionic acid, an enteric bacterial metabolic end-product, impairs social behavior in the rat: Implications for an animal model of autism." *Neuropharmacology.* 2008; 54:901–11.

98   Shultz SR, MacFabe DF, Martin S, et al. "Intracerebroventricular injections of the enteric bacterial metabolic product propionic acid impair cognition and sensorimotor ability in the Long–Evans rat: further development of a rodent model of autism." *Behavioural Brain Research.* 2009; 200:33–41.

99   Sudo N, Chida Y, Aiba Y, et al. "Postnatal microbial colonization programs the hypothalamic-pituitary-adrenal system for stress response in mice." *The Journal of Physiology.* 2004; 558:263–75.

100 Verdu EF, Bercik P, Verma-Gandhu M, et al. "Specific probiotic therapy attenuates antibiotic induced visceral hypersensitivity in mice." *Gut.* 2006; 55:182–90.

101 Wakefield AJ, Stott C. "Autism, an epicenter in the brainstem." *The Autism File.* 2010; 37:120–9.

102 Whiteley P, Haracopos D, Knivsberg AM, et al. "The ScanBrit randomised, controlled, single-blind study of a gluten- and casein-free dietary intervention for children with autism spectrum disorders." *Nutritional Neuroscience.* 2010; 13:87–100.

   Knivsberg AM, Reichelt KL, Høien T, et al. "A randomised, controlled study of dietary intervention in autistic syndromes." *Nutritional Neuroscience.* 2002; 5:251–61.

   Walker-Smith J, Davies SE, Murch SH, et al. "Ileo-caecal lymphoid nodular hyperplasia non-specific ileo-colitis with regressive behavioural disorder and food intolerance: A case study." *Journal of Pediatric Gastroenterology and Nutrition.* 1997; 25:48.

103 De Magistris L, Familiari V, Pascotto A, et al. "Alterations of the intestinal barrier in patients with autism spectrum disorders and in their first-degree relatives." *Journal of Pediatric Gastroenterology and Nutrition.* 2010; 51: 418–24.

104 Anthony A, Ashwood P, Wakefield AJ. "Histopathology of the lower gastrointestinal tract in autistic children: The influence of dietary restriction." Unpublished audit.

105 Doctors and parents/guardians were aware of the treatment.

106 Sandler RH, Finegold SM, Bolte ER, et al. "Short-term benefit from oral vancomycin treatment of regressive-onset autism." *Journal of Child Neurology.* 2000; 15:429–35.

107 Deykin EY, MacMahon B. "Viral exposure and autism." *American Journal of Epidemiology.* 1979; 109:628–38

   Ring A, Barak Y, Ticher A, et al. "Evidence for an infectious etiology in autism." *Pathophysiology.* 1997; 4:1485–88.

108 Uhlmann V, Martin CM, Sheils O, et al. "Potential viral pathogenic mechanism for new variant inflammatory bowel disease." *Molecular Pathology.* 2002; 55:84–90.

109 Wakefield AJ. "Enterocolitis, autism and measles virus." *Molecular Psychiatry.* 2002; 7:S44–6.

110 Hornig M, Briese T, Buie T, et al. "Lack of association between measles virus vaccine and autism with enteropathy: A case-control study." *PLoS ONE.* 2008; 3:e3140.

111 http://www.medpagetoday.com/Neurology/Autism/10772.

112 Kushak RI, Lauwers GY, Winter HS, et al. "Intestinal disaccharidase activity in patients with autism: Effect of age, gender, and intestinal inflammation." *Autism.* 2011; 15:285–94.

113 Land JM, Morgan-Hughes JA, Hargreaves I, et al. "Mitochondrial disease: A historical, biochemical, and London perspective." *Neurochemical Research.* 2004; 29:483–91.

114 Poling JS, Frye RE, Shoffner J, et al. "Developmental regression and mitochondrial dysfunction in a child with autism." *Journal of Child Neurology.* 2006; 21:170–2.

115 Oliveria G, Ataide A, Marques C, et al. "Epidemiology of autism spectrum disorder in Portugal: Prevalence, clinical characterization, and medical conditions." *Developmental Medicine and Child Neurology.* 2007; 49:726–33.

116 Elliott HR, Samuels DC, Eden JA, et al. "Pathogenic mitochondrial DNA mutations are common in the general population." *The American Journal of Human Genetics.* 2008; 83:254–60.

117 Rossignol DA, Frye RE. "Mitochondrial dysfunction in autism spectrum disorders: a systematic review and meta-analysis." *Molecular Psychiatry.* Advance onlinepublication:Jan25,2011.doi:10.1038/mp.2010.136.http://www.nature.com/mp/journal/vaop/ncurrent/full/mp2010136a.html.

118 Yel L, Brown LE, Su K, et al. "Thimerosal induces neuronal cell apoptosis by causing cytochrome c and apoptosis-inducing factor release from mitochondria." *International Journal of Molecular Medicine.* 2005; 16:971–7.

119 Transcript of the Proceedings of the April 11, 2008, Meeting of the Vaccine Safety Working Group of the National Vaccine Advisory Committee (NVAC). http://www.ageofautism.com/2008/07/top-mitochondri.html.

120 http://www.umdf.org/site/c.otJVJ7MMIqE/b.5472191/k.BDB0/Home.htm.

121 Transcript of the Proceedings of the April 11, 2008, Meeting of the Vaccine Safety Working Group of the National Vaccine Advisory Committee (NVAC). http://www.ageofautism.com/2008/07/top-mitochondri.html.

122 Kirby D. (November 11, 2008). "'Revolutionary' news from medicine: 1 in 200 people carry mitochondrial disease mutation." *The Huffington Post.* Retrieved from: http://www.huffingtonpost.com/david-kirby/revolutionary-news-from-m_b_118307.html; and Kirby D. (November 28, 2008). "New study: 'Mitochondrial autism' is real; vaccine triggers cannot be ruled out." *The Huffington Post.* Retrieved from: http://www.huffingtonpost.com/david-kirby/new-study---mitochondrial_b_147030.html.

123 Centers for Disease Control and Prevention. ISO Scientific Agenda for NVAC Vaccine Safety Working Group, April 4, 2008, p. 33.

Chapter 3

1   "Sooner or later we must all sit down to a feast of consequences" (Robert Louis Stevenson).

2   Dourado I, Cunha S, Teixeira MG, et al. "Outbreak of aseptic meningitis associated with mass vaccination with a Urabe-containing measles-mumps-rubella vaccine." *American Journal of Epidemiology*. 2000; 151:524–30.

3   *Federal Register*, Vol. 70, No. 94, Tuesday, May 17, 2005. Rules and Regulations, page 28386. "93.103 Research misconduct: (b) Falsification is manipulating research materials, equipment, or processes, or changing or omitting data or results that the research is not accurately represented in the research record." Retrieved from: http://ori.hhs.gov/sites/default/files/42_cfr_parts_50_and_93_2005.pdf.

4   The Verstraeten Study was the first study the CDC carried out to examine the association between thimerosal and neurodevelopmental outcomes including autism. "Some of the major concerns included 1) many of the statistical analyses were carried out post hoc after an initial set of analyses were run, 2) the study protocol evolved over time, and 3) the CDC did not share many of the internal study findings with individuals and constituents outside the CDC" (Thompson's statement to Congressman Bill Posey).

5   Family Background and Other Data Collection: Information extracted from the child's school record included child's date of birth, sex, birth state, and *race*. [Exhibit 2, page 7, emphasis added] The Analysis Plan, "Statistical Analyses," states that "race" data were available for the entire sample: The only variable that will be assessed as a potential confounder using the *entire sample* will be the child's *race*. [Exhibit 2, page 8, emphasis added]. Thus, "race" data came explicitly from the "school record" and not from the Georgia birth certificate/Georgia birth records and was available for the "entire sample."

6   For the subset of children with Georgia birth records, sub-analyses will be performed in which potential confounding variables from the birth certificate will be used to adjust the estimated association between the MMR vaccine and autism. The variables that will be assessed as potential confounders will be birth weight, APGAR scores, gestational age, birth type, parity, maternal age, maternal race/ethnicity, and maternal education.

7   "Although the birth certificate sample results in Table 3 were adjusted for maternal and birth characteristics, the ORs were not different from unadjusted results for the birth certificate sample (data not shown), indicating that there was little to no confounding effect by these factors." DeStefano

F, Bhasin TK, Thompson WW, et al. "Age at first measles-mumps-rubella vaccination in children with autism and school-matched control subjects: A population-based study in metropolitan Atlanta." *Pediatrics.* 2004; 113:259–66.

8   Retrieved from: http://www.morganverkamp.com/august-27-2014-press-release-statement-of-william-w-thompson-ph-d-regarding-the-2004-article-examining-the-possibility-of-a-relationship-between-mmr-vaccine-and-autism/.

9   Thompson to Hooker, May 24, 2014.

10 He had twenty-one awards for scientific excellence, eighty-one major scientific publications, and 107 conference abstracts.

11 "The mantra should be that CDC once again didn't share controversial analyses and results and the CDC can no longer be trusted to do vaccine safety work" (e-mail to Wakefield and Hooker).

   "The CDC can't be trusted to police itself" (e-mail to Wakefield and Hooker).

   "The CDC can no longer be trusted to conduct vaccine safety science" (Thompson in recorded telephone conversation with Hooker).

   Hooker: "You agree with me that vaccine safety science should be out of the CDC?" Thompson: "Absolutely" (Thompson in recorded telephone conversation with Hooker).

   "The CDC has set the research back ten years because the CDC is so paralyzed when it comes to anything to do with autism" (Thompson in recorded telephone conversation with Hooker).

Chapter 4

1   Rona RJ, Kiel T, Summers C, et al. "The prevalence of food allergy: A meta-analysis." *Journal of Allergy and Clinical Immunology.* 2007; 120:638–46.

2   Ward CM, Geng L, Jyonouchi H. "Fetal sensitization to cow's milk protein and wheat: Cow's milk protein and wheat-specific TNF-alpha production by umbilical cord blood cells and subsequent decline of TNF-alpha production by peripheral blood mononuclear cells following dietary intervention." *Pediatric Allergy and Immunology.* 2007; 18:276–80.

3   Fergusson DM, Horwood LJ, Shannon FT. "Early solid feeding and recurrent eczema: A 10-year longitudinal study." *Pediatrics.* 1990; 86:541–6.

   A prospective study of over 1200 infants demonstrated a direct relationship between the number of solid foods introduced into the diet by four months of age and the subsequent development of atopic dermatitis, with a three-fold increase in recurrent eczema at ten years of age in infants who had received four or more different solid foods before four months of age.

Halken S. "Prevention of allergic disease in childhood: Clinical and epidemiological aspects of primary and secondary allergy prevention." *Pediatric Allergy and Immunology*. 2004; 15 Suppl 16:4–5, 9–32.

4   Urticaria refers to a raised, itchy area of skin that is usually a sign of an allergic reaction.

5   An eosinophil is a type of white blood cell involved in allergic and other immune responses that releases histamine and other potentially toxic molecules when activated. The name comes from the characteristic intense red staining seen under the microscope when the dye eosin is used.

6   Wakefield AJ, Ashwood P, Limb K, et al. "The significance of ileo-colonic lymphoid nodular hyperplasia in children with autistic spectrum disorder." *European Journal of Gastroenterology and Hepatology*. 2005; 17:827–36.

Krigsman A, Boris M, Goldblatt A, et al. "Clinical presentation and histologic findings at ileocolonoscopy in children with autistic spectrum disorder and chronic gastrointestinal symptoms." *Autism Insights*. 2010; 2:1–11.

7   Chen B, Girgis S, El-Matary W. "Childhood autism and eosinophilic colitis." *Digestion*. 2010; 81:127–9.

Wakefield AJ, Anthony A, Murch SH, et al. "Enterocolitis in children with developmental disorders." *The American Journal of Gastroenterology*. 2000; 95:2285–95.

8   Food allergens eliciting a wheal (a raised mark on the skin) that is at least 3 mm greater than the saline control injection are considered positive. See: Sampson HA. "Food allergy. Part 2: diagnosis and management." *Journal of Allergy and Clinical Immunology*. 1999; 103:981–9.

9   See www.foodallergytest.com for additional explanation.

10   http://www.truetest.com/PhysicianPDF/HCP23_FinnCh%20details.pdf.

11   Wood RA. "The natural history of food allergy." *Pediatrics*. 2003; 111:1631–7.

12   Hadjivassiliou M, Gibson A, Davies-Jones GA, et al. "Does cryptic gluten sensitivity play a part in neurological illness?" *Lancet*. 1996; 347:369–71.

13   Ibid.

14   Wakefield AJ, Stott C, Limb K. "Gastrointestinal co-morbidity, autistic regression and measles-containing vaccines: Positive re-challenge and biological gradient effects." *Medical Veritas*. 2006; 3:796–802.

15   Hadjivassiliou M, Grünewald R, Sharrack B, et al. "Gluten ataxia in perspective: epidemiology, genetic susceptibility and clinical characteristics." *Brain*. 2003; 126:685–91.

16   Hadjivassiliou M, Boscolo S, Davies-Jones GA, et al. "The humoral response in the pathogenesis of gluten ataxia." *Neurology*. 2002; 58:1221–6.

17   Alaedini A, Okamoto H, Briani C, et al. "Immune cross-reactivity in celiac disease: Anti-gliadin antibodies bind to neuronal synapsin I." *The Journal of Immunology*. 2007; 178:6590–5.

18   Hadjivassiliou M, Maki M, Sanders DS, et al. "Autoantibody targeting of brain and intestinal transglutaminase in gluten ataxia." *Neurology*. 2006; 66:373–7.

19   Hadjivassiliou M, Davies-Jones GA, Sanders DS, et al. "Dietary treatment of gluten ataxia." *Journal of Neurology, Neurosurgery and Psychiatry*. 2003; 74:1221–4.

20   Goldberg D. "A psychiatric study of patients with diseases of the small intestine." *Gut*. 1970; 11:459–65.

   Ciacci C, Iavarone A, Mazzacca G, et al. "Depressive symptoms in adult coeliac disease." *Scandinavian Journal of Gastroenterology*. 1998; 33:247–50.

   Addolorato G, Capristo E, Ghittoni G, et al. "Anxiety but not depression decreases in coeliac patients after one-year gluten-free diet: A longitudinal study." *Scandinavian Journal of Gastroenterology*. 2001; 36:502–6.

21   Carta MG, Hardoy MC, Boi MF, et al. "Association between panic disorder, major depressive disorder, and celiac disease: A possible role for thyroid autoimmunity." *Journal of Psychosomatic Research*. 2002; 53:789–93.

22   Ljungman G, Myrdal U. "Compliance in teenagers with celiac disease: A Swedish follow-up study." *Acta Paediatrica*. 1993; 82:235–8.

23   Hernanz A, Polanco I. "Plasma precursor amino acids of central nervous system monoamines in children with celiac disease." *Gut*. 1991; 32:1478–81.

24   Fasano A, Catassi C. "Current approaches to diagnosis and treatment of celiac disease: an evolving spectrum." *Gastroenterology*. 2001; 120:636–51.

25   Fabiani E, Taccari LM, Ratsch IM, et al. "Compliance with gluten-free diet in adolescents with screening-detected celiac disease: A 5-year follow-up study." *Journal of Pediatrics*. 2000; 136:841–3.

26   Pynnönen PA, Isometsä ET, Verkasalo MA, et al. "Gluten-free diet may alleviate depressive and behavioural symptoms in adolescents with coeliac disease: A prospective follow-up case-series study." *BMC Psychiatry*. 2005; 5:14.

27   Goodwin MS, Cowen MA, Goodwin TC. "Malabsorption and cerebral dysfunction: A multivariate and comparative study of autistic children." *Journal of Autism and Schizophrenia*. 1971; 1:48–62.

28   Genuis SJ, Bouchard TP. "Autism presenting as celiac disease." *Journal of Child Neurology*. 2010; 25:114–9.

29 Randolph TG. "Allergy as a causative factor of fatigue, irritability, and behavior problems of children." *Journal of Pediatrics*. 1947; 31:560–72.

30 Ibid.

31 Ibid.

32 Ibid.

33 Mayron LW. "Allergy, learning, and behavior problems." *Journal of Learning Disabilities*. 1979; 12:32–42.

Atkins FM. "Food allergy and behavior: definitions, mechanisms, and a review of the evidence." *Nutrition Reviews*. 1986; 44(Suppl):104–12.

34 Atkins FM. "Food allergy and behavior: Definitions, mechanisms, and a review of the evidence." *Nutrition Reviews*. 1986; 44(s3):104–12.

35 "Treatment in the hyperkinetic syndrome." *Lancet*. 1985; 325:540–5.

36 Kahn A, Rebuffat E, Blum D, et al. "Difficulty in initiating and maintaining sleep associated with cow's milk allergy in infants." *Sleep*. 1987; 10:116–21.

37 Basso AS, Pinto FAC, Russo M, et al. "Neural correlates of IgE-mediated food allergy." *Journal of Neuroimmunology*. 2003; 140:69–77.

38 Theoharides TC. "Autism spectrum disorders and mastocytosis." *International Journal of Immunopathology and Pharmacology*. 2009; 22:859–65.

39 Theoharides TC, Angelidou A, Alysandratos KD, et al. "Mast cell activation and autism." *Biochimica et Biophysica Acta*. Dec 28, 2010. [Epub ahead of print]

40 Asadi S, Zang B, Weng Z, et al. "Luteolin and thiosalicylate inhibit $HgCl_2$ and thimerosal-induced VEGF release from human mast cells." *International Journal of Immunopathology and Pharmacology*. 2010; 23:1015–20.

41 Breakey J. "The role of diet and behaviour in childhood." *Journal of Paediatrics and Child Health*. 1997; 33:190–4.

42 Kaplan BJ, McNicol J, Conte RA, et al. "Dietary replacement in preschool-aged hyperactive boys." *Pediatrics*. 1989; 83:7–17.

43 Egger J, Carter CM, Graham PJ, et al. "Controlled trial of oligoantigenic treatment in the hyperkinetic syndrome." *Lancet*. 1985; 1:540–5.

Pollock I, Warner JO. "Effect of artificial food colors on childhood behavior." *Archives of Disease in Childhood*. 1990; 65:74–7.

Carter CM, Urbanowicz M, Hemsley R, et al. "Effects of a few food diet in attention deficit disorder." *Archives of Disease in Childhood*. 1993; 69:564–8.

Rowe KS, Rowe KJ. "Synthetic food coloring and behavior: A dose-response effect in a double-blind, placebo-controlled, repeated-measures study." *Journal of Pediatrics*. 1994; 125(5 Pt 1):691–8.

Boris M, Mandel FS. "Foods and additives are common causes of the attention deficit hyperactive disorder in children." *Annals of Allergy*. 1994; 72:462–8.

Schmidt MH, Mocks P, Lay B, et al. "Does oligoantigenic diet influence hyperactive/conduct-disordered children—a controlled trial?" *European Child and Adolescent Psychiatry*. 1997; 6:88–95.

44   Arnold LE. "Treatment alternatives for attention deficit hyperactivity disorder." *NIH Consensus Development Conference on Diagnosis and Treatment of Attention Deficit Hyperactivity Disorder*. November 16–18, 1998. National Institutes of Health, Bethesda, MD.

45   Rice, turkey, lamb, vegetables, fruits, margarine, vegetable oil, tea, pear juice, and water.

46   Pelsser LMJ, Frankena K, Toorman J, et al. "A randomized controlled trial into the effects of food on ADHD." *European Child and Adolescent Psychiatry*. 2009; 18:12–19.

47   Pelsser LM, Frankema K, Toorman J, et al. "Effects of a restricted elimination diet on the behaviour of children with attention-deficit hyperactivity disorder (INCA study): A randomized controlled trial." *Lancet*. 2011; 377:495–503.

48   Ibid.

49   IgA antibodies to casein, α-lactalbumin and β-lactoglobuin and IgG and IgG to casein.

50   Lucarelli S, Frediani T, Zingoni AM, et al. "Food allergy and infantile autism." *Panminerva Medica*. 1995; 37:137–41.

51   Horror autotoxicus, literally meaning the horror of self-toxicity, was a term coined by the great German bacteriologist and immunologist Paul Ehrlich (1854-1915) to describe the body's innate aversion to immunological self-destruction. However, the immune system can upon occasion attack itself and does so in autoimmune disorders.

52   Infections, toxic chemicals, and dietary peptides binding to lympho-cyte receptors and tissue enzymes are major instigators of autoimmunity in autism. See: Vojdani A, Pangborn JB, Vojdani E, et al. "Infections, toxic chemicals and dietary peptides binding to lymphocyte receptors and tissue enzymes are major instigators of autoimmunity in autism." *International Journal of Immunopathology and Pharmacology*. 2003; 16:189–99.

53   Vojdani A, Bazargan M, Vojdani E, et al. "Heat shock protein and gliadin peptide promote development of peptidase antibodies in children with autism and patients with autoimmune disease." *Clinical and Diagnostic Laboratory Immunology*. 2004; 3:515–24.

54 Vojdani A, Campbell B, Anyanwub E, et al. "Antibodies to neuron-specific antigens in children with autism: possible cross reaction with encephalitogenic proteins from milk, *Chlamydia pneumonia* and *Streptococcus* group A." *Journal of Neuroimmunology.* 2002; 129:168–77.

55 Ashwood P, Anthony A, Pellicer AA, et al. "Intestinal lymphocyte populations in children with regressive autism: Evidence for extensive mucosal immunopathology." *Journal of Clinical Immunology.* 2003; 23:504–17.

   Wakefield AJ, Puleston J, Montgomery SM, et al. "Entero-colonic encephalopathy, autism and opioid receptor ligands." *Alimentary Pharmacology and Therapeutics.* 2002; 16:663–74.

   Ashwood P, Anthony A, Torrente F, et al. "Spontaneous mucosal lymphocyte cytokine profiles in children with regressive autism and gastrointestinal symptoms: Mucosal immune activation and reduced counter regulatory interleukin-10." *Journal of Clinical Immunology.* 2004; 24:664–73.

56 Jyonouchi H, Sun S, Itokazu N. "Innate immunity associated with inflammatory responses and cytokine reduction against common dietary proteins in patients with autism spectrum disorder." *Neuropsychobiology.* 2002; 46:76–84.

57 Jyonouchi H, Geng L, Ruby A, et al. "Dysregulated innate immune responses in young children with autism spectrum disorders: Their relationship to gastrointestinal symptoms and dietary intervention." *Neuropsychobiology.* 2005; 51:77–85.

58 Jyonouchi H, Geng L, Ruby A, et al. "Evaluation of an association between gastrointestinal symptoms and cytokine production against common dietary proteins in children with autism spectrum disorders." *Journal of Pediatrics.* 2005; 146:605–10.

59 Casein, β-Lactoglobulin, and α-Lactalbumin.

60 Jyonouchi H, Geng L, Ruby A, et al. "Dysregulated innate immune responses in young children with autism spectrum disorders: Their relationship to gastrointestinal symptoms and dietary intervention." *Neuropsychobiology.* 2005; 51:77–85.

61 Knivsberg AM, Reichelt KL, Høien T, et al. "A randomised, controlled study of dietary intervention in autistic syndromes." *Nutritional Neuroscience.* 2002; 5:251–61.

62 Whiteley P, Haracopos D, Knivsberg AM, et al. "The ScanBrit randomised, controlled, single-blind study of a gluten- and casein-free dietary intervention for children with autism spectrum disorders." *Nutritional Neuroscience.* 2010; 13:87–100.

63 Ibid.

64   Jyonounchi H, Geng L, Cushing-Ruby A, et al. "Mechanisms of non-IgE mediated adverse reaction to common dietary proteins (DPs) in children with autism spectrum disorders (ASD)." *Journal of Allergy and Clinical Immunology.* 2004; 113:S208.

65   Jyonouchi H, Sun S, Itokazu N. "Innate immunity associated with inflammatory responses and cytokine production against common dietary proteins in patients with autism spectrum disorder." *Neuropsychobiology.* 2002; 46:76–84.

66   Jyonuchi H, Geng L, Ruby A, et al. "Suboptimal responses to dietary intervention in children with autism spectrum disorder and non-IgE-mediated food allergy." In *Autism Research Advances,* Zhao LB (Ed). (pp. 169–184). Hauppauge, NY: Nova Science Publishers, Inc., 2007.

67   Jyonouchi H. "Food allergy and autism spectrum disorders: Is there a link?" *Current Allergy and Asthma Reports.* 2009; 9:194–20.

Chapter 5

1   Meadow R. "Münchausen syndrome by proxy: The hinterland of child abuse." *Lancet.* 1977; II:343–5.

2   http://www.drbilllong.com/About.html.

3   Long WR. "Münchausen syndrome by proxy/factitious disorder by proxy: A critical assessment for judges and lawyers." Available at: http://www.autism.com/pdf/families/MBSP_unabridged.pdf.

4   John Batt. *Stolen Innocence—A Mother's Fight for Justice: The Authorised Story of Sally Clark.* United Kingdom: Ebury Publishing, 2004. See http://www.sallyclark.org.uk/.

5   Fleming PJ, Blair PS, Bacon C, et al. (Eds.) *Sudden Unexpected Death in Infancy.* The CESDI SUDI Studies. London: Stationery Office, 2000.

6   https://docs.google.com/viewer?url=http%3A%2F%2Fwww.statslab.cam.ac.uk%2F~apd%2FSallyClark_report.doc.

7   Rosenberg DA. "Web of deceit: A literature review of Münchausen syndrome by proxy." *Child Abuse and Neglect.* 1987; 11:547–63.

8   Taylor B, Miller E, Lingam R, et al. "Measles, mumps, rubella, vaccination and bowel problems or developmental regression in children with autism: population-based study." *British Medical Journal.* 2002; 324:393–6.

9   Referred to in *Diagnostic and Statistical Manual of Mental Disorders, Fourth Edition* as "Factitious Disorder by Proxy."

10   Emphasis added.

11   Ibid.

12   Ibid.

13   Dr. Eric Mart is a psychologist licensed in New Hampshire, Massachusetts, and Vermont and a board-certified forensic psychologist through the American Board of Professional Psychology.

14   Rosenberg DA. "Münchausen syndrome by proxy: Medical diagnostic criteria." *Child Abuse and Neglect*. 2003; 27:421–30.

15   Long WR. "Münchausen syndrome by proxy/factitious disorder by proxy: A critical assessment for judges and lawyers." Available at: http://www.autism .com/pdf/families/MBSP_unabridged.pdf.

16   Ibid.

17   Rosenberg DA. "Münchausen syndrome by proxy: Medical diagnostic criteria." *Child Abuse and Neglect*. 2003; 27:421–30.

18   The Judge Rotenberg Educational Center in Massachusetts required residents with autism to wear backpacks holding a device that delivered a moderate shock to their arms or legs. The device was activated when they misbehaved. A previous legal decision by the state of Massachusetts allowed the center to continue with its practice for a certain amount of time (under close scrutiny). See Rudy LJ. (December 26, 2007). "Aversive therapy for autism: A tool for good or evil?" Available at: http://autism.about.com/b/2007/12/26/ aversive-therapy-for-autism-a-tool-for-good-or-evil.htm.

Fortunately, Disability Rights International filed an urgent appeal with the United Nations insisting that the practices at JRC were torture. The UN Special Rapporteur on Torture agreed. The US Justice Department opened an investigation of the center. In May 2011, the director of the Judge Rotenberg Center resigned in the face of criminal charges. Matthew Israel, founder and director of JRC, was charged with misleading a grand jury and destroying evidence in relation to an incident in 2007 in which a prank phone call to the center from a person posing as an employee led to two children with disabilities being given dozens of electrical shocks for absolutely no reason. One of these children was restrained and given seventy-seven shocks over three hours. Israel accepted a court settlement requiring him to resign as director and sentencing him to five years of probation.

19   Ip P. "Fever of the imagination—a case of Münchausen Syndrome by proxy." *Hong Kong Paediatr Journal*. 1996; 1:189–91.

20   In Briquet's syndrome, first described by Paul Briquet in 1859, patients feel that they have been sickly most of their lives and complain of a multitude of symptoms referable to numerous different organ systems. This conviction of illness persists despite repeatedly negative and unrevealing consultations, hospitalizations, and diagnostic procedures, and patients continue to seek medical care, to take prescription medicines, and to submit to

needless diagnostic procedures. http://www.brown.edu/Courses/BI_278/Other/Clerkship/Didactics/Readings/Somatization.pdf.

21 Long WR. "Münchausen syndrome by proxy/factitious disorder by proxy: A critical assessment for judges and lawyers." Available at: http://www .autism.com/pdf/families/MBSP_unabridged.pdf. Page 16.

22 *Gustafson v. Mazer*, 54 P3d 743 (Wash. App. 2002). Ibid, p. 744.

23 Long WR. "Münchausen syndrome by proxy/factitious disorder by proxy: A critical assessment for judges and lawyers." Available at: http://www .autism.com/pdf/families/MBSP_unabridged.pdf. Page 16.

24 *Arizona Department of Economic Security et al. v. Anon*, page 51.

25 Ibid, page 34.

26 Ibid, page 27.

27 Equivalent of a surgical resident in the US.

Chapter 6

1 *Gustafson v. Mazer*, 54 P3d 743 (Wash. App. 2002).

2 *Arizona Department of Economic Security et al. v. Anon*. November 1, 2010. Page 13.

3 Thoracic outlet syndrome.

4 http://www.nanstiel.com/media/TheArizona5.mov [last accessed February 2012].

5 The founder of the network formerly known as DAN!, the late Dr. Bernard Rimland, was among the first to pioneer biomedical approaches for the treatment of autism as a medical rather than a behavioral disorder. The former DAN! conferences are now referred to as Autism Research Institute (ARI) conferences.

6 Campbell DB, Sutcliffe JS, Ebert PJ, et al. "A genetic variant that disrupts *MET* transcription is associated with autism." *Proceedings of the National Academy of Sciences of the United States of America*. 2006; 103:16834–9.

    Sacco R, Militerni R, Frolli A, et al. "Clinical, morphological, and biochemical correlates of head circumference in autism." *Biological Psychiatry*. 2007; 62:1038–47.

    Conciatori M, Stodgell CJ, Hyman SL, et al. "Association between the *HOXA1* A218G polymorphism and increased head circumference in patients with autism." *Biological Psychiatry*. 2001; 55:413–9.

    Persico AM, Militerni R, Bravaccio C, et al. "Lack of association between serotonin transporter gene promoter variants and autistic disorder in two ethnically distinct samples." *American Journal of Medical Genetics.* 2000; 96:123–7.

    D'Amelio M, Ricci I, Sacco R, et al. "Paraoxonase gene variants are associated with autism in North America, but not in Italy: possible regional specificity in gene–environment interactions." *Molecular Psychiatry.* 2005; 10:1006–16.

    Vojdani A, Mumper E, Granpeesheh D, et al. "Low natural killer cell cytotoxic activity in autism: the role of glutathione, IL-2 and IL-15." *Journal of Neuroimmunology.* 2008; 205:148–54.

7   *Arizona Department of Economic Security et al. v. Anon.* 10.29.2010. page 158.

8   www.medicinenet.com/script/main/art.asp?articlekey=100210 [last accessed June 2011]. Also available at www.clinicaltrials.gov [last accessed February 2012].

9   *Arizona Department of Economic Security et al. v. Anon.* 10.29.2010. page 141.

10 American Academy of Pediatrics Committee on Environmental Health. "Screening for elevated blood lead levels." *Pediatrics.* 1998; 101:1072–8.

Chapter 7

1   May 2005. Urinary lead level was 54 mcg/g creatinine (normal 0–5).

2   Dr. Rice to Dr. Sipes, August 22, 2006.

3   Dr. Rice provided Dr. Sipes with a copy of the DSM-IV criteria for this condition.

4   Dr. Rice to Dr. Sipes, August 22, 2006.

5   Childhood disintegrative disorder was first described by Theodore Heller, a remedial educator in Vienna. He described a new syndrome—*dementia infantilis* (later to become CDD)—in the *Journal for Research and Treatment of Juvenile Feeblemindedness.* (1908; 2:141–165). CDD is a pervasive developmental disorder that fulfills behavioral criteria for childhood autism/autistic disorder, but where the pattern of onset is different. CDD requires documented normal or near-normal development up to twenty-four months of age with subsequent regression and loss of skills in at least two of the following: expressive/receptive language, play, social/adaptive skills, continence, and motor skills.

6   E-mail from the mother to Dr. Rice, March 4, 2009.

7   Purpura is a purplish discoloration of the skin produced by small bleeding vessels near the surface. Purpura may also occur in the mucous membranes, especially of the mouth and in the internal organs. Purpura is not a disease per se but is indicative of an underlying cause of bleeding.

8   Henoch–Schönlein purpura (HSP) is an inflammation of small vessels (vasculitis) whose major manifestations include arthritis, non-thrombocy-topenic (normal blood platelet levels) purpura, abdominal pain, and renal disease. HSP was first recognized by Heberden in 1801. The association between purpura and arthritis was described by Schönlein in 1837. Henoch added descriptions of GI involvement in 1874 and renal involvement in 1899. See Ballinger S. "Henoch-Schönlein purpura." *Current Opinion in Rheumatology.* 2003; 15:591–4.

9   Hamlet. Act IV, Scene V.

10   Medical record of Dr. Cooper, December 14, 2008.

11   This result is consistent with the development of a progressive anemia from December 30, 2008 (12.1 g/dl) to December 31, 2008 (10.7g/dl) to January 1, 2009 (8.3g/dl). The latter count was associated with a low platelet count of 96 K/ml (normal 140–450) and a low albumin of 2.3g/L (normal 3.5–5.2). The same day, a repeat test showed a resolution of the anemia (12.3 g/dl) but no explanation as to whether he was transfused or whether the initial result was the result of a lab error.

12   Medical record of Dr. Shishov, December 31, 2008.

13   Dr. Ursea to Dr. Sipes, January 8, 2009.

14   For example, see Dr. Ede to Dr. Sipes, January 31, 2009.

15   Rettig P, Cron RQ. "Methotrexate used as a steroid-sparing agent in non-renal chronic Henoch-Schönlein purpura." *Clinical and Experimental Rheumatology.* 2003; 21:767–9.

16   C-reactive protein (CRP) 9.8mg/L (normal <8.0), February 24, 2009.

17   CPS document listing allegations (undated and unsigned), Dr. Stephens, *Arizona Department of Economic Security et al. v. Anon.* October 29, 2010, page 110, and e-mail from Heather Williams to colleagues, April 23, 2010.

18   The stool guaiac test finds hidden (occult) blood in the stool. A stool sample is applied to the guaiac paper. When hydrogen peroxide is dripped onto the guaiac paper, it oxidizes the alpha-guaiaconic acid to a blue colored quinone. Normally, when no blood and no peroxidases or catalases from vegetables are present, this oxidation occurs very slowly. Heme, a component of hemoglobin found in blood, catalyzes this reaction, giving a result in about two seconds. Therefore, a positive test result is one where there is a quick and intense blue color change of the film.

19   *The Arizona Department of Economic Security et al. v. Anon.* November 1, 2010. Page 192.

20   Father was a special education teacher.

21   Medical record of Dr. Weiss, February 24, 2010.

22   Ibid.

23   Ibid.

24   Child 1's anti-tetanus antibody level = 0.14 [>0.15 = protective].

25   Specific antibody deficiency indicates a failure of the immune system to mount a protective antibody response to exposure to an organism and is typically assessed using vaccine responses.

26   Medical record of Dr. Carter, February 25, 2009.

27   Ibid.

28   CRP 9.8 g/dl (normal upper limit in blood at PCH = 9.5 g/dl), hemoglobin 19.2 g/dl and hematocrit 54.2 indicative of dehydration.

29   Medical record of Dr. Carter, February 26, 2009.

30   Ibid.

31   Gupta S, Aggarwal S, Heads C. "Brief report: Dysregulated immune system in children with autism: Beneficial effects of intravenous immune globulin on autistic characteristics." *Journal of Autism and Developmental Disorders.* 1996; 439–52.

    Gupta S. "Immunological treatments for autism." *Journal of Autism and Developmental Disorders.* 2000; 30:475–9.

    Boris M, Goldblatt A, Edelson SM. "Improvement in children with autism treated with intravenous gamma globulin." *Journal of Nutritional and Environmental Medicine.* 2005; 15:169–76.

32   Medical record of Dr. Carter, February 26, 2009.

33   *The Arizona Department of Economic Security v. Anon.* November 1, 2010. Page 19.

34   American Psychiatric Association. *Diagnostic and Statistical Manual of Mental disorders.* DSM IV-TR, 4th Edition, text revision. Washington, DC: American Psychiatric Association, 2000.

35   Rosenberg DA. "Münchausen Syndrome by Proxy: Medical diagnostic criteria." *Child Abuse and Neglect.* 2003; 27:421–30.

36   *The Arizona Department of Economic Security v. Anon.* November 1, 2010. Page 12.

37   Weiss PF, Feinstein JA, Luan X, et al. "Effects of corticosteroid on Henoch-Schönlein Purpura: A systematic review." *Pediatrics.* 2007; 120:1079–87. The authors found that treatment with steroids was associated with reduced duration of abdominal symptoms for patients with HSP (odds ratio [OR], 5.42; 95% confidence interval [CI], 1.60–18.29).

38   *The Arizona Department of Economic Security v. Anon*. November 1, 2010. For example, Page 77.

Chapter 8

1   Expert report of Dr. McDonough-Means, October 2010.
2   Ibid.
3   Ibid.
4   Medical record of Dr. Schneider, July 5, 2005.
5   The cerebellum (Latin for *little brain*) is a region of the brain that plays an important role in motor control. It is also involved in some cognitive functions such as attention and language, and probably in some emotional functions such as regulating fear and pleasure responses. Its movement-related functions are the most clearly understood, however. The cerebellum does not initiate movement, but it contributes to coordination, precision, and accurate timing. It receives input from sensory systems and from other parts of the brain and spinal cord, and integrates these inputs to fine tune motor activity. Because of this fine-tuning function, damage to the cerebellum does not cause paralysis, but instead produces disorders in fine movement, equilibrium, posture, and motor learning. http://en.wikipedia.org/wiki/Cerebellum.
6   Incoordination revealed by asking the patient to undertake a rapidly repeating movement like rotating the hand back and forth or tapping a rhythm on a surface.
7   Medical record of Dr. Schneider, July 5, 2005.
8   For example, Selvin-Tasta A, Loidl CF, López-Costa JJ, et al. "Chronic lead exposure induces astrogliosis in hippocampus and cerebellum." *Neurotoxicology*. 1994; 15:389–401.
9   Rapoport M, van Reekum R, Mayberg H. "The role of the cerebellum in cognition and behavior: a selective review." *The Journal of Neuropsychiatry and Clinical Neurosciences*. 2000; 12:193–8.
10   110 µg/g creatinine (normal <5).
11   Medical record of Dr. Schneider, October 12, 2005.
12   Expert report of Dr. McDonough-Means, October 2010.
13   The complaint included the hand going blue in certain positions. This is suggestive of an autonomic (sympathetic) nerve involvement.
14   Telephone interview with the parents, December 19, 2010.
15   Interview with Teri Holloway, January 2011.
16   This document is no longer available, having been lost.

17   Medical record of Dr. Carter, March 16, 2010.

18   Ibid.

19   Interview with Teri Holloway, January 2011.

20   A "condition" that affects the family of an infant or child who has suffered what the parents believe is a "close call" with death and thereafter perceived as vulnerable to serious injury or accidents. See http://medical-dictionary .thefreedictionary.com/vulnerable+child+syndrome.

21   Joint between the collarbone and the shoulder blade.

22   Telephone interview with parents, December 19, 2010.

23   E-mail from Dr. Carter to colleagues, January 26, 2010.

24   Ibid.

25   Social work record of Nicole Ordway, March 19, 2010.

26   Methylenetetrahydrofolate reductase (MTHFR).

27   Social work report of Jennifer Slatteri, March 17, 2010.

28   Paşca SP. Dronca E, Kaucsár T, et al. "One carbon metabolism disturbances and the C677T MTHFR gene polymorphism in children with autism spectrum disorders." *Journal of Cellular and Molecular Medicine.* 2009; 13:4229–38.

      Boris M, Goldblatt A, Galanko J, et al. "Association of MTHFR gene variants with autism." *Journal of American Physicians and Surgeons* 2004; 9:106–8.

      Adams M, Lucock M, Stuart J, et al. "Preliminary evidence for involvement of the folate gene polymorphism 19 bp deletion-DHFR in occurrence of autism." *Neuroscience Letters.* 2007; 422:24–9.

      Filiano JJ, Goldenthal MJ, Rhodes CH, et al. "Mitochondrial dysfunction in patients with hypotonia, epilepsy, autism, and developmental delay: HEADD syndrome." *Journal of Child Neurology.* 2002; 17:435–9.

      Weissman JR, Kelley RI, Bauman ML, et al. "Mitochondrial disease in autism spectrum disorder patients: A cohort analysis." *PLoS One.* 2008; 3:e3815.

      Oliveira G, Diogo L, Grazina M, et al. "Mitochondrial dysfunction in autism spectrum disorders: A population-based study." *Developmental Medicine and Child Neurology.* 2005; 47:185–9.

Chapter 9

1   Medical record of Dr. McCarthy, December 24, 2002.

2   Medical record of Dr. McCarthy, June 3, 2003.

3   Ibid.

4   Report of Dr. Friedman on Child 3, September 3, 2003.

5   Wakefield AJ, Puleston JM, Montgomery SM, et al. "Review article: The concept of entero-colonic encephalopathy, autism and opioid receptor ligands." *Alimentary Pharmacology and Therapeutics*. 2002; 16:663–74.

6   Medical record of Dr. Schneider, April 19, 2004.

7   On SAGE testing, Child 3 had a non-IgE-mediated allergy to milk, peanuts, soy, wheat, corn, oregano, cabbage, celery, cucumber, peach, pinto beans, pineapple, plums, dill, strawberries, mushrooms, food dyes, and food additives.

8   Knivsberg AM, Reichelt KL, Høien T, et al. "A randomised, controlled study of dietary intervention in autistic syndromes." *Nutritional Neuroscience*. 2002; 5:251–61.

    Whitely P, Haracopos D, Knivsberg AM, et al. "The ScanBrit randomised, controlled, single-blind study of a gluten- and casein-free dietary intervention for children with autism spectrum disorders." *Nutritional Neuroscience*. 2010; 13:87–100.

9   0.185 µg/g (normal <0.09).

10 The cerebral cortex at the back of the brain.

11 Canales P, Mery VP, Larrondo FJ, et al. "Epilepsy and celiac disease: Favorable outcome with a gluten-free diet in a patient refractory to antiepileptic drugs." *Neurologist*. 2006; 12:318–21.

    Pratesi R, Modelli IC, Martins RC, et al. "Celiac disease and epilepsy: Favorable outcome in a child with difficult to control seizures." *Acta Neurologica Scandinavica*. 2003; 108:290–3.

    Mavroudi A, Karatza E, Papastavrou T, et al. "Successful treatment of epilepsy and celiac disease with a gluten-free diet." *Pediatric Neurology*. 2005; 33:292–5.

12 LKS or acquired epileptic aphasia is characterized by the subacute onset of an isolated language disturbance associated with an epileptiform electroencephalogram and/or a few seizures. In classic reports, the child's language and all other development is normal before the onset of the convulsive disorder.

13 LKS–variant, a term coined by Connelly et al., includes children with autistic regression with epileptiform EEGs (particularly during sleep). Striking improvement in language function in patients with LKS and LKSV after treatment with immunomodulating agents has been reported by some authors, but not all. Because of this response, Connelly et al. investigated the frequency of autoantibodies to brain in both disorders in LKS and LKS-variant. Child 3 was positive for anti-brain antibodies in this testing.

Connolly AM, Chez MG, Pestronk A, et al. "Serum autoantibodies to brain in Landau-Kleffner variant, autism, and other neurologic disorders." *Journal of Pediatrics.* 1999; 134:607–13.

14   The records of Dr. Bradstreet were not available for review.

15   In common with his other siblings (except Child 5), he had received a diagnosis of functional antibody deficiency from Dr. Hellmers.

16   New York: Skyhorse Publishing, 2010. ISBN 978-1-61608-169-0.

17   Medical record of Dr. Blitz-Wetterland, August 31, 2010.

18   Ibid.

19   Ibid.

20   Whitely P, Haracopos D, Knivsberg AM, et al. "The ScanBrit randomised, controlled, single-blind study of a gluten- and casein-free dietary intervention for children with autism spectrum disorders." *Nutritional Neuroscience.* 2010; 13:87-100.

Chapter 10

1   Outward angulation of the ankle joint.

2   From the report of Dr. McDonough-Means.

3   By chelation challenge.

4   89 μg/gm creatinine.

Chapter 11

1   7.6 ug/gm creatinine (normal <5).

2   Father was a special education teacher.

3   Medical record of Dr. Weiss, February 24, 2009.

Chapter 12

1   *Arizona Department of Economic Security et al. v. Anon.* Court transcript November 1, 2010. Page 70.

2   E-mail from Heather Williams. April 23, 2010.

3   E-mail from Ms. Williams to colleagues, March 23, 2010.

4   Ibid.

5   Ibid.

6   Ibid.

7   Ibid.

8   Ibid.

9   Ibid.

10   Ibid.

11   E-mail from Dr. S. Stephens to colleagues, May 27, 2010.

12   "The child is father." *Time*. July 25, 1960. Last accessed March 4, 2011.

13   Bettelheim B. *The Empty Fortress: Infantile Autism and the Birth of the Self.* New York: Free Press, 1967.

14   E-mail from Ms. Williams to colleagues, March 23, 2010.

15   Report of Dr. Susan Stephens, June 10, 2010.

16   Ibid.

17   Bold as per original document.

18   Report of Dr. Susan Stephens, June 10, 2010.

19   Ibid.

20   Ibid.

21   *Arizona Department of Economic Security et al. v. Anon.* October 29, 2010. Page 75.

22   Wakefield AJ, Murch SH, Anthony A, et al. "Ileal lymphoid nodular hyperplasia, non-specific colitis, and pervasive developmental disorder in children." *Lancet.* 1998; 351:637–41.

23   Child 1. Elevated* 8-Oxo-deoxyguanosine (oxidative DNA damage), and elevated* 8-Oxo-guanosine (oxidative DNA damage), and elevated* urinary isoprostane F2-α. (April 12, 2008).

        Child 2. Elevated* 8-Oxo-deoxyguanosine (oxidative DNA damage), and elevated* 8-Oxo-guanosine (oxidative DNA damage), and elevated* 8-iso-PGF2-α. (June 10, 2008).

        Child 3. Elevated* 8-Oxo-guanosine (oxidative DNA damage) (December 26, 2007).

        *In excess of the normal range.

        Child 5. Urinary isoprostane F2-α 270 ng/gCr (normal 100-200). Urinary 8-hydroxy deoxyguanosine (8OHdG) 31 nmole/gCr (normal 12-25), urinary 8-hydroxy guanosine (8OHG) 118 nmole/gCr (normal 20-40), 8OHdG:8OHG ration 3.8 (normal < 2).

24   Admission history on Child 2, taken by Dr. Carter on March 16, 2010. Page 1.

25   *Arizona Department of Economic Security et al. v. Anon.* October 29, 2010. Page 24.

26   Ibid. Page 100.

27   Ibid. Pages 100–101.

28   Ibid. Page 24.

29   Medical record of Dr. Carter, March 16, 2010.

30   E-mail from Dr. Carter to colleagues, April 26, 2010.

31   Report of Dr. Stephens, June 10, 2010.

32   Ibid.

33 The stool guaiac test finds hidden (occult) blood in the stool. A stool sample is applied to the guaiac paper. When hydrogen peroxide is dripped onto the guaiac paper, it oxidizes the alpha-guaiaconic acid to a blue colored quinone. Normally, when no blood and no peroxidases or catalases from vegetables are present, this oxidation occurs very slowly. Heme, a component of hemoglobin found in blood, catalyzes this reaction, giving a result in about two seconds. Therefore, a positive test result is one where there is a quick and intense blue color change of the film. Clinical record of Dr. Weiss, February 24, 2009.

34 See Chapter 3.

35 E-mail from Ms. Williams to colleagues, April 23, 2010.

36 Emphasis added.

37 *Arizona Department of Economic Security et al. v. Anon.* October 29, 2010. Page 110.

38 Ibid. Page 126.

39 Ibid. November 1, 2010, page 208.

40 Report of Dr. Stephens, October 7, 2010.

41 Ibid.

42 Ibid.

43 Kane K. "Drug error, not chelation therapy, killed boy, expert says." *Pittsburgh Post-Gazette.* January 18, 2006. Retrieved from: http://www .post-gazette.com/pg/06018/639721.stm.

 Abubakar Tariq Nadama died August 23 in his Butler County doctor's office because he was given the wrong chelation agent, Disodium EDTA instead of Calcium Disodium EDTA. The generic names are Versinate and Endrate.

44 Rimland B. "The safety and efficacy of chelation therapy in autism." *Autism Research Institute.* Retrieved from: www.autism.com/pro_chelationsafety.asp

45 Report of Dr. Stephens, October 7, 2010.

46 Ibid.

47 Bold as per Dr. Stephen's report, October 7, 2010.

48 *Arizona Department of Economic Security et al. v. Anon.* November 1, 2010. Page 90.

49 Ibid. Page 90.

50 Ibid. Page 231.

51 Report of Dr. Stephens, October 7, 2010.

52 Ibid.

53 Ibid.

54 Ibid.

55 Ibid.

56 On the second occasion, she wrote "An educational diagnosis of autism."

57 *Arizona Department of Economic Security et al. v. Anon.* November 1, 2010. Page 102.

58 Ibid. Page 191.

59 Ibid. Page 97.

60 Ibid.

61 Ibid. Page 69.

62 Ibid. Page 78.

63 Ibid. Page 129.

64 On the basis of her statements of June 9, 2010, summarized by Dr. Stephens.

65 *Arizona Department of Economic Security et al. v. Anon.* November 1, 2010. Page 130.

66 Drs. Stephens, Carter, Sanders and Ms. Williams.

67 Medical report of Dr. McDonough-Means. October 2010.

68 *Arizona Department of Economic Security et al. v. Anon.* October 29, 2010.

69 Wolpert J, Knutsen AP. "Natural history of selective antibody deficiency to bacterial polysaccharide antigens in children." *Pediatric Asthma Allergy.* 1998; 12:183–91.

70 *Arizona Department of Economic Security et al. v. Anon.* November 1, 2010. Page 97.

71 Ibid. Page 96.

72 Boris M, Goldblatt A, Edelson AM. "Improvement in children with autism treated with intravenous gamma globulin." *Journal of Nutritional and Environmental Medicine.* 2005; 15:169–76. In an open-label study of twenty-six children with autism, significant improvement occurred in autistic children receiving monthly IVIG. Baseline and monthly aberrant behavior checklists.

There is a reasonable rationale considering the risk/reward ratio to utilize IVIG therapy in children with autism. A well-controlled placebo double-blind study would be important to further clarify the use of IVIG in autism and its duration of benefits.

As recently as 2010, Chez wrote: "Initially reported by Plioplys in 1999, a series of 10 children was observed after receiving 400 mg/kg of intravenous immunoglobulin (IVIG) and 1 out of 10 children dramatically improved in their autistic findings. Similar results were described in 2000 by Gupta, and Gupta et al; in an open-label prospective study, they gave repeated doses of IVIG and improvement occurred in 10% to 20% of the patients who were treated. Other authors have also reported a positive IVIG response in autism, but no one has reported curing or totally reversing autism symptoms."

Chez MG, Guido-Estrada N. "Immune therapy in autism: Historical experience and future directions with immunomodulatory therapy." *Neurotherapeutics*. 2010; 7:293–301.

73   *Arizona Department of Economic Security et al. v. Anon*. November 1, 2010. Page 88.

74   Canfield RL, Henderson CR Jr, Cory-Slechta DA, et al. "Intellectual impairment in children with blood lead concentrations below 10μg per deciliter." *The New England Journal of Medicine*. 2003; 348:1517–26.

75   *Arizona Department of Economic Security et al. v. Anon*. November 1, 2010. Page 105.

76   *Arizona Department of Economic Security et al. v. Anon*. November 1, 2010. Page 105.

77   Dr. Ede reviewed Child 1 on a monthly basis. On January 31, 2009, concerned with the adverse effects of long-term steroid therapy, he started Child 1 on methotrexate.

78   *Arizona Department of Economic Security et al. v. Anon*. October 29, 2010. Page 96.

79   Ibid. Page 88.

80   Ibid. Page 117.

81   *Arizona Department of Economic Security et al. v. Anon*. October 29, 2010. Page 117.

82   Ibid.

83   Ibid. Page 83.

84   Emphasis added.

85   Ibid.

86   *Arizona Department of Economic Security et al. v. Anon*. October 29, 2010. Page 129.

87   *Arizona Department of Economic Security et al. v. Anon*. October 29, 2010. Page 133.

88   Macbeth. Act 1, Scene 1.

89   Macbeth. Act 1, Scene 1.

Chapter 13

1   Interview with the mother, January 2011.

2   In the Superior Court of the State of Arizona in and for the County of Yavapai. January 6, 2011.

3   *Arizona Department of Economic Security et al. v. Anon.* November 1, 2010. Page 132.

4   Rosenberg DA. "Web of deceit: A literature review of Münchausen syndrome by proxy." *Child Abuse and Neglect.* 1987; 11:547–63.

5   DSM–IV-TR. 2000; page 513. MSBP renamed as Facitious Disorder by Proxy (FDBP).

6   Rosenberg DA. "Münchausen syndrome by proxy: medical diagnostic criteria." *Child Abuse and Neglect.* 2003; 27:421–30.

7   Hon. Robert M. Brutinel. Findings of fact and conclusions of law. January 6, 2011. Case no. redacted.

8   Undated summary of allegations from CPS.

9   Undated report from CPS.

10   Report of Susan Symington, September 7, 2010.

11   Ibid.

12   James SJ, Melnyk S, Jernigan S, et al. "Metabolic endophenotype and related genotypes are associated with oxidative stress in children with autism." *American Journal of Medical Genetics B Neuropsychiatr Genet.* 2006; 141B:947–56.

     Bradstreet JJ, El-Dahr J, Anthony A, et al. "Detection of measles virus genomic RNA in cerebrospinal fluid of children with regressive autism: A report of three cases." *Journal of American Physicians and Surgeons.* 2004; 9:38–45.

     Rossignol DA, Bradstreet JJ. "Evidence of mitochondrial dysfunction in autism and implications for treatment." *American Journal of Biochemistry and Biotechnology.* 2008; 4:208–17.

     Adams JB, Baral M, Geis E, et al. "Safety and efficacy of oral DMSA therapy for children with autism spectrum disorders: Part A—medical results." *BMC Clinical Pharmacology* 2009; 9:16. Retrieved from: http://www.biomedcentral.com/1472-6904/9/16.

13   Patch testing usually involves the use of glycerinated food extracts or fresh food preparations in a Finn Chamber. See http://www.truetest.com/PhysicianPDF/HCP23_FinnCh%20details.pdf.

14   *Arizona Department of Economic Security et al. v. Anon.* November 18, 2010. Page 12.

15   Ibid. Page 12.

16   If any references to food allergies are to be found, they are not in the records of doctors. The mother states that she only ever referred to sensitivities and not allergies when discussing dietary matters in all but Child 3.

17   Report of Dr. Stephens, October 7, 2010.

18 Ibid.

19 Report of Dr. Sanders, September 27, 2010.

20 Ibid.

21 *Arizona Department of Economic Security et al. v. Anon.* October 27, 2010. Page 37.

22 See Part 1, Chapter 3.

23 Emphasis added.

24 Jyonouchi H. "Autism spectrum disorders and allergy: Observation from a pediatric allergy/immunology clinic." *Expert Review of Clinical Immunology.* 2010; 6:397–411.

25 This point was reinforced by Dr. McDonough-Means in testimony:

   Q. "So those [allergic] gut reactions, would those show up on traditional allergy testing?"

   A. "No."

   Based upon her review of the records, she confirmed that in her opinion the five children had these gut problems. *Arizona Department of Economic Security et al. v. Anon.* November 1, 2010. Page 133.

26 Report of Susan Symington, September 7, 2010.

27 Report of Dr. Stephens, October 7, 2010.

28 Report of Dr. Sanders, September 27, 2010.

29 *Arizona Department of Economic Security et al. v. Anon.* October 29, 2010. Page 102.

30 Wood RA. "The natural history of food allergy." *Pediatrics.* 2003; 111:1631–7.

   Sampson HA. "Food allergy. Part 2: diagnosis and management." *Journal of Allergy and Clinical Immunology.* 1999; 103:981–9.

31 *Arizona Department of Economic Security et al. v. Anon.* November 18, 2010. Page 14.

Chapter 14

1 E-mail from Dr. Jodi Carter to Heather Williams, April 26, 2010.

2 Ibid.

3 Ibid.

4 E-mail from Heather Williams to colleagues, April 23, 2010.

5 Meadow R. "Mothering to death." *Archives of Disease in Childhood.* 1999; 80:359–62. See also Sally Clark, retrieved from http://www.innocent .org.uk/cases/sallyclark/, and Dawid AP, Sally Clark appeal, retrieved from: https://docs.google.com/viewer?url=http%3A%2F%2Fwww.statslab .cam.ac.uk%2F~apd%2FSallyClark_report.doc.

6 Orange JS, Hossny EM, Weiler CR, et al. "Use of intravenous immunoglobulin in human disease: A review of evidence by members of the Primary Immunodeficiency Committee of the American Academy of Allergy, Asthma and Immunology." *Journal of Allergy and Clinical Immunology*. 2006; 117: S525–53.

7 These include anaphylaxis, Stevens-Johnson syndrome, hypotension, myocardial infarction, thrombosis, cytopenia, hemolysis, stroke, seizure, loss of consciousness, acute respiratory distress syndrome, pulmonary edema, acute bronchospasm, and transfusion-associated lung injury.

8 Mother's recollection in 2011 of Dr. McCarthy's statement. Interview February 6, 2011.

9 Medical record by Dr. Ursea, August 8, 2008.

10 Medical record, January 6, 2010.

11 Medical record, July 31, 2009.

12 Dr. Ursea to Dr. Sipes, January 26, 2010.

13 Dr. Ursea to Dr. Sipes, February 13, 2009.

14 Dr. Ursea to Dr. Sipes, June 19, 2009.

15 Emphasis added.

16 Medical record by Dr. Carter, February 25, 2009.

17 Emphasis added.

18 E-mail from Dr. Carter to colleagues, April 26, 2010.

19 See Part 3, Chapter 2. Admission record of Child 1 to PCH. February 25, 2009.

20 Letter from Dr. Hellmers, addressed "To Whom it May Concern." January 29, 2009.

21 Dr. Longhurst, PCH records, February 25, 2009.

22 Medical record by Jason Samuel, February 24, 2009.

23 Medical record by Dr. Carter, February 26, 2009.

24 Further medical record by Dr. Carter, February 26, 2009.

25 Medical record by Dr. McCarthy (see Table 1).

26 Letter from Dr. Hellmers addressed "To Whom it May Concern." January 29, 2009.

27 Emphasis added.

28 Memo from Emily to Dr. Hellmers, February 26, 2010.

29 Medical record by Dr. Carter, March 16, 2010.

30 Medical record by Dr. Ursea, March 27, 2009, June 19, 2009, and January 26, 2010.

31 Medical record, January 26, 2010.

32 Medical record by Dr. Theresa Murdoch, March 16, 2010.

33　Medical record by Dr. Carter, March 16, 2010.

34　Medical record by Dr. Ursea June 19, 2009.

35　Medical record by Dr. Hellmers, April 8, 2009.

36　Dr. Rice, July 22, 2008.

37　Dr. Rice, November 18, 2008.

38　Medical record by Dr. Ursea, January 26, 2010.

39　*Arizona Department of Economic Security et al. v. Anon.* October 29, 2010. Page 70.

40　Ibid.

41　E-mail from Heather Williams to colleagues, April 23, 2010.

42　Ibid.

43　Ibid.

44　Ibid.

45　Emphasis added.

46　E-mail from Heather Williams to colleagues, April 23, 2010.

47　E-mail from Dr. Carter to colleagues, April 26, 2010.

48　*Arizona Department of Economic Security et al. v. Anon.* November 18, 2010. Page 68.

49　E-mail from Heather Williams to colleagues, April 23, 2010.

50　Ibid.

51　E-mail from Dr. Stephens to colleagues, May 27, 2010.

52　Ibid.

53　Arizona State Immunization Information System.

54　Presumably tetanus toxoid vaccine.

55　E-mail from Dr. Stephens to colleagues, May 27, 2010.

56　Report of Dr. Mary Sanders, September 27, 2010.

57　Ibid.

58　Heather Williams, Dr. Jodi Carter, Dr. Mary Stephens, Dr. Albert Jacobsen, John Destephano (ADES), D. Kimsey (ADES), and Ginny Debartolomo.

59　Second report of Dr. Stephens, October 7, 2010.

60　Ibid.

61　Ibid.

62　Ibid.

63　MacBeth. Act 1, Scene 1.

64　Records of Dr. Katherine McCarthy, 100 Weatheridge Drive, Camillus, NY 13031.

65　Lederle.

66   Merck and Co., Inc. (Merck Sharp and Dohme).

67   Varicella zoster (chickenpox) vaccine.

68   Records of Dr. Katherine McCarthy, 100 Weatheridge Drive, Camillus, NY 13031.

69   SmithKline Beecham (now GlaxoSmithKline).

70   Connaught Laboratories.

71   Rotavirus vaccine.

72   Wyeth Lederle.

73   Health Services Association Immunization Flow Sheet MR# 430650.

74   Health Services Association Immunization Flow Sheet MR# 430649.

Chapter 15

1   Dr. Sanders, PhD, is Clinical Associate Professor in the Department of Child and Adolescent Psychiatry and the Program Director of the Comprehensive Care Unit at Stanford University, where she teaches and works with inpatients with eating disorders. She has specialized in the treatment of eating disorders for the past twenty years at Stanford. She also works in the outpatient clinic at Stanford and is a therapist in an ongoing treatment outcome study through Stanford Child Psychiatry. She has written extensively and presented nationally on the subject of the evaluation and treatment of eating disorders and also in the field of child abuse, specifically in the area of Münchausen by proxy.

2   Mary Sanders, PhD. Retrieved from: http://med.stanford.edu/profiles/psychiatry/frdActionServlet?choiceId=facProfileandfid=7383.

3   Sanders MJ, Bursch B. "Forensic assessment of illness falsification, Münchausen by proxy, and factitious disorder, NOS." *Child Maltreatment.* 2002; 7:112–24.

4   Letter from Michael Kruley, Health and Human Services, Office for Civil Rights, to complainant Ms. Shauna Taylor, May 16, 2011.

5   Meadow SR. "Münchausen syndrome by proxy." *Medico-Legal Journal.* 1995; 63:89–104.

6   Sanders MJ, Bursch B. "Forensic assessment of illness falsification, Münchausen by proxy, and factitious disorder, NOS." *Child Maltreatment.* 2002; 7:112–24.

7   Ibid.

8   Long WR. "Münchausen syndrome by proxy/factitious disorder by proxy: a critical assessment for judges and lawyers." July 12, 2008. Retrieved from: http://www.autism.com/pdf/families/MBSP_unabridged.pdf.

Pankratz L. "Problems with the diagnosis of factitious disorder by proxy in forensic settings." *American Journal of Forensic Psychology*. 1999; 17:69–82. And http://journal.9med.net/qikan/article.php?id=177168.

9   According to Dr. Mart, defense expert in the Arizona 5 case.

10 *Arizona Department of Economic Security et al. v. Anon.* October 27, 2010. Page 26.

11 Report of Dr. Sanders, September 27, 2010.

12 Emphasis added.

13 Sanders MJ, Bursch B. "Forensic assessment of illness falsification, Münchausen by proxy, and factitious disorder, NOS." *Child Maltreatment*. 2002; 7:112–24.

14 *Arizona Department of Economic Security et al. v. Anon.* October 27, 2010, page 62.

15 Report of Dr. Sanders, September 27, 2010.

16 Ibid.

17 *Arizona Department of Economic Security et al. v. Anon.* October 27, 2010, page 63.

18 License number 171641, granted by the Education Department of the State of New York on June 25, 1984.

19 *Arizona Department of Economic Security et al. v. Anon.* October 27, 2010, page 63.

20 *Arizona Department of Economic Security et al. v. Anon.* October 27, 2010, page 82.

21 *Arizona Department of Economic Security et al. v. Anon.* October 27, 2010, page 76.

22 Ibid.

23 Ibid.

24 Interview, April 19, 2011, 3:47 CST.

25 Chapter 3.

26 Report of Dr. Sanders, September 27, 2010.

27 Lovaas OI. "Behavioral treatment and normal educational and intellectual functioning in young autistic children." *Journal of Consulting and Clinical Psychology*. 1987; 55:3–9.

Sitholey P, Agarwal W, Pargaonkar A. "Rapid and spontaneous recovery in autistic disorder." *Indian Journal of Psychiatry*. 2009; 51:209–11.

Gajzago G, Prior M. "Two cases of 'recovery' in Kanner syndrome." *Archives of General Psychiatry*. 1974; 31:264–8.

Perry R, Cohen I, DeCarlo R. "Case study: deterioration, autism, and recovery in two siblings." *Journal of the American Academy of Child and Adolescent Psychiatry.* 1995; 34:232–7.

28 http://www.medicinenet.com/script/main/art.asp?articlekey=100210 [last accessed June 2010]. Also available at www.clinicaltrials.gov [last accessed February 2012].

29 Report of Dr. Sanders, September 27, 2010.

30 Ibid.

31 Ibid.

32 Ibid.

33 Sanders MJ, Bursch B. "Forensic assessment of illness falsification, Münchausen by proxy, and factitious disorder, NOS." *Child Maltreatment.* 2002; 7:112–24.

34 *Arizona Department of Economic Security et al. v. Anon.* October 27, 2010, page 86.

35 Ibid.

36 Ibid.

37 Emphasis added.

38 Sanders MJ, Bursch B. "Forensic assessment of illness falsification, Münchausen by proxy, and factitious disorder, NOS." *Child Maltreatment.* 2002; 7:112–24.

39 Report of Dr. Sanders, September 27, 2010.

40 Emphasis added.

41 Sanders MJ, Bursch B. "Forensic assessment of illness falsification, Münchausen by proxy, and factitious disorder, NOS." *Child Maltreatment.* 2002; 7:112–24.

42 Bass C, Adshead G. "Fabrication and induction of illness in children: The psychopathology of abuse." *Advances in Psychiatric Treatment.* 2007; 13: 169–77.

43 *Arizona Department of Economic Security et al. v. Anon.* October 27, 2010. Page 32.

44 Sanders MJ, Bursch B. "Forensic assessment of illness falsification, Münchausen by proxy, and factitious disorder, NOS." *Child Maltreatment.* 2002; 7:112–24.

45 Ibid.

46 *Arizona Department of Economic Security et al. v. Anon.* October 27, 2010, page 29.

47 Ibid. Page 66.

Chapter 16

1   www.mctplaw.com/vaccine-injury/vaccine-case-results/dtap-mmr-hepa-pearson.pdf.

2   Ibid.

3   Rutter M, Bailey A, Bolton P, et al. "Autism and known medical conditions: myth and substance." *The Journal of Child Psychology and Psychiatry*. 1994; 35:311–22.

4   http://www.uscfc.gov/sites/default/files/Abell.BANKS.02-0738V.pdf
     Attkisson S. "Vaccine watch." *CBS News Investigates*. June 19, 2008. Retrieved from: http://www.cbsnews.com/8301-501263_162-4194102-501263.html.

5   Holland M, Conte L, Krakow R, et al. "Unanswered questions from the Vaccine Injury Compensation Program: A review of compensated cases of vaccine-induced brain injury." *Pace Environmental Law Review*. 2011; 28:480. Available at: http://digitalcommons.pace.edu/pelr/vol28/iss2/6.

6   The Vaccine Injury Table lists and explains injuries/conditions that are presumed to be caused by vaccines. It also lists time periods in which the first symptom of these injuries/conditions must occur after receiving the vaccine. If the first symptom of these injuries/conditions occurs within the listed time periods, it is presumed that the vaccine was the cause of the injury or condition unless another cause is found. For example, if you received the tetanus vaccine and had a severe allergic reaction (anaphylaxis) within four hours after receiving the vaccine, then it is presumed that the tetanus vaccine caused the injury if no other cause is found. http://www.hrsa.gov/vaccinecompensation/table.htm.

7   Richler J, Luyster R, Risi S, et al. "Is there a 'regressive phenotype' of autism spectrum disorder associated with the measles-mumps-rubella vaccine? A CPEA study." *Journal of Autism and Developmental Disorders*. 2006; 36:299–316.
     DeStefano F, Bhasin TK, Thompson WW, et al. "Age at first measles-mumps–rubella vaccination in children with autism and school-matched control subjects: A population-based study in metro-politan Atlanta." *Pediatrics*. 2004; 113:259–66.
     Edwardes M, Baltzan M. "MMR immunization and autism." *Journal of the American Medical Association*. 2001; 285:2852–3.
     Dales L, Hammer SJ, Smith NJ. "Time trends in autism and MMR immunization coverage in California." *Journal of the American Medical Association*. 2001; 285:1183–5.

Stott C, Blaxill M, Wakefield AJ. "MMR and autism in perspective: The Denmark story." *Journal of American Physicians and Surgeons*. 2004; 9:89–91.

8   Schultz ST, Klonoff-Cohen HS, Wingard DL, et al. "Acetominophen (paracetamol) use, measles-mumps-rubella vaccination, and autistic disorder: The results of a parent survey." *Autism*. 2008; 12:293–307.

9   Petrik MS, Wong MC, Tabata RC, et al. "Aluminum adjuvant linked to Gulf War illness induces motor neuron death in mice." *NeuroMolecular Medicine*. 2007; 9:83–100.

10   DeSoto MC, Hitlan RT. "Sorting out the spinning of autism: Heavy metals and the question of incidence." *Acta Neurobiologiae Experimentalis (Wars)*. 2010; 70:165–76.

11   Crawford J. "U.S. Supreme Court rejects vaccine lawsuit." KXLH.com, February 24, 2011. Retrieved from: http://www.kxlh.com/news/u-s-supreme-court-rejects-vaccine-lawsuit/.

12   Institute of Medicine. *Adverse Effects of Vaccines: Evidence and Causality*. National Academy of Sciences, August 25, 2011. Available at: http://www.iom.edu/Reports/2011/Adverse-Effects-of-Vaccines-Evidence-and-Causality.aspx (Read full report.)

13   http://www.uscfc.uscourts.gov/omnibus-autism-proceeding; Cedillo v. Secretary of Health and Human Services Case No. 98-916V; Hazlehurst v. Secretary of Health and Human Services Case No. 03-654V; Snyder v. Secretary of Health and Human Services Case No. 01-162V.

14   Wakefield AJ, Stott C, Limb K. "Gastrointestinal comorbidity, autistic regression and measles-containing vaccines: positive re-challenge and biological gradient." *Medical Veritas*. 2006; 3:796–802.

15   Report of Dr. Stephens, October 7, 2010.

16   See Part 4, Building a Case.

17   Macbeth. Act 1, Scene 5.

18   Dr. Jacobsen to Dr. Sipes, July 15, 2010.

19   www.hrsa.gov/vaccinecompensation/statistics_report.htm [last accessed June 2011].

20   *Wisconisn v. Yoder*, 92 S. Ct. 1526, (1541-1542) (1972).

21   *Santosky v. Kramer*, 455 U.S. 753, 754 (1982).

22   Kupiszewski J. Objection to State's motion and request to vaccinate the children. July 20, 2010.

23   Ibid.

24   *Diana v. Rubin*, 217 Ariz. 131, 134, 171 P.3d 200, 203 (App. 2007).

25 Young AA. ADES's reply to father and mother's objections to ADES' motion for immunizations. August 3, 2010.

26 Report of Dr. Sanders, September 27, 2010.

27 Ibid.

28 Medical records of Dr. McCarthy, September 11, 2003.

29 *Arizona Department of Economic Security v. Anon.* Hon. Robert M Brutinel. Findings of fact and conclusions of law. January 6, 2011, Case No. JD21100.

30 Macbeth. Act 1, Scene 3.

31 The measles rubella was used in a one-off mass vaccination campaign of approximately eight million school children in the UK in November 1994.

32 Howson CP, Howe CJ, Fineberg HV (Eds). *Adverse Effects of Pertussis and Rubella Vaccines.* Washington, DC: National Academy Press, 1991, p. 158.

33 Stratton K, Gable A, Shetty P, et al. "Immunization safety review: Measles-mumps-rubella vaccine and autism" (Draft). Washington, DC: National Academy Press, 2001.

34 Wakefield AJ, Stott C, Limb K. "Gastrointestinal co-morbidity, autistic regression and measles-containing vaccines: Positive re-challenge and biological gradient." *Medical Veritas.* 2006; 3:796–802.

35 $p < 0.0001$.

36 $p = 0.009$.

37 Rutter M, Taylor E, Hersor L. *Child and Adolescent Psychiatry.* London: Blackwell Scientific Publications, 1994, pp. 581–682.

38 $p = 0.002$.

39 0.04.

40 $p < 0.01$.

41 $p < 0.05$.

42 $p < 0.001$.

43 $p < 0.05$.

44 Wakefield AJ, Stott C, Limb K. "Gastrointestinal comorbidity, autistic regression and measles-containing vaccines: Positive re-challenge and dose-response effects." *Medical Veritas.* 2006; 3:796–802.

45 An emerging brain injury and associated dysfunction.

46 Plesner AM. "Gait disturbance after measles, mumps, and rubella vaccine." *Lancet.* 1995; 345:316.

47 Doctors are required by law to report adverse reactions.

48 Plesner AM, Hansen FJ, Taudorf K, et al. "Gait disturbance interpreted as cerebellar ataxia after MMR vaccination at 15 months of age: A follow-up study." *Acta Paediatrica.* 2000; 89:58–63.

49   Apoptosis or cell "suicide." Yel L, Brown LE, Su K, et al. "Thimerosal induces neuronal cell apoptosis by causing cytochrome c and apoptosis-inducing factor release from mitochondria." *International Journal of Molecular Medicine*. 2005; 16:971–7.

Suárez-Fernández MB, Soldado AB, Sanz-Medel A, et al. "Aluminum-induced degeneration of astrocytes occurs via apoptosis and results in neuronal death." *Brain Research*. 1999; 835:125–36.

50   Horizontal transmission refers to spread excluding mother to child during pregnancy, childbirth or breastfeeding. Vertical transmission refers to spread from mother to child, for example, *in utero*, *intra partum*, or through breast-feeding.

51   Report of Dr. Sanders, September 27, 2010.

52   Breslin NP, Nash C, Hilsden RJ, et al. "Intestinal permeability is increased in a proportion of spouses of patients with Crohn's disease." *The American Journal of Gastroenterology*. 2001; 96:2934–8.

Söderholm JD, Olaison G, Lindberg E, et al. "Different intestinal permeability patterns in relatives and spouses of patients with Crohn's disease: An inherited defect in mucosal defense?" *Gut*. 1999; 44:96–100.

Alic M. "Is exposure to a patient with Crohn's disease an environmental factor for developing the disease?" *Gut*. 1999; 45:631–2.

Comes MC, Gower-Rousseau C, Colombel JF, et al. "Inflammatory bowel disease in married couples: 10 cases in Nord Pas de Calais region of France and Liège county of Belgium." *Gut*. 1994; 35:1316–8.

Rhodes JM, Marshall T, Hamer JD, et al. "Crohn's disease in two married couples." *Gut*. 1985; 26:1086–7.

Sustento-Reodica N, Ruiz P, Rogers A, et al. "Recurrent Crohn's disease in transplanted bowel." *Lancet*. 1997; 349:688–91.

Harpaz N, Schiano T, Ruf AE, et al. "Early and frequent histological recurrence of Crohn's disease in small intestinal allografts." *Transplantation*. 2005; 80:1667–70.

53   Kohler KA, Banerjee K, Hlady WG, et al. "Vaccine-associated paralytic poliomyelitis in India during 1999: Decreased risk despite massive use of oral polio vaccine." *Bulletin of the World Health Organization*. 2002; 80:210–6.

54   Millson DS. "Brother-to-sister transmission of measles after measles, mumps, and rubella immunisation." *Lancet*. 1989; 1:271.

55   Campbell AG. "Brother-to-sister transmission of measles after MMR immunisation." *Lancet*. 1989; 1:442.

56   Sawada H, Yano S, Oka Y, et al. "Transmission of Urabe mumps vaccine between siblings." *Lancet*. 1993; 342:371.

57   Yazbak FE, Diodati CJ. "Postpartum live virus vaccination: Lessons from veterinary medicine." *Medical Hypotheses*. 2002; 59:280–2.

58   Haggarty RJ, Meyer RJ, Lenihan E, et al. "Studies on an attenuated measles-virus vaccine. VII: Clinical, antigenic, and prophylactic effects in home dwelling children." *The New England Journal of Medicine*. 1960; 263:178–80.

Smith W, Evans DG, Gaisford W, et al. "Vaccination against measles: A study of clinical reactions and serological responses of young children." *British Medical Journal*. 1965; 1:817–23.

Katz SL, Kempe HC, Black FL, et al. "Studies on an attenuated measles-virus vaccine: VII General summary and evaluation of the results of vaccination." *The New England Journal of Medicine*. 1960; 263:180–4.

Lepow ML, Gray N, Robbins FC. "Studies on an attenuated measles-virus vaccine. V. Clinical, antigenic and prophylactic effects of vaccine in institutionalised and home-dwelling children." *The New England Journal of Medicine*. 1960; 263:170–3.

Katz SL, Enders JF, Holloway A. "Studies on an attenuated measles-virus vaccine. II. Clinical, virologic and immunological effects of vaccine in institutionalized children." *The New England Journal of Medicine*. 1960; 263:159–62.

59   Rota PA, Khan AS, Durigon E, et al. "Detection of measles virus RNA in urine specimens from vaccine recipients." *Journal of Clinical Microbiology*. 1995; 33:2485–8.

Jenkin GA, Chibo D, Kelly HA, et al. "What is the cause of a rash after measles-mumps-rubella vaccination?" *Medical Journal of Australia*. 1999; 171;194–5.

60   Chibo D, Riddell M, Catton M, et al. "Studies of measles viruses circulating in Australia between 1999 and 2001 reveals a new genotype." *Virus Research*. 2003; 91:213–21.

61   Pütz MM, Bouche FB, de Swart RL, et al. "Experimental vaccines against measles in a world of changing epidemiology." *International Journal for Parasitology*. 2003; 33:525–45.

Outlaw MC, Pringle CR. "Sequence analysis within an outbreak of measles virus in the Coventry area during spring/summer 1993." *Virus Research*. 1995; 39:3–11.

Christensen LS, Scholler S, Schierup MH, et al. "Sequence analysis of measles virus strains during the pre- and early-vaccination era in Denmark reveals a considerable diversity of ancient strains." *Acta Pathologica, Microbiologica et Immunologica Scandinavica*. 2002; 110:113–22.

Muller CP, Mulders MN. "Molecular epidemiology in measles control." In T. Leitner (Ed.), *The Molecular Epidemiology of Human Viruses* (pp. 237–72), Boston, MA: Kluwer Academic Publishers, 2002.

Wairagkar N, Rota PA, Liffick S, et al. "Characterization of measles sequences from Pune, India." *Journal of Medical Virology.* 2002; 68: 611–4.

Riddell MA, Rota JS, Rota PA. "Review of the temporal and geographical distribution of measles virus genotypes in the prevaccine and postvaccine eras." *Virology Journal.* 2005; 2:87–92.

Bellini WJ, Rota PA. "Genetic diversity of wild-type measles viruses: implications for global measles elimination programs." *Emerging Infectious Diseases.* 1998; 4:29–35.

Rota PA, Bellini WJ. "Update on the global distribution of genotypes of wild type measles viruses." *International Journal of Infectious Diseases.* 2003; 187:S270-S276.

Pedersen IR, Mordhorst CH, Ewald T, et al. "Long-term antibody response after measles vaccination in an isolated arctic society in Greenland." *Vaccine.* 1986; 4:173–8.

Pedersen IR, Mordhorst CH, Glikmann G, et al. "Subclinical measles infection in vaccinated seropositive individuals in arctic Greenland." *Vaccine.* 1989; 7:345–8.

62   Christensen LS, Scholler S, Schierup MH, et al. "Sequence analysis of measles virus strains during the pre- and early-vaccination era in Denmark reveals considerable diversity of ancient strains." *Acta Pathologica, Microbiologica et Immunologica Scandinavica.* 2002; 110:113–22.

63   Chen P, Miller GF, Powell DA. "Colitis is a female tamarin (Saguinus mystax)." *Contemporary Topics in Laboratory Animal Science.* 2000; 39:47–9.

64   Zdziarski JM, Sarich NA, Witecki KE, et al. "Molecular analysis of SV-40-CAL, a new slow growing SV-40 strain from the kidney of a caged new world monkey with fatal renal disease." *Virus Genes.* 2004; 29:183–90.

65   Tierney P. *Darkness in El Dorado: How Scientists and Journalists Devastated the Amazon.* New York, NY: WW Norton and Company, 2000.

66   Inga Steinworth Goetz, Uriji Jami!: *Life and Belief of the Forest Waika in the Upper Orinoco,* trans. Peter Furst (Caracas: Association Cultural Humboldt, 1969), p. 56.

67   Alfredo Aherowe, Yanomami, elected representative of the United Shabonos of the Upper Orinoco, testimony to the Comision Indigena del Congreso de Venezuela, Caracas, Venezuela, November 8, 2000.

Neel JV, Asch T, Chagnon N. Yanomama. *A multidisciplinary study*. (43-minute video documentary) Washington, DC: Department of Energy, 1971.

Hill J. Tierney's use of the Asch sound tapes as evidence. In *El Dorado Task Force Papers*, Vol II (p. 139). Virginia: American Anthropological Association, 2002.

68 Pütz MM, Bouche FB, de Swart RL, et al. "Experimental vaccines against measles in a world of changing epidemiology." *International Journal for Parasitology*. 2003; 33:525–45.

69 Ashwood P, Anthony A, Pellicer AA, et al. "Intestinal lymphocyte populations in children with regressive autism: Evidence for extensive mucosal immunopathology." *Journal of Clinical Immunology*, 2003; 23:504–17.

Gupta S, Samra D, Agrawal S. "Adaptive and innate immune responses in autism: Rationale for therapeutic use of intravenous immunoglobulin." *Journal of Clinical Immunology*. 2010; 30:90–6.

Warren RP, Foster A, Margaretten NC. "Reduced natural killer cell activity in autism." *Journal of the American Academy of Child and Adolescent Psychiatry*. 1987; 26:333–5.

Vojdani A, Mumper E, Granpeesheh D, et al. "Low natural killer cell cytotoxic activity in autism: the role of glutathione, IL-2 and IL-15." *Journal of Neuroimmunology*. 2008; 205:148–54.

70 Chi-square and Fishers Exact tests used.

71 In order to exclude the possibility that the presence of inflammation might be influenced by differences in the interval between first exposure to a measles vaccine and colonoscopy, this relationship was examined. There was no difference in the relevant interval between those who did not have acute ileo-colonic inflammation.

To exclude the possibility that the presence of acute and/or chronic inflammation is influenced by age, the larger cohort of the first 148 children with ASD who had undergone ileo-colonoscopy at the RFH were studied. There was no statistical correlation between age and presence of (i) acute inflammation, (ii) chronic inflammation, and (iii) ileal LNH.

Chapter 17

1 Skinner BF. *The Behavior of Organisms: An Experimental Analysis*. New York: Appleton-Century-Crofts, 1938.

2 *Arizona Department of Economic Security et al. v. Anon*. Joint Notice of Filing Findings of Fact and Conclusion of Law. Kupiszewski J. 2011. Page 13.

3   Report on Dr. Stephens, June 10, 2010.

4   Ibid.

5   *Callous Disregard: Autism and Vaccines—The Truth Behind a Tragedy.* New York: Skyhorse Publishing, 2010.

6   *Arizona Department of Economic Security et al. v. Anon.* October 27, 2010, pages 46, 52.

7   The meeting was a mediation, held on March 4. Two assistant attorney generals were there, CPS, Jane (the court appointed special advocate), the guardian ad litem, the children's attorney, the grandparents and their attorney, the parents and their attorneys, and the court mediator.

8   *Arizona Department of Economic Security et al. v. Anon.* November 1, 2010, page 56.

9   United Nations. *The Universal Declaration of Human Rights.* Available at: http://www.un.org/en/documents/udhr/index.shtml.

10   E-mail from Ms. Williams to colleagues, April 23, 2010.

11   *The Diagnostic and Statistical Manual of Mental Disorders.*

12   E-mail report by Ms. Williams on conversation with Dr. Carter, April 23, 2010.

13   Emphasis added.

14   Diagnostic criteria for 301.83, Borderline Personality Disorder: A pervasive pattern of instability of interpersonal relationships, self-image, and affects, and marked impulsivity beginning by early adulthood and present in a variety of contexts, as indicated by five (or more) of the following:

(1)   frantic efforts to avoid real or imagined abandonment.

(2)   a pattern of unstable and intense interpersonal relationships characterized by alternating between extremes of idealization and devaluation.

(3)   identity disturbance: markedly and persistently unstable self-image or sense of self.

(4)   impulsivity in at least two areas that are potentially self-damaging (e.g., spending, sex, substance abuse, reckless driving, binge eating): Do not include suicidal or self-mutilating behavior covered in Criterion 5.

(5)   recurrent suicidal behavior, gestures, or threats, or self-mutilating behavior.

(6)   affective instability due to a marked reactivity of mood (e.g., intense episodic dysphoria, irritability, or anxiety usually lasting a few hours and only rarely more than a few days).

(7)   chronic feelings of emptiness.

(8)   inappropriate, intense anger or difficulty controlling anger (e.g., frequent displays of temper, constant anger, recurrent physical fights).

(9)   transient, stress-related paranoid ideation or severe dissociative symptoms.

15   "[Husband's name] and I have both been diagnosed with Post-traumatic Stress Disorder (PTSD), and a diagnosis of a personality disorder is supposed to first rule out other causes, such as PTSD, brain injury, etc., which was not ruled out when making the personality disorder diagnosis; I had a brain injury, and [husband's name] had meningitis, as well as PTSD from the service."

16   *Arizona Department of Economic Security et al. v. Anon.* November 3, 2010, page 108.

17   A person or thing that one particularly dislikes.

18   Hiller A. "Vaccines continue to bolster pharma market." *PharmPro.* December 2, 2010. Retrieved from: http://www.pharmpro.com/articles/2010/12/busines-Vaccines-Continue-to-Bolster-Pharma-Market/.

19   *Arizona Department of Economic Security et al. v. Anon.* November 18, 2010, pages 55–57.

20   Ibid. Pages 157–158.

Epilogue

1   Holland M, Conte L, Krakow R, et al. "Unanswered questions from the Vaccine Injury Compensation Program: A review of compensated cases of vaccine-induced brain injury." *Pace Environmental Law Review.* 2011; 28:480. Available at: http://digitalcommons.pace.edu/pelr/vol28/iss2/6.

2   Emphasis added.

3   Marie Witman.

4   Bethlem Royal Hospital, London, one of the first specialist hospitals for the mentally ill and home of the Institute of Psychiatry. Origin of the word "bedlam" describing chaos or madness.

5   Leo Kanner.

6   Montagnier L, Vialard D. *Les Combats de la Vie.* Paris: JC Lattès, 2008.

7   *Age of Autism.* "Bill Gates: They kill children . . . take action!" *Age of Autism,* February 13, 2011. Available at: http://www.ageofautism.com/2011/02/are-you-a-baby-killer-take-action.html.

8   Kim YS, Leventhal BL, Koh YJ, et al. "Prevalence of autism spectrum dis-orders in a total population sample." *The American Journal of Psychiatry.* 2011; 168:904–12.

9   Bethell CD, Kogan MD, Strickland BB, et al. "A national and state profile of leading health problems and healthcare quality for US children: Key insurance disparities and across-state variations." *Academic Pediatrics.* 2011; 11:S22–S33. Children's Health Insurance Program Reauthorization Act Supplement.

10   The family tomb bears the name "De Gas," which was changed from its original form to "Degas" by the artist.

11   www.autismmediachannel.com.

12   Chriswell M. "EPA whistleblower Dr. David Lewis: 10 years of fighting." *Whistleblowers Protection Blog.* August 11, 2008. Available at: http://www.whistleblowersblog.org/2008/08/articles/environmental-1/epa-whistleblower-dr-david-lewis-10-years-of-fighting/.

13   University College London. "UCL and Glaxo to develop drug–antibody treatment for rare disease." *UCL News.* March 24, 2009.

      "Pentraxin Therapeutics Ltd, a UCL spin-off company, and GlaxoSmithKline (GSK) are collaborating to develop the world's first dual drug–antibody treatment for the rare and often fatal condition amyloidosis. [...]

      'We are delighted to enter into this alliance,' said Mike Owen, Senior Vice-President of Biopharmaceutical Research at GSK. 'Our biopharma-ceutical and clinical development capabilities and Professor Pepys's team's knowledge of the disease provide a synergistic collaboration that will greatly enhance our chances of success.'" Retrieved from: http://www.ucl.ac.uk/news/news-articles/0903/09032401.

Postscript

1   Arizona Supreme Court Foster Care Review Board Findings and Recom-mendations. Review date May 23, 2011.